THE WASHINGTON MANUAL®

Pulmonary Medicine

Subspecialty Consult

SECOND EDITION

THE WASHINGTON MANUAL®

Pulmonary Medicine

Subspecialty Consult

SECOND EDITION

Editors

Adrian Shifren, MD
Assistant Professor of Medicine
Pulmonary and Critical Care
Washington University School of Medicine
St. Louis, Missouri

Derek E. Byers, MD, PhD
Assistant Professor of Medicine
Pulmonary and Critical Care
Washington University School of Medicine
St. Louis, Missouri

Chad A. Witt, MD
Assistant Professor of Medicine
Pulmonary and Critical Care
Washington University School of Medicine
St. Louis, Missouri

Series Editors

Thomas M. De Fer, MD, FACP
Professor of Medicine
Director, Internal Medicine Clerkship and the ACES Program
Division of Medical Education, Department of Medicine
Washington University School of Medicine
St. Louis, Missouri

Thomas Ciesielski, MD
Instructor in Medicine, Fellow in Patient Safety and Quality
Division of Medical Education/ Department of Internal Medicine
Washington University School of Medicine
St. Louis, Missouri

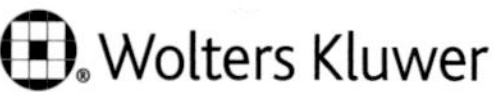

Philadelphia • Baltimore • New York • London
Buenos Aires • Hong Kong • Sydney • Tokyo

Executive Editor: Rebecca Gaertner
Senior Product Development Editor: Kristina Oberle
Production Project Manager: Bridgett Dougherty
Design Coordinator: Stephen Druding
Senior Manufacturing Coordinator: Beth Welsh
Editorial Coordinator: Katie Sharp
Prepress Vendor: Aptara, Inc.

9 8 7 6 5 4 3 2 1

Printed in China

Library of Congress Cataloging-in-Publication Data

Names: Shifren, Adrian, editor. | Byers, Derek E., editor. | Witt, Chad A., editor.
Title: The Washington manual pulmonary medicine subspecialty consult / editors, Adrian Shifren, Derek E. Byers, Chad A. Witt.
Other titles: Pulmonary medicine subspecialty consult | Washington manual subspecialty consult series.
Description: Second edition. | Philadelphia : Wolters Kluwer, [2017] | Series: Washington manual subspecialty consult series | Includes bibliographical references and index.
Identifiers: LCCN 2016020149 | ISBN 9781451114171
Subjects: | MESH: Lung Diseases | Pulmonary Medicine–methods | Respiratory Function Tests | Handbooks
Classification: LCC RC756 | NLM WF 39 | DDC 616.2/4–dc23
LC record available at https://lccn.loc.gov/2016020149

LWW.com

CCS0616

Contributors

Amber A. Afshar, MD
Fellow
Department of Medicine
Division of Cardiology
Washington University School of Medicine
St. Louis, Missouri

Jennifer Alexander-Brett, MD, PhD
Instructor in Medicine
Department of Medicine
Division of Pulmonary and Critical Care Medicine
Washington University School of Medicine
St. Louis, Missouri

Adam Anderson, MD
Fellow
Department of Medicine
Division of Pulmonary and Critical Care Medicine
Washington University School of Medicine
St. Louis, Missouri

Jonathan Baghdadi, MD
Hospitalist
Department of Internal Medicine
New York University
New York, New York

Brad Bemiss, MD
Fellow
Department of Medicine
Division of Pulmonary and Critical Care Medicine
Washington University School of Medicine
St. Louis, Missouri

Sanjeev Bhalla, MD
Professor of Radiology
Department of Radiology
Washington University School of Medicine
St. Louis, Missouri

James Bosanquet, MD
Fellow
Department of Medicine
Division of Pulmonary and Critical Care Medicine
Washington University School of Medicine
St. Louis, Missouri

Richard D. Brasington, MD
Professor of Medicine
Department of Medicine
Division of Rheumatology
Washington University School of Medicine
St. Louis, Missouri

Steven L. Brody, MD
D & H Moog Professor of Pulmonary Disease
Department of Medicine
Division of Pulmonary and Critical Care Medicine
Washington University School of Medicine
St. Louis, Missouri

Daniel J. Brown, MD
Fellow
Department of Medicine
Division of Pulmonary and Critical Care Medicine
Washington University School of Medicine
St. Louis, Missouri

Mario Castro, MD, MPH, FCCP
Alan A. and Edith L. Wolff Distinguished Professor
Department of Medicine
Division of Pulmonary and Critical Care Medicine
Washington University School of Medicine
St. Louis, Missouri

Murali M. Chakinala, MD
Associate Professor of Medicine
Department of Medicine
Division of Pulmonary and Critical Care Medicine
Washington University School of Medicine
St. Louis, Missouri

Jake M. Chanin, MD
Fellow
Department of Cardiology
Cornell University
Ithaca, New York

Alexander C. Chen, MD
Associate Professor of Medicine and Surgery
Department of Medicine
Division of Pulmonary and Critical Care Medicine
Washington University School of Medicine
St. Louis, Missouri

Catherine Chen, MD
Fellow
Department of Medicine
Division of Pulmonary and Critical Care Medicine
Washington University School of Medicine
St. Louis, Missouri

Praveen R. Chenna, MD
Assistant Professor of Medicine
Department of Medicine
Division of Pulmonary and Critical Care Medicine
Washington University School of Medicine
St. Louis, Missouri

Daniel R. Crouch, MD
Assistant Professor of Medicine
Department of Pulmonary Medicine
University of California San Diego
San Diego, California

Carlos C. Daughaday, MD
Professor of Medicine
Department of Medicine
Division of Pulmonary and Critical Care Medicine
Washington University School of Medicine
St. Louis, Missouri

John Dickinson, MD
Fellow
Department of Medicine
Division of Pulmonary and Critical Care Medicine
Washington University School of Medicine
St. Louis, Missouri

Cristina Vazquez Guillamet, MD
Fellow
Department of Medicine
Division of Infectious Diseases
Washington University School of Medicine
St. Louis, Missouri

Robert Guzy, MD
Fellow
Department of Medicine
Division of Pulmonary and Critical Care Medicine
Washington University School of Medicine
St. Louis, Missouri

Ramsey Hachem, MD
Professor of Medicine
Department of Medicine
Division of Pulmonary and Critical Care Medicine
Washington University School of Medicine
St. Louis, Missouri

Warren Isakow, MD
Associate Professor of Medicine
Department of Medicine
Division of Pulmonary and Critical Care Medicine
Washington University School of Medicine
St. Louis, Missouri

Brian C. Keller, MD
Fellow
Department of Medicine
Division of Pulmonary and Critical Care Medicine
Washington University School of Medicine
St. Louis, Missouri

Alfred H. J. Kim, MD, PhD
Assistant Professor of Medicine
Department of Medicine
Division of Rheumatology
Washington University School of Medicine
St. Louis, Missouri

Marin H. Kollef, MD, FACP, FCCP
Professor of Medicine
Department of Medicine
Division of Pulmonary and Critical Care Medicine
Washington University School of Medicine
St. Louis, Missouri

Barbara Lutey, MD
Assistant Professor of Medicine
Department of Medicine
Division of Medical Education
Washington University School of Medicine
St. Louis, Missouri

Mark Mangano, MD
Diagnostic Radiology Resident
Massachusetts General Hospital
Boston, Massachusetts

Hannah Otepka Mannem, MD
Fellow
Department of Medicine
Division of Pulmonary and Critical Care Medicine
University of Pittsburgh School of Medicine
Pittsburgh, Pennsylvania

Amy McQueen, PhD
Assistant Professor of Medicine
Department of Medicine
Division of General Medical Sciences
Washington University School of Medicine
St. Louis, Missouri

Michael D. Monaco, MD
Instructor in Medicine
Department of Medicine
Division of Hospitalist Medicine
Washington University School of Medicine
St. Louis, Missouri

Desh Nandedkar, MD
Assistant Professor of Medicine
Division of Pulmonary, Critical Care and Sleep Medicine
Icahn School of Medicine at Mount Sinai Medical Center
New York, New York

Amit Patel, MD
Fellow
Department of Medicine
Division of Gastroenterology
Washington University School of Medicine
St. Louis, Missouri

David Picker, MD
Fellow
Department of Medicine
Division of Pulmonary and Critical Care Medicine
Washington University School of Medicine
St. Louis, Missouri

Daniel B. Rosenbluth, MD
Tracey C. and William J. Marshall Professor of Medicine
Department of Medicine
Division of Pulmonary and Critical Care Medicine
Washington University School of Medicine
St. Louis, Missouri

Tonya D. Russell, MD
Associate Professor of Medicine
Department of Medicine
Division of Pulmonary and Critical Care Medicine
Washington University School of Medicine
St. Louis, Missouri

Carlos A. Q. Santos, MD
Assistant Professor of Medicine
Department of Medicine
Division of Infectious Diseases
Washington University School of Medicine
St. Louis, Missouri

Adrian Shifren, MD
Assistant Professor of Medicine
Department of Medicine
Division of Pulmonary and Critical Care Medicine
Washington University School of Medicine
St. Louis, Missouri

Sandeep Sodhi, MD
Fellow
Department of Medicine
Division of Cardiovascular Medicine
Washington University School of Medicine
St. Louis, Missouri

Peter G. Tuteur, MD
Associate Professor of Medicine
Department of Medicine
Division of Pulmonary and Critical Care Medicine
Washington University School of Medicine
St. Louis, Missouri

Sundeep Viswanathan, MD
Cardiologist, Private Practice
The Medical Center of Aurora
Aurora, Colorado

Chad A. Witt, MD
Assistant Professor of Medicine
Department of Medicine
Division of Pulmonary and Critical Care Medicine
Washington University School of Medicine
St. Louis, Missouri

Roger D. Yusen, MD, MPH, FCCP
Associate Professor of Medicine
Department of Medicine
Division of Pulmonary and Critical Care Medicine
Washington University School of Medicine
St. Louis, Missouri

Chairman's Note

It is a pleasure to present the second edition of the *Pulmonary Subspecialty Consult Manual*, which is part of *The Washington Manual*® Subspecialty Consult Series. This pocket-size book provides a comprehensive approach to the diagnosis and management of a variety of acute and chronic lung diseases. This manual is an excellent medical reference for students, residents, interns, and other practitioners who need access to practical clinical subspecialty information to diagnose and treat patients with asthma, COPD, interstitial lung disease, pulmonary hypertension, cystic fibrosis, pulmonary infections, as well as other common pulmonary conditions. Medical knowledge continues to increase at an astounding rate, which creates a challenge for physicians to keep with up the biomedical discoveries, genetic and genomic information, and novel diagnostic and therapeutic strategies that can positively impact patients with lung diseases. The *Pulmonary Subspecialty Consult Manual* addresses this challenge by concisely and practically providing current scientific information for clinicians to aid them in the diagnosis, investigation, and treatment of common acute and chronic lung diseases.

I want to personally thank the authors, who include house officers, fellows, and attending physicians at Washington University School of Medicine and Barnes-Jewish Hospital. Their commitment to patient care and education is unsurpassed, and their efforts and skill in compiling this subspecialty manual are evident in the quality of the final product. In particular, I would like to acknowledge our editors, Drs. Adrian Shifren, Derek E. Byers, and Chad A. Witt, who have worked tirelessly to produce another outstanding edition of this manual, as well as our series editors, Thomas M. De Fer and Thomas M. Ciesielski. I would also like to thank Dr. Melvin Blanchard, Professor of Medicine and Chief of the Division of Medical Education in the Department of Medicine at Washington University School of Medicine, for his advice and guidance. The *Pulmonary Subspecialty Consult Manual* will provide practical knowledge that can be directly applied at the bedside and in outpatient settings to improve patient care.

Sincerely,
Victoria Fraser, MD
Adolphus Busch Professor and Chairman
Department of Medicine
Washington University School of Medicine
St. Louis, Missouri

Preface

This is the second edition of the *Washington Manual® Pulmonary Medicine Subspecialty Consult*. The book is intended to provide medical students, residents, and fellows a handbook for the evaluation of patients with pulmonary disease. The book is designed to reflect "real-life" clinical experiences. To effectively address our target audience, many of the chapters have been written with the input of medical residents or medical subspecialty fellows. Most of the chapters have been coauthored by an attending physician with expertise in the relevant field to ensure that both accurate and relevant information are provided.

A book such as this is always a collaborative effort. We would like to express our thanks for the commitment of the key individuals who helped prepare the second edition: the residents, fellows, and faculty from across departments and divisions at the Washington University School of Medicine who contributed chapters. We are indebted to Becky Light, whose ability to keep this project on track was nothing short of remarkable. We also thank Katie Sharp for her assistance with publication formalities.

Lastly, the editors appreciate the great collaboration that we shared and the love and patience of our families that allowed us to complete this work.

AS
DEB
CAW

Contents

The Chest Radiograph

1

Mark Mangano, Adrian Shifren,
and Sanjeev Bhalla

GENERAL PRINCIPLES

- The CXR is ubiquitous in medicine and remains among the hardest of diagnostic studies to master. The key to proficiency lies in reviewing all CXRs ordered. Close interaction with radiology staff is invaluable in building ones' skills and honing in on a specific diagnosis.
- Using a constant search pattern will allow for systematic and comprehensive analyses.
- Ideally, CXRs should be interpreted without knowledge of the clinical context to allow an unbiased and objective evaluation of the study. However, similar to any diagnostic test, evaluating the CXR in the context of the clinical scenario is very important and allows a focus on specific areas of the study and a detailed search for associated pathologic findings.
- At the Mallinckrodt Institute of Radiology (MIR), we try to initially read all CXRs without any clinical history. The clinical information is reviewed after the initial perusal so as to avoid bias at first glance and ensure subtle, clinically relevant issues are not overlooked.
- The importance of prior CXRs for comparison cannot be stressed enough. Understanding a finding often relies on knowing whether it is acute, subacute, or chronic. An area of consolidation, for example, could represent a community-acquired pneumonia on a CXR. If the area is stable from 1 year ago, low-grade adenocarcinoma or radiation changes become more likely.
- In our daily practice we often rely on old films. They are cheaper and lower in radiation than a CT and often provide greater information.

INITIAL ASSESSMENT

Patient Position and Study Quality

- Initial evaluation begins with assessment of patient position and quality of the study.
- This evaluation includes assessing the film for:
  - Rotation
  - Degree of inspiration
  - Patient position
  - Radiation dose

Patient Rotation

- A common method of assessing for the presence of rotation is to evaluate the relationship of the medial heads of the clavicles to the spinous processes of the vertebral bodies. When truly straight, each clavicular head will be equidistant to the adjacent spinous process.
- If the patient is rotated, the mediastinal borders will be altered. Rotation can be confused for mediastinal widening. Lack of appreciation for patient rotation can result in needless workup of perceived mediastinal changes.

Degree of Inspiration

- The degree of inspiration will affect the density of the lungs.
- As a general rule, the diaphragm should be crisp and the peak should be rounded.
- For those who prefer counting ribs, 10 posterior ribs and 6 anterior ribs should be seen on an inspiratory study.

Patient Position

- Erect versus supine positioning is pertinent to verify, as it will alter the interpretation of air–fluid interfaces, blood flow distribution, and caliber of the pulmonary vessels. Cephalization, for example, can be appreciated only on an upright film.
- The air–fluid level in the gastric fundus often allows one to understand whether the CXR is upright, supine, or decubitus.

Radiation Dose

- Radiation dose of a CXR has become more challenging in the digital era.
- As a general rule, the optimally exposed CXR allows visualization of the vertebral bodies and disk spaces through the mediastinal structures and also allows visualization of the pulmonary vessels through the heart and diaphragm.
- With new digital techniques, postprocessing allows the technologist to manipulate the image to achieve this same effect. The reader, therefore, must be careful that he/she can see through both the heart and mediastinum but that the image does not look too pixilated. Should pixilation occur, the reader must be aware that an insufficient radiation dose was used.

CXR Views

- There are a number of different variations of a CXR that may be obtained to evaluate thoracic pathology. These include the posteroanterior (PA) view, the lateral (LAT) view, the anteroposterior (AP) view, and the lateral decubitus (LD) view. Some centers also make use of end-expiratory (EE) views.
- All of these views share the concept of a point source which results in a fan x-ray beam. The result is magnification of structures which are farther from the detector. A good analogy is the shadow created by your hand on a classroom desk from an overhead light bulb. If you lift your hand off the desk, the shadow becomes bigger and fuzzier.

Posteroanterior View

The **PA view** is acquired with the patient in a standing position during full inspiration. The patient faces the detector, which is in contact with the anterior chest wall. The x-ray beam is directed toward the cassette from a distance of 6 ft, which results in minimal magnification of the heart.

Lateral View

- The **LAT** view is also taken with the patient standing during full inspiration at a distance of 6 ft. The arms are lifted. By convention, the patient's left side is placed in contact with the detector, and the beam is directed from right to left to reduce magnification of the heart.
- LAT views are useful for evaluating lesions behind the heart, diaphragm, or mediastinum that may be hidden on PA views.
- The left diaphragm can be differentiated from the right diaphragm on this view by locating the loss of the left diaphragmatic border when in contact with the cardiac silhouette or by locating the right posterior ribs (which will appear magnified and larger since they are farther from the cassette).
- It is important to note that magnification is about the same between the PA and LAT views. If a lesion is found on one view, the relationship with a landmark (e.g., aortic arch) can be used to localize it on the other.

Anteroposterior Views

- **The AP views** are usually taken with portable machines and are most often used to image the chest in patients who cannot have formal PA and LAT views, such as intensive care unit or intraoperative patients.
- These studies are conducted with the cassette behind the patient, in contact with his/her back. The x-rays are directed from front to back, often at a distance of <6 ft. The patient is often in a sitting or supine position and unable to perform a full inspiration.
- AP views often result in increased lung attenuation (from lack of complete inspiration) and increased magnification of mediastinal and cardiac structures (from increased distance between these structures and the cassette).
- It is important to understand that magnification of anterior structures occurs in the AP view to prevent inappropriate interpretation of an enlarged mediastinum or cardiac silhouette.

Lateral Decubitus Views

- **LD views** are taken with the patient lying on the ipsilateral side. For example, a left LD is taken with the left side down.
- There are four clinical situations in which a decubitus view might be helpful.
    - When evaluating whether the ipsilateral effusion is mobile
    - When evaluating whether a contralateral pneumothorax is present
    - When the contralateral lung has a concomitant pneumonia with an effusion
    - When the ipsilateral lung collapses normally. If it does not, one might suspect a radiolucent foreign body

End-Expiratory Views

- **EE views** are occasionally used to detect a subtle pneumothorax. The EE view should accentuate a pneumothorax as the EE radiograph will make the lung artificially whiter.
- Care must be taken to avoid mixing inspiratory and expiratory images when following a pneumothorax on serial images. The expiratory images will exaggerate the size of the pneumothorax.

GENERAL APPROACH TO CXR INTERPRETATION

- A systematic approach to the CXR reduces the risk of missed pathology. Subtle pathologies can be missed for two reasons. Only the process that is suspected is noted. Or, an obvious but previously unexpected finding commands the viewer's attention.
- There are as many systems for evaluating CXRs as there are physicians. The schema used here is arranged so that often-neglected areas are addressed first, and more common areas that may divert attention are addressed last.
- The PA CXR is addressed in detail, but any view can be read in a similar or slightly modified fashion.

Osseous Structures

The first structures surveyed are the **osseous structures** of the thorax, including the ribs (anterior and posterior aspects), the sternum (including signs of previous sternal splitting surgeries), the shoulder girdle (including the clavicles and scapulae), and the spine (both the vertebrae and the disk spaces). The skeletal survey should look for clues to understanding the other findings, including fractures, metastases, or previous surgery.

Upper Abdomen

Next, the **upper abdomen** is inspected. On an upright film any gas collections are evaluated, including the stomach bubble and the colon. Displacement of these structures may be indicative of organomegaly. An abnormal shape of the gas may be indicative of free intraperitoneal gas. The upright PA film is the study of choice for evaluating the presence of free air in the abdomen which is seen as a thin crescent under the diaphragm.

The Diaphragm

The **diaphragm** is evaluated next. The hemidiaphragms are smooth hemispherical structures, with the right diaphragm being 2–3 cm higher than the left owing to the presence of the liver below. The hemidiaphragms should be evaluated for shape (flattened in hyperinflation), sharpness (obscured with pleural effusions), and general symmetry (eventration, paralysis, or hernia through the hemidiaphragm leads to asymmetry).

The Mediastinum

Evaluation of the **mediastinum** usually follows, and is one of the more complex parts of the CXR evaluation because it includes so many thoracic structures.

Mediastinal Lines

The nine key lines of the mediastinum should be assessed for any focal distortion or displacement.

- The interfaces of the lungs, the anterior and posterior junction lines
- The right paratracheal stripe
- The left subclavian artery reflection
- The concave aorticopulmonary window
- The descending aorta
- The left and right paravertebral lines
- The azygoesophageal recess

Mediastinal Borders

- The nine lines are followed by the right and left mediastinal borders.
- The right border is formed (from bottom to top) by the right atrium, the ascending aorta, and superior vena cava.
- The left border is formed (from bottom to top) by the left ventricle, left atrial appendage, main pulmonary artery, and aortic knob.
- Both global cardiac and chamber enlargement should be noted. Global cardiac enlargement can be determined by calculating the cardiothoracic ratio—the width of the cardiac shadow on a PA view should be less than half the internal width of the bony thorax at its widest point. Any ratio >50% usually signifies cardiac enlargement.
- Although chamber enlargement is often the cause of an enlarged cardiac shadow, a pericardial effusion gives a similar appearance and should always be considered, especially when there is an acute change in apparent cardiac size.
- The LAT film can be especially helpful in differentiating chamber enlargement versus pericardial effusion. On an LAT film the pericardium is usually seen as a 2-mm stripe between two lucent arcs. In the presence of an effusion, this stripe is thickened. This finding is fairly specific and is often referred to as the sandwich or Oreo cookie sign.

Mediastinal Masses

- Mediastinal masses are often noted on this portion of the evaluation. The mediastinum is broken up into three different compartments, anterior, middle, and posterior for convenience of differential diagnosis. While various methods for dividing the mediastinum exist, a commonly used method is to define the compartments as follows:
  - **Anterior mediastinum** as the compartment between the sternum and an imaginary line drawn directly anterior to the trachea and posterior to the inferior vena cava. The differential for anterior mediastinal masses is usually headed by thymic lesions (thymoma and germ cell tumors) and lymphoma.

- ◦ **Middle mediastinum** as the compartment from the trachea to a vertical line drawn 1 cm behind the anterior edge of the vertebral bodies. The differential for middle mediastinal masses most commonly includes foregut duplication cysts (esophageal or bronchogenic) or lymphadenopathy, but a hiatal hernia should be considered if an air–fluid level is present.
- ◦ **Posterior mediastinum** as the remaining space. Most posterior mediastinal masses are neurogenic in nature usually schwannoma or neurofibroma.

The Aorta

The **aorta** should also be evaluated on the CXR. All of its portions (ascending, arch, and descending) should be evaluated for enlargement (possible aneurysm), calcification (atherosclerotic disease), and tortuosity (hypertensive disease).

The Hila

The hila are then evaluated. Their shape, size, and density are important and may indicate the presence of disease. The left hilum should be higher than the right owing to the fact that the left pulmonary artery courses above the left mainstem bronchus and the right pulmonary artery arises below the right mainstem bronchus.

The Pleural and Extrapleural Spaces

- The **pleural space** (between the parietal and visceral pleurae) and **extrapleural spaces** (between the parietal pleura and chest wall) are also carefully inspected.
- First, the pleura along the diaphragm is inspected from the cardiophrenic to the costophrenic angles. Next, the pleura lining the lateral margin of the lung is followed upward to the apex, and then over and down the mediastinal contour to the cardiophrenic angle where the inspection began.
- By following the pleural markings, the fissures of the lungs (including fluid collecting or tracking into them) and even accessory fissures can be evaluated.
- Careful examination of these spaces allows for the detection of small pleural effusions, pneumothoraces, pleural thickening or calcification, and masses.
- LAT films are more sensitive than PA films for the detection of small pleural effusions. Whereas ~175 mL of fluid is needed to produce blunting of the costophrenic angles on PA views, as little as 75 mL can be detected in the costophrenic angle on an LAT view.

Extrapulmonary Masses

- Extrapulmonary masses (pleural and extrapleural) can be difficult to distinguish from pulmonary masses on PA films.
- A number of features may assist in differentiating between the two types of masses.
  - ◦ First, a second view can be obtained (a mass overlying the lungs on a PA view may be noted to be extrapulmonary on an LAT view).
  - ◦ Second, the interface between the lesion and the lung is sharp with an extrapulmonary mass because they are superimposed structures.
  - ◦ Third, the angle between the chest wall and an extrapulmonary lesion is obtuse (>90 degrees).
- The incomplete border sign can be useful as well. In this sign, only 270 degrees of a round mass are seen. This comes from the fact that the last 90 degrees is the portion that is arising from the pleura or chest wall. As a general rule this sign denotes an extrapulmonary mass.

Medical Devices

Medical devices should also be carefully evaluated. Commonly encountered medical appliances include endotracheal tubes (ETs), nasogastric tubes, central venous catheters (including dialysis catheters), Swan–Ganz catheters, pacing and defibrillating devices, coronary artery stents, chest tubes, various peritoneal shunts, and surgical staple lines or wires.

Endotracheal Tubes

ET tips should be assessed for proper location, ideally 4 cm from the carina in the midtrachea with a minimal safe distance of 2 cm from the carina. Malpositioned ET tubes may ventilate only one lung if advanced too far, leading to contralateral lung collapse, or may enter the pharynx or dislodge into the esophagus if placed too superiorly. ET tubes move with changes in chin position. When the patient flexes, the tip advances. In other words, the "hose follows the nose."

Nasogastric Tubes

Nasogastric tubes should be evaluated for proper positioning.

Central Access Devices

- Central venous catheters need to be evaluated for proper course and tip placement in the superior vena cava, with special attention for pneumothorax after placement.
- Swan–Ganz catheter tips should be assessed for proper location in the pulmonary artery, and should not be advanced any more distally than the proximal interlobar pulmonary arteries (tip should remain within mediastinal shadow). Improper placement can lead to complications such as pulmonary infarction, pulmonary artery perforation, or pneumothorax.

Lungs

The **lungs** are the last to be evaluated. A focused, consistent approach is best. Working from bottom to top, the lungs are compared to each other. With the exception of the slightly elevated right hemidiaphragm and the asymmetric cardiac shadow, the lungs should be similar in appearance at each level of inspection. Any differences in the density of the film or the vascular markings are an indication of possible pulmonary pathology.

Final Steps

Again, it must be emphasized that once the evaluation is complete, it is essential to **evaluate old films and compare them with the current study**. This comparison allows for a more detailed understanding of the pathology being evaluated and may affect management in a significant fashion (e.g., a rapidly growing mass will be managed differently than a mass that has been stable for a number of years). Before concluding the CXR assessment, the study should be reviewed with a radiologist or the final report should be reviewed. This way any subtle findings can be addressed and reviewed.

COMMONLY USED FINDINGS FOR EVALUATING LUNG DISEASE

Radiographic Densities

- The key to understanding findings on a CXR relies on understanding the five main densities detected by radiography. Air, Fat, Fluid, Calcium, Metal. The densities are listed from darkest (air) on a radiograph to the whitest (metal). Metal attenuates the x-ray beam the most while air attenuates it the least.
- Only by juxtaposing two different densities, (e.g., heart and lung) can one see borders. Knowledge of normal borders allows for distinction from pathology. When a normal border is lost or a new border is present, pathology is suspected.

Radiographic Signs

Another basic tenet is the understanding that certain findings are frequently associated with a specific disease process. This association is often referred to as a sign.

TABLE 1-1 ANATOMIC LOCATIONS OF SILHOUETTE SIGNS

Lung Pathology	Silhouette Sign (Loss of Border)
Right upper lobe	Ascending aorta and right tracheal lung interface
Right middle lobe	Right heart border
Right lower lobe	Right diaphragm
Left upper lobe	Aortic knob
Lingula	Left heart border
Left lower lobe	Left diaphragm and descending aorta

The Silhouette Sign

- One common reason for ordering CXRs is to exclude pneumonia. The silhouette sign can be useful for this indication.
- Normally, the lungs attenuate the x-ray beam less than the heart and mediastinum. As a result the lungs appear black and provide nice contrast with the white central structures. When the lung becomes filled with fluid (as in a pneumonia), the border with the heart is effaced. This loss of the normal border is known as the silhouette sign.
- This silhouette will vary on the location of lung pathology; see Table 1-1 for anatomic locations of silhouette signs.

Luftsichel Sign

A hyperlucent crescent adjacent to the aorta, often indicative of a hyperexpanded left lower lobe associated with left upper lobe collapse. This finding has been labeled the **luftsichel** sign (meaning air crescent in German). Often, the luftsichel sign is easier to appreciate on a CXR than the actual lobar collapse itself.

Air Bronchogram Sign

- Often times the bronchi are visualized within a consolidation. This finding is known as the air bronchogram sign. Consolidation refers to filling of the alveoli by fluid. The air bronchogram sign can be explained by the contrast of the air-filled bronchi (dark) against the consolidation (white). Inflammation adjacent to the airway may result in dilatation of the airway (akin to an ileus). This feature may accentuate the air bronchogram.
- When acute this may be indicative of pulmonary edema, pneumonia, or pulmonary hemorrhage.
- When more chronic, one needs to think about low-grade adenocarcinoma or an inflammatory air–space process such as organizing pneumonia, radiation pneumonitis, or eosinophilic pneumonia.

Lobar Collapse

- Helpful findings in identifying lobar collapse (lobar atelectasis) include movement of lung fissures and crowding of pulmonary vessels or bronchi. Less specific signs include airway deviation, mediastinal shift, changes in adjacent lung density, and narrowing of the rib spaces. These findings occur because lobar collapse is associated with volume loss.
- Although pneumonia, lobar collapse, and pleural effusion may all appear white on a CXR, only lobar collapse will have volume loss. The distinction is important in guiding the appropriate management (pulmonary toilet vs. thoracentesis).
- Volume loss is important to differentiate from volume gain because it is indicative of a different differential diagnosis.
- There are helpful findings indicating volume gain.
    - Mediastinal shift **away** from the lesion
    - Airway deviation **away** from the lesion

Pneumothorax

- Another common indication for CXR is the evaluation of pneumothorax. Certain radiologic findings can help with identification.
- There are two essential signs of a pneumothorax.
  - Presence of a white visceral pleural line
  - Absence of lung markings peripheral to this pleural line.
- There are other radiologic findings that may be helpful.
  - Total or subtotal lung collapse
  - The deep sulcus sign (larger costophrenic recess on the side of the pneumothorax potentially with an inverted diaphragm)
  - Displacement of mediastinal structures
- Pneumothorax will move with changes in patient position. As a result, the pneumothorax is better seen apically on an upright view and better seen over the diaphragm and costophrenic angle on a supine view.
- In fact, this mobility can be useful in distinguishing a medial pneumothorax from a pneumomediastinum. The medial pneumothorax should move with a change in position.
- In larger patients skin rolls are often confused with a pleural line. These are differentiated by the fact that skin rolls form a dark line due to intervening gas in the fold.

Diffuse Lung Disease

- Evaluation of diffuse lung disease is also a common clinical question and its proper understanding relies on the interpretation of the predominant pattern on CXR.
- Diffuse disease can present as a generalized linear (reticular) pattern, a nodular pattern, a reticulonodular pattern, or a consolidative pattern.
- Although much has been written about trying to distinguish interstitial from alveolar disease, this can be very tricky on CXR alone. As a general rule, reticular processes tend to be interstitial.
- Knowing the chronicity of the process is extremely helpful, as acute diffuse reticular disease is usually secondary to pulmonary edema or viral pneumonia. More chronic reticular disease suggests a more chronic disease, such as fibrosis.
- When the pattern assumes a more nodular form, pneumonia and malignancy are more likely.

Chest Computed Tomography

2

Mark Mangano and Sanjeev Bhalla

GENERAL PRINCIPLES

- The cross-sectional orientation and contrast sensitivity of CT are well suited for detecting, describing, and distinguishing among diseases of the thorax.
- Common indications for a CT scan of the chest are broken into two main categories: those patients with abnormal CXR findings requiring further evaluation, and those patients with a normal CXR but with suspicion for occult disease.
  - Common abnormal radiographic findings prompting a follow-up CT include staging of bronchogenic carcinoma; evaluation of a nodule, mass, or opacity; and characterization of infiltrative lung disease, mediastinal, pleural, or chest wall abnormalities.
  - Common radiographically occult diseases include the evaluation of potential metastases, suspected aortic dissection, hemoptysis, bronchiectasis, infiltrative lung disease, endocrine abnormalities, or source of infection.
- Similar to the interpretation of CXR, it is important not to bias your interpretation of the CT scan based solely on the patient's known clinical history. While an understanding of the clinical scenario is important to focus on specific areas of the study, careful attention must be paid to the entirety of the examination to avoid missing pertinent findings.
- Comparison to prior CT studies is also essential to both characterize the time progression of lesions, and to determine whether subtle findings truly represent pathology.

INITIAL ASSESSMENT

Ordering a CT

- Not all chest CT examinations are performed in the same way. For efficient throughput, many CT departments use a variety of protocols to scan the thorax. These protocols are created to convey to the technologists information on radiation technique, reconstruction techniques, and methods of contrast use and enhancement. The protocols are usually based on clinical scenarios, such as aortic dissection, pulmonary embolism, or interstitial lung disease, and providing a meaningful indication for the examination will help ensure that the proper protocol is used.
- There are several important aspects to be considered when preparing the patient for a CT scan, including the area to be scanned, the use of contrast, and the patient's ability to tolerate the contrast.

Body Region

- The region of the body to be scanned should be documented, and will typically consist of a combination of the chest, abdomen, and pelvis. This decision will be made by the referring physician based on clinical context and may be adjusted by the radiologist as needed.
- Increasingly, insurance restrictions do not allow for the changing of the region to be scanned by anyone but the referring clinician. Hence, careful thought at the time of writing the order can save added work later.

- A chest CT tends to scan from the thoracic inlet through the adrenal gland.
- An abdomen CT tends to cover the dome of the diaphragm through the iliac crests.
- A pelvic CT scans from the iliac crest through the pubic symphysis.

Contrast

- The appropriate use of contrast is necessary to understand when ordering a CT study. A scan can be ordered with contrast, without contrast, and with and without contrast and is dependent on the indication for the study.
- Contrast can be administered intravenously (most common) or orally (rare for thoracic conditions). As a general rule, IV contrast is indicated for patients with suspected hilar, mediastinal, or pleural abnormalities and in patients with potential vascular abnormalities such as a pulmonary embolus. It can help distinguish lymph nodes from hilar vessels, underscore the vascular component of arteriovenous malformations, and identify the enhancing rim characteristic of empyemas.
- A noncontrast scan is generally indicated for assessing lung disease, ruling out pulmonary metastases, and for assessing nodules.
- A chest CT scan with and without contrast is typically only indicated for evaluation and differentiation of an aortic dissection or intramural hematoma, initial evaluation of pulmonary arteriovenous malformations, or characterization of a known mediastinal mass.
- There are four important considerations to understand if a patient can receive contrast: renal function, allergy, vascular access, and volume status.
- Since contrast agents are excreted by the kidneys and may cause changes in renal hemodynamics or tubular toxicity, it is important to assess renal function prior to ordering a contrast-enhanced study, as contrast may result in irreparable damage to a borderline set of kidneys.
  - Many centers use a serum creatinine level because of its ease in acquisition and it can be converted via a simple equation to creatinine clearance, which is an estimation of the glomerular filtration rate (GFR). Normal creatinine clearance ranges from 100 to 160 mL/min with physiologic variation by age. Generally, IV contrast should be avoided in patients with a clearance of <30 mL/min.
  - Of note, patients on dialysis can receive contrast media since the contrast will be filtered in their next dialysis session.
- It is also important to assess for a history of a reaction to contrast media when preparing a patient for CT. Patients should be specifically asked about iodinated contrast material, as many do not consider contrast a type of medication.
  - Shellfish allergy alone is not a contraindication to the use of IV contrast.
  - The severity of any reaction to contrast agents should also be characterized.
  - Generally, a patient with a history of itching or hives following prior contrast administration can receive premedication, whereas a patient with a history of prior serious contrast reactions such as laryngeal edema or anaphylaxis should not receive contrast despite premedication. The reactions can be somewhat idiosyncratic and tend to get more severe over time.
  - Premedication typically consists of a combination of corticosteroid and antihistamine. These medications may produce side effects of increased intraocular pressure or urinary retention, so a history of glaucoma or prostate enlargement should also be obtained.
- When ordering a study with contrast, the vascular access of the patient is an important and potentially limiting consideration. Although convention may vary by institution, typically central access or peripheral antecubital access with a 20-gauge line or larger is required. Specific questions about access requirements are best addressed through consultation with the radiology department.
- It is also important to remember that contrast is a bolus of fluid volume. Because of the osmolality, the contrast dose is equivalent to over 1 L of normal saline and may cause

problems for patients with pulmonary edema or cardiac issues. **As a general guideline, if the patient could not tolerate a 1-L bolus of saline, they should not receive IV contrast.**

CT Scans and Protocols

In the modern era, all thoracic CTs are performed on helical, multidetector CT machines. The term "spiral CT," which gained popularity as a synonym for the PE protocol CT, is not helpful, as most scans are performed helically or spirally.

High-Resolution CT

- High-resolution CT (HRCT) is a scanning protocol often used to diagnose diffuse lung diseases, bronchiectasis, emphysema, and focal lung lesions.
- HRCT does not require contrast and obtains detailed images that are comparable to gross tissue inspection.
- HRCT uses thin slices to improve resolution and view the fine details of the pulmonary parenchyma.
- In many centers, HRCT is performed in both inspiration and expiration.

Low-Dose CT

- Low-dose CT reduces the total radiation dose and is accomplished by lowering the tube current or kilovolt peak during the scan, which still results in readable images in the majority of patients.
- This type of scan is typically indicated for lung cancer screening, in children, or if multiple follow-up examinations are required.
- Low-dose CT may be limited by parameters such as patient size.

Other Protocols

Various protocols also exist for the evaluation of pulmonary embolus, aortic dissection, and thoracic aorta pathology. The appropriate use of these protocols is best clarified through consultation with a radiologist.

Preparing the Patient

- Patients can be hesitant about CT scans, which usually stem from lack of knowledge about the radiation dose and specifics of the procedure. It is helpful to relate the radiation exposure to that of natural background radiation, where one conventional chest CT is approximately equal in exposure to 3 years of natural background radiation.
- It is also helpful to explain to patients that the scan can be interrupted or terminated at any time if problems arise and that they will be able to communicate with the radiographer in the control room through an intercom.
- Claustrophobic patients may find it helpful to close their eyes during the examination.
- Patients should also be aware of the need for controlled breathing throughout the study, as this reduces image noise due to diaphragmatic movement.
- All clothing with zippers and all metallic objects should be removed to prevent confusion when interpreting the image.
- Patients should be made NPO 4 hours prior to their scheduled scan. IV contrast material can occasionally be proemetic. Four hours allow the stomach to be cleared of contents so the risk of aspiration can be reduced.

GENERAL APPROACH TO CT INTERPRETATION

- When starting the CT analysis, prior imaging studies and the clinical history should be examined to focus the interpretation and the differential diagnosis.
- The use of prior imaging to aid in the interpretation of the current chest CT cannot be stressed enough, as it is extremely useful in determining the time course of certain lesions and bringing subtle abnormalities to light.

- The characterization of lesions into acute or chronic is also essential to narrow the differential diagnosis and help rule out malignancy.

Window Levels and Window Width

- CT has much better contrast discrimination than a standard CXR. Levels of CT attenuation that are often able to be differentiated include (from dark to light): air, fat, fluid, muscle, enhancing organ, bone, and metal. The density levels of these items are assigned values known as a hounsfield unit (HU). The density of water is arbitrarily set to a value of 0 HU and the scale increases/decreases with corresponding radiodensity.
- Chest CT scans will often load with multiple series to view. These series are typically broken up by windowing technique or the use of contrast.
    - Since the human eye is unable to differentiate between the 2000 shades of gray that can be seen on a CT scan, windowing is used in areas of the body with similar density.
    - Windowing narrows the HU pixel range that will be displayed (decreases the potential number of shades of gray) so that each shade can be differentiated easier by the human eye. With fewer shades of gray to be displayed, contrast between the fine tissue details is maximized. Areas with density above the designated window range will appear white, and those with density below the range will appear black. The zero point or center of the window range is also adjusted and is analogous to the brightness of the image.
- Routine window settings for chest CT include one for the lung parenchyma, bone, and the mediastinum.

Basic Anatomy

- Identification of the correct anatomical structures must first start with understanding of patient positioning.
- When viewing a CT scan, imagine that you are standing at the patient's feet looking toward the head as he or she lies supine on a table. This way the patient's left side is on image right, and right side is on image left.
- The patient is also supine, so the vertebral column is at the bottom of the image and the chest wall is at the top.
- There may be circumstances where an image is taken in the prone position, where image right is the patient's right and image left is the patient's left. The top of the image is the vertebral column, and the bottom is the chest wall.
- Knowledge of the positioning is not only important for identifying anatomy, but also aids in distinguishing gravity-related changes (i.e., dependent atelectasis) from pathologic findings such as inflammation or fibrosis.
- Images can also be reconstructed in the coronal and sagittal planes. The coronal plane is as if you are looking at the patient from the front, and the sagittal plane is as if you were looking at the patient from the left side.
- Differentiating an expiratory CT from an inspiratory CT may also be required, and is best done through inspection of the shape of the trachea on corresponding levels. In the expiratory CT, the membranous portion of the trachea will flatten so that the trachea does not resemble an "O" as it does during inspiration.
- The identification of normal structures on the chest CT is required to be able to identify any abnormal structures or pathology. This is best carried out by grouping structures into the mediastinum, hila and lungs, pleura, chest wall, and diaphragm.

Mediastinal Anatomy

- The mediastinum is the tissue compartment situated between the lungs, bounded anteriorly by the sternum and posteriorly by the spine.
- Superiorly, structures are identified with reference to the trachea. The esophagus lies posterior to the trachea at this level, and the great arterial branches of the aorta lie anterior

and lateral to the walls of the trachea. At this level the great arterial branches will be seen from anatomic right to left as the innominate artery (brachiocephalic artery), left carotid artery, and left subclavian artery.

- Anterior to these great arterial vessels will be the great veins with the left brachiocephalic vein coursing across the mediastinum as the most anterior great vessel.
- The thyroid gland can also be identified caudally near the level of the thoracic inlet. Because of its iodine content, the thyroid is usually very bright.
- In the subaortic mediastinum, the aorta, superior vena cava, pulmonary arteries, and lymph node groups are important to identify. Usually, the aortic arch is easily identified crossing from the anterior to posterior mediastinum lateral to the trachea. The superior vena cava is seen anterior and to the anatomic right of the trachea.
- The thymus may also be seen anterior to the aortic arch and posterior to the sternum. Other notable structures at this level are the main pulmonary arteries and the azygous vein, which can be seen passing over the right main bronchus and emptying into the superior vena cava.
- Important lymph node groups to identify and assess for enlargement or pathology include the paratracheal chain, subcarinal nodes, and aortopulmonary window nodes. Lymph nodes with a short axis >1 cm are considered enlarged, with an exception in subcarinal nodes where >1.3 cm is considered enlargement.
- The paracardiac mediastinum includes the chambers of the heart and origins of the great vessels. The main pulmonary artery can be seen arising most anterior and rising from the right ventricle. It can be followed to its split into left and right pulmonary branches.
- The superior vena cava can also be visualized as it enters the right atrium. Identification of the aortic root as it projects out of the left ventricle can be helpful since coronary arteries may be seen as they originate near the aortic valve cusps, and can be assessed for calcification. The aortic root originates between the main pulmonary artery and right atrium.
- The most posterior portion of the heart is the left atrium, and most anterior is the right ventricle. The remaining heart chambers can be identified with relation to these structures and their outflow tracts. The inferior vena cava may also be identified caudally near the diaphragm as it courses into the right atrium.
- Assessment of the retrosternal space for the internal mammary arteries and veins, and lymph nodes may aid in diagnosis.
- Enlarged vessels may indicate superior vena cava obstruction, and enlarged lymph nodes always indicate pathology (most commonly breast cancer or lymphoma).

Hila and Lung Anatomy

- The anatomy of the pulmonary hila is visualized well on CT, which aids in the diagnosis of endobronchial lesions, surrounding masses, and vascular lesions. Contrast enhancement also helps to identify a hilar mass or lymph node enlargement.
- CT evaluates these structures so well and the anatomy is relatively consistent among individuals, so it is important to identify the normal anatomy to be able to distinguish abnormal pathology.
- Vascular anatomy often follows airway anatomy, so evaluation of these structures can take place concomitantly. The anatomy of the right and left hila with a focus on airway anatomy will be reviewed here separately.
- The right hilum can be tracked as the right bronchus branches from the trachea at the level of the carina.
- The right pulmonary artery passes anterior and inferior to the bronchus at this level. The right bronchus is, therefore, known as "eparterial."
- The right upper lobe bronchus will first be seen branching off ~1 cm distal to the carina with the right superior pulmonary vein directly anterior to this structure. This upper lobe bronchus will further branch into anterior, posterior, and superior segmental branches.

- After the upper lobe bronchus branches, the right airway will continue as bronchus intermedius. At the lower level of bronchus intermedius, the right middle lobe bronchus arises anteriorly just caudal to the right pulmonary artery and can be followed branching into medial and lateral segments.
- Distal to the branching of the middle lobe bronchus, bronchus intermedius becomes the right lower lobe bronchi and gives rise to the superior segment and the basal segmental bronchi (anterior, medial, lateral, and posterior). These segments vary in their appearance and are not always visible on CT.
- The left hilum can also be tracked as the left main bronchus courses from the trachea at the level of the carina. The left pulmonary artery passes superior to the left main bronchus at this level and will then descend posteriorly.
- The left main bronchus takes a longer course than the right before branching, and first branches off as the left upper lobe bronchus, which courses anterolaterally from its origin.
- The left superior pulmonary veins are anteromedial to the bronchus at this level. The upper lobe bronchus further branches into a lingular bronchus (which gives rise to superior and inferior segments) and anterior and apicoposterior segments.
- The left lower lobe bronchus is relatively symmetrical with the right lower lobe bronchus, and branches into a superior segment and three basal segments (anteromedial, lateral, and posterior).

Pleural, Diaphragm, and Chest Wall Anatomy

- The pleura, diaphragm, and chest wall are visualized well on chest CT imaging, and are most efficiently evaluated with soft tissue (mediastinal) windows.
- When assessing the pleura and diaphragm, it is important to remember that the diaphragmatic space extends well below the lung bases and scans must continue all the way down to this angle to be completely assessed.
- The visceral and parietal layers of the pleura are not normally visible on CT. The parietal (superficial) and visceral (deep) layers lie internal to the ribs and the innermost intercostal muscles and are separated from these structures by a layer of extrapleural fat.
- Identification of the diaphragmatic crura is also important to avoid mistaking them with enlarged lymph nodes or masses, as they can take on a rounded appearance. The crura are tendinous structures that extend inferiorly from the diaphragm to attach to the vertebral column.
- There are several physiologic openings in the diaphragm that should also be identified. These include the aortic hiatus, esophageal hiatus, and foramen of the inferior vena cava.
  - The aortic hiatus is most posterior and is bounded anteriorly by the crura and posteriorly by the spine. It is usually found at vertebral level T12. The azygous and hemiazygous veins, thoracic duct, intercostal arteries, and splanchnic nerves also pass through the aortic hiatus.
  - The esophageal hiatus is more anterior in the diaphragm and is located in the muscular part of the diaphragm. It arises around the level of the T10 vertebrae and also contains both vagal nerve trunk branches.
  - The foramen of the inferior vena cava arises around the level of the T8 vertebrae and is anterior and to the right of the esophageal hiatus.
- Gross inspection of the chest wall is important to identify any abnormalities that may also be clues to the diagnosis. Knowledge of the anatomy of the axillary space is particularly helpful in identifying abnormal lymph nodes and other pathology.
- When patients are scanned with both arms by their side, the axilla is bordered by the fascial coverings of pectoralis major and minor anteriorly; the chest wall and serratus anterior medially; the latissimus dorsi, teres major, and subscapularis posteriorly; and the biceps brachii and coracobrachialis laterally.
  - The axillary space also contains physiologic lymph nodes, axillary vessels, and nerves such as the brachial plexus and intercostals.

  - Normal lymph nodes in this region can be as large as 1.5 cm in the short axis, but with the appropriate clinical context lymph nodes >1 cm may be cause for concern.
  - Pathologic lymph nodes are best identified by direct comparison for symmetry in the axillae.
- Inspection of the supraclavicular area, breasts, and superior sulci should also take place with a concern for enlarged lymph nodes and masses.

APPROACH FOR READING CHEST CT

- With knowledge of the key anatomy, an organized approach for evaluating the chest CT is required to identify all findings. It is important to adhere to a regimen every time a chest CT is evaluated, as obvious findings may take attention away from less obvious findings that are equally important.
- Specific evaluation of the lung parenchyma will be discussed in the following section. Inspection should begin with the transaxial images in the soft tissue window.
- Because the beginner often neglects the soft tissues of the thoracic wall, these tissues should be evaluated first, followed by the mediastinum.
- Images should then be switched to the transaxial lung window with evaluation of the lung parenchyma, pleura, and bones.

Soft Tissue Window

- Inspection of the thoracic wall will occur first in the soft tissue window. Close attention should be paid to the axilla and breasts for enlarged lymph nodes and masses.
- The mediastinum should then be evaluated for pathologic masses or anatomical abnormalities. It may be easiest to orient yourself relative to the aortic arch or trachea.
- Cranially from the aortic arch (supra-aortic mediastinum), careful attention should be paid to the presence of enlarged lymph nodes, thyroid lesions or enlargement, and vessel abnormalities. When evaluating the space caudally from the aortic arch to the superior aspect of the heart (subaortic mediastinum), focus should be paid to the aortopulmonary window, subcarinal space, and anterior aortic space for the presence of enlarged lymph nodes.
- As you extend caudally into the paracardiac mediastinum, the hilar region should be assessed for configuration and vessel caliber, lobulation, and enlargement.
- The heart should also be assessed for signs of coronary atherosclerosis or dilations, and the descending aortic space evaluated for pathologic lymph node enlargement.
- When analyzing lymphadenopathy or a mass on CT, pay attention to the location and the attenuation of the abnormality. Both will be helpful in generating differential diagnoses and will be useful in communicating with other specialists. A fatty mass in the anterior mediastinum, for example, is less likely to be malignant than one in the middle mediastinum.

Lung Window

- The lung window is very wide and allows for assessment of the parenchyma, pleura, and bones.
- The lung parenchyma should be assessed first with evaluation for the normal branching pattern and caliber of vessels along with the interlobar fissures and presence of bullae.
- Careful attention should be paid for any nodules (<3 cm), masses (>3 cm), consolidation, or infiltrate.
- The pleura should then be assessed for the presence of abnormalities such as thickening, enhancement, calcification, plaques, pleural fluid, or pneumothorax.
- Finally the bones (ribs, scapula, and vertebrae) should be evaluated for normal marrow structure, spinal stenosis, or signs of osteoarthritis such as osteophyte formation. Focal lytic or sclerotic processes and fractures should also be identified.

Basic Lung Parenchymal Patterns

- Narrowing the differential diagnosis of lung disease on CT also requires an organized schema and is best delineated by characterizing the dominant pattern, distribution within the secondary lobule, and distribution within the lung.
- The dominant pattern is assessed first with other findings serving to narrow the differential diagnosis. This dominant finding should be grouped into reticular, nodular, high attenuation, or low attenuation patterns.

Reticular Pattern

The reticular pattern displays too many lines and is usually from thickened interlobular septae.

- Smooth septal line thickening is most often due to interstitial pulmonary edema (Kerley B lines) or lymphangitic carcinomatosis. Occasionally, it may be seen with viral pneumonias.
- Nodular septal line thickening is most often due to sarcoidosis, silicosis, or lymphangitic carcinomatosis.
- Irregular septal line thickening is a finding most often seen with fibrosis (usually nonspecific interstitial pneumonia).

Nodular Pattern

With a nodular pattern, the distribution of the nodules is key to narrowing the differential diagnosis, and identifying pleural nodules can help with this process.

- If no pleural nodules are present, it is likely a centrilobular distribution, with the most likely differential diagnosis consisting of hypersensitivity pneumonitis, infection, respiratory bronchiolitis, and bronchioloalveolar carcinoma.
- The presence of a tree-in-bud pattern of irregular and often nodular branching structures most identifiable in the lung periphery can narrow this differential diagnosis to endobronchial spread of infection (usually mycobacterial or bacterial) or airway disease associated with infection (bronchiectasis, cystic fibrosis, or allergic bronchopulmonary aspergillosis [ABPA]).
- If pleural nodules are present with a random distribution, the likely differential diagnosis is miliary TB, fungal infection, sarcoidosis, or the hematogenous spread of metastases.
- Otherwise nodules are considered perilymphatic and are characteristic of sarcoidosis, silicosis, and lymphangitic carcinomatosis.

High Attenuation Pattern

- A high attenuation pattern can be characterized as ground glass opacity (GGO) or consolidation with a large degree of overlap between the two.
- GGO occurs when there is a hazy increase in lung opacity without obscuring the underlying vessels, and is broken down into acute versus chronic.
  - Acute GGO occurs in cases such as pulmonary edema, pneumonia, or pulmonary hemorrhage.
  - Chronic GGO may be due to organizing pneumonia, hypersensitivity pneumonitis, chronic eosinophilic pneumonia, alveolar proteinosis, lung fibrosis, and bronchoalveolar carcinoma.
  - The location of GGO in the lung is helpful in distinguishing these etiologies.
- **Crazy paving** is another term used to describe the distribution of GGO and occurs when it is combined with smooth septal thickening, resembling a pattern of paving stones or irregular shapes and lines. The differential diagnosis is similar to GGO. Of note, however, is the classic association of this pattern with alveolar proteinosis.

- Consolidation refers to filling in of the alveolar air spaces with loss of visualization of the pulmonary vessels.
  - As with GGO, the differential is very much based on the chronicity of the finding.
  - When chronic, one must consider atypical infection, bronchioloalveolar carcinoma, inflammatory pneumonia (organizing pneumonia or eosinophilic pneumonia), or congenital lesions (such as sequestration).

Low-Attenuation Pattern

- A low attenuation pattern occurs due to emphysema, cystic lung disease, honeycombing, or bronchiectasis.
- Cystic lung disease is defined as radiolucent areas with a wall thickness <4 mm and is most often due to pneumatoceles, honeycombing, Langerhans cell histiocytosis (LCH), lymphocytic interstitial pneumonia, or lymphangioleiomyomatosis.
- Honeycombing occurs with usual interstitial pneumonia (UIP), interstitial fibrosis, or end stage sarcoidosis.
- Bronchiectasis can occur with cystic fibrosis, ABPA, immune deficiency, or a prior infection causing focal bronchiectasis. With bronchiectasis, care should be taken to exclude a central obstructing mass.
- Mosaic attenuation refers to scattered dark (low attenuation) areas within normal lung akin to a tile mosaic. Visualization of attenuated vasculature in the darker areas helps to prevent confusion with GGO.
- In mosaic attenuation, the darker areas are abnormal secondary to:
  - Small airways disease (most notably bronchiolitis obliterans).
  - Small vessels disease (most notably chronic pulmonary embolism).

Pulmonary Function Testing 3

Adam Anderson and Adrian Shifren

GENERAL PRINCIPLES

- Pulmonary function tests (PFTs) are an integral part of a pulmonary evaluation and management.
- PFTs can be divided into spirometry (measurement of air movement in and out of the lungs), diffusing capacity (measure of gas exchange within the lungs), and plethysmography (measurement of lung volumes).
- The availability of user-friendly pulmonary function testing devices has resulted in widespread use of on-site PFTs by community physicians and an increased need for formal training in collecting and interpreting valid pulmonary function measurements.
- PFTs are best interpreted in relation to an individual's clinical presentation and not in isolation. All parts of the PFTs should be used when evaluating a patient.
- It is important to remember that PFTs **do not** make pathologic diagnoses such as emphysema or pulmonary fibrosis. They provide physiologic measurements identifying ventilatory defects and, in doing so, support the existence of the relevant disease process and aid in the evaluation of its treatment.
- This text assists with evaluation of basic spirometry, diffusing capacity, and lung volumes and will allow the reader to identify common ventilatory defects using the data provided by PFTs.

NORMAL VALUES AND REFERENCE RANGES

- The results of PFTs are interpreted by comparing them to reference values representing normal healthy subjects.
- These normal or **predicted values** take into account many variables, most importantly age, height, gender, race/ethnicity, and to a lesser extent, weight.
- However, they neglect other influencing variables that may have effects, including air pollution, socioeconomic status, and others.

Percent Predicted Method

- Traditionally, but without scientific basis, pulmonary function labs have arbitrarily set normal ranges for each predicted value.
- The lower and upper limits of normal for each predicted value are set as 80% and 120% of the predicted value, respectively.
- The measured values for each pulmonary function variable are compared with the predicted values of each variable and expressed as "percent of predicted."
- Measured values that fall within the 80–120% range of predicted values are considered normal.
- This method is used in this text because it permits easy instruction and is still in widespread use.

Fifth Percentile Method

- An alternative method for defining normal range of each predicted (normal) value uses a percentile-based approach.
- Using this method, measured values less than the 5th percentile or greater than the 95th percentile within a healthy population are considered abnormal.
- The percentile method can lead to more precise diagnoses of chronic obstructive pulmonary disease (COPD), especially in the elderly.[1] The percent predicted method may over-diagnose COPD in elderly patients.[2]

STANDARDIZATION OF PULMONARY FUNCTION TESTS

- To obtain useful information from PFTs, the adequacy of both the testing equipment and the test results needs to be scrutinized.
- The American Thoracic Society (ATS) publishes guidelines for the standardization of spirometry, including recommendations on equipment calibration, validation of results, measurement of parameters, and acceptability and reproducibility criteria for the data obtained.[3,4]
- Because most PFTs are obtained from dedicated PFT labs, this text describes the standardized criteria for interpretation of PFT data and excludes details on equipment setup and testing techniques.
- Only when all the acceptability and reproducibility criteria are met can PFTs be interpreted with confidence.
- If acceptability and reproducibility criteria are not met, further testing needs to be performed to assess maximum function.
- Up to eight patient efforts may be performed; after this, patient fatigue affects the data obtained.
- The best results are always used for interpretation.

Acceptability Criteria

PFTs should initially be assessed for acceptability that is best determined by studying the flow-volume loops. Acceptability criteria for PFTs include the following:

- Freedom from artifacts (coughing, glottic closure, early termination leak, variable effort)
- Good starts (i.e., the initial portion of the curve that is most dependent on patient effort is free from artifact)
- Satisfactory expiratory time (at least 6 seconds of expiration on the volume–time curve, or at least 1-second plateau in the volume–time curve)

Reproducibility Criteria

Once the minimum of three acceptable flow-volume loops has been obtained, the reproducibility of the PFTs should be assessed. Reproducibility criteria for PFTs include the following:

- The two largest forced vital capacity (FVC) measurements should be within 0.2 L of each other.
- The two largest forced expiratory volumes in 1 second (FEV_1) measurements should be within 0.2 L of each other.

NORMAL PULMONARY FUNCTION TESTS

Flow-Volume Loops

- Normal PFTs are defined by a normal-shaped flow-volume loop (Fig. 3-1).[5]
- The flow-volume loop is the plot of the FVC maneuver.

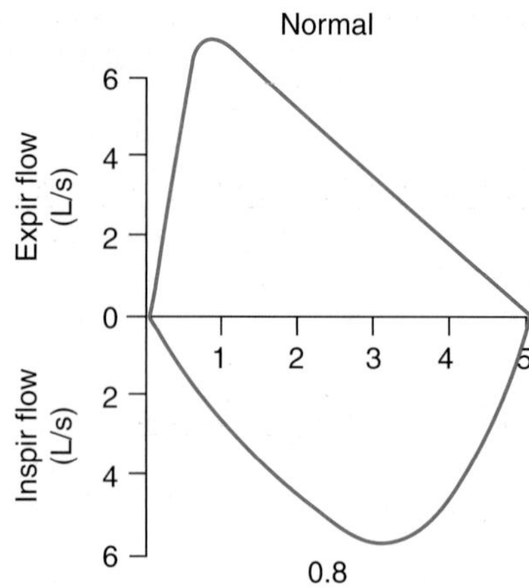

FIGURE 3-1. Normal flow-volume loop. (From Hyatt RE, Scanlon PD, Nakamura M. *Interpretation of Pulmonary Function Tests*. 4th ed. Philadelphia, PA: Lippincott Williams & Wilkins; 2014. © Mayo Foundation for Medical Education and Research.)

- The FVC maneuver involves the patient taking a maximum inspiration followed by a maximum and forceful expiration.
- The flow-volume loop portion of pulmonary function testing is also known as spirometry.
- The expiratory limb of a normal flow-volume loop has a rapid peak and a gradual decline in flow back to zero.
- The inspiratory limb should have a rounded shape.

FEV_1 and FVC

- Normal pulmonary function is also defined by the measured values for the FVC and the FEV_1.
- **FVC** is defined as the maximum volume of air that is **forcefully** exhaled after a maximum inspiration.
- **FEV_1** is defined as the maximum volume of air exhaled during the first second of the FVC.
- The measured values for FEV_1 and FVC are compared to the predicted values for FEV_1 and FVC as a percent of predicted. **Values of 80–120% are considered normal.**

Lung Volumes

- Lung volumes are measured separately from the flow-volume loop.
- Like the FEV_1 and FVC, measured lung volumes are compared to the predicted values for that volume as a percent predicted.
- Lung volumes between 80% and 120% are considered normal.
- The most important lung volumes for this discussion are total lung capacity (**TLC**), residual volume (**RV**), and slow vital capacity (**SVC**).
  - **TLC** is defined as the volume of air in the lung after complete maximal inspiration and a value of 80–120% of predicted is normal.
  - **RV** is defined as the volume of air left in the lungs after complete maximal expiration and a value of 80–120% of predicted is normal.

  - **SVC** is defined as the maximal volume of air that can be exhaled with **normal** effort after a maximum inspiration. (It is similar to the FVC except performed without full force.) A value of 80–120% of predicted is normal.

EVALUATING PULMONARY FUNCTION TEST PATTERNS

There are normal, obstructive, and restrictive patterns observed on PFTs, which will be discussed in detail. The following algorithm will allow for characterization of the disease pattern (Fig. 3-2).[6,7]

OBSTRUCTIVE VENTILATORY DEFECTS

- An obstructive ventilatory defect (**OVD**) exists when there is a disproportionate decrease in the FEV_1 when compared to the FVC. **An FEV_1:FVC ratio of <70% defines an OVD.**
- The FVC may be reduced in an OVD, but the FEV_1 is always reduced to an even greater degree.
- The ATS cautions against diagnosing an OVD in individuals who have a decreased FEV_1:FVC ratio but normal measured FEV_1 and FVC, because this pattern can on occasion be seen in healthy subjects.
- OVDs indicate airflow limitation and imply airway narrowing.
- In emphysema, for example, the narrowing is believed to be the result of decreased elastic support of smaller airways owing to alveolar septal destruction, whereas in chronic bronchitis, mucosal inflammation and excess mucus production are the etiologies.
- Once the diagnosis of an OVD has been made, the defect needs to be fully characterized by performing the following:
  - Quantifying the severity of the OVD
  - Assessing the reversibility of the obstruction
  - Determining whether there is hyperinflation
  - Determining whether there is air trapping

Quantifying an Obstructive Ventilatory Defect

Quantifying the severity of the OVD is done by comparing the measured FEV_1 to the predicted FEV_1 as a percent (Table 3-1).

Assessing for Bronchodilator Reversibility

- Assessing for reversibility of an obstruction requires spirometry be performed both before and after bronchodilator administration.
- An increase in the postbronchodilator FEV_1 *or* FVC (calculated from prebronchodilator values) of **both** ≥12% **and** ≥200 mL defines a positive bronchodilator response and indicates reversibility of an airway obstruction.
- Thus, reversibility is said to be present when, compared with prebronchodilator values:
  - **Postbronchodilator FEV_1 improves by both 12% and 200 mL, OR**
  - **Postbronchodilator FVC improves by both 12% and 200 mL**
- These criteria are best applied when active therapy is not present (e.g., no albuterol for 4 hours).
- The lack of reversibility during a PFT does not prohibit a clinical response to bronchodilator therapy.
- Although asthma is typically a reversible OVD, bronchodilator responsiveness during a PFT is not pathognomonic for asthma.

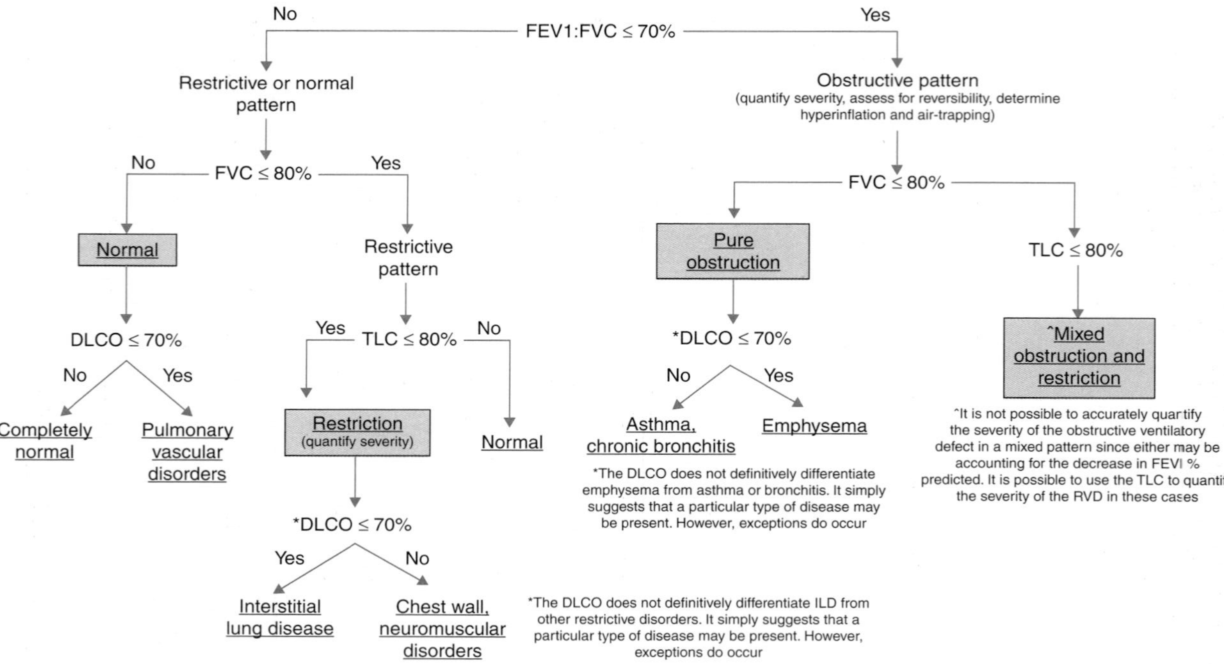

FIGURE 3-2. Evaluation of pulmonary function tests. DLCO, diffusing capacity for carbon monoxide; FVC, forced vital capacity; TLC, total lung capacity. (Data from Pellegrino R, Viegi G, Brusasco V, et al. Interpretive strategies for lung function tests. *Eur Respir J.* 2005;26:948–68; and Al-Ashkar F, Mehra R, Mazzone PJ, et al. Interpreting pulmonary function tests: recognize the pattern and the diagnosis will follow. *Cleve Clin J Med.* 2003;70(10):866, 868, 871–73.)

TABLE 3-1 QUANTIFYING AND CLASSIFYING THE SEVERITY OF AN OBSTRUCTIVE VENTILATOR DEFECT

Severity	FEV% of Predicted
Mild	>70%
Moderate	60–69%
Moderately severe	50–59%
Severe	35–49%
Very severe	<35%

Determining If Hyperinflation Is Present

- **Hyperinflation** denotes that at maximum inspiration or expiration the lungs are at a greater volume than is expected for an individual. In physiologic terms, the individual's TLC *or* RV is increased.
- The presence of **hyperinflation** is determined by comparing the measured TLC *or* RV to the predicted TLC *or* RV as a percent:
    - **TLC >120% of predicted, or**
    - **RV >120% of predicted**
- **Some sources consider hyperinflation to be present only when the TLC >120% of predicted, and air trapping to be present when the RV >120% of predicted.**

Determining If Air Trapping Is Present

- **Air trapping** denotes that during forced (rapid) expiration, there is dynamic collapse of airways with resultant incomplete exhalation of air compared with nonforced (slow) expiration. In physiologic terms, the individual's FVC is smaller than the SVC.
- Air trapping occurs because forced expiration causes worsening of airway obstruction as a result of higher positive intrathoracic pressures.
- An increase in the SVC by **both** ≥12% **and** ≥200 mL compared with the FVC indicates air trapping. **SVC ≥ FVC by both 12% and 200 mL.**
- **Some sources consider air trapping to be present when the RV >120% of predicted.**

The Flow-Volume Loop in Obstructive Ventilatory Defects

- OVDs change the shape of the flow-volume curve. The expiratory curve still has a rapid initial peak, but the terminal portions of the expiratory flow drop progressively with worsening obstruction.
- As a result, the expiratory limb of the curve takes on a progressively increasing concavity. Eventually, there is also a decrease in the peak expiratory flow at the initial portion of the curve.
- In severe disease, there is an initial rapid but reduced peak followed by a precipitous drop in flow and a very gradual taper of the flow to zero (Fig. 3-3).[5]
- Where lung volumes are measured the curve will also shift leftward, indicating that all lung volumes have increased, consistent with air trapping and hyperinflation.

UPPER AIRWAY OBSTRUCTION

- The OVDs discussed so far all represent obstruction at the level of smaller, more distal airways. Obstruction of the larger, more central airways (trachea and major bronchi) presents differently and is most easily identified on inspection of the inspiratory and expiratory limbs of the flow-volume loop.

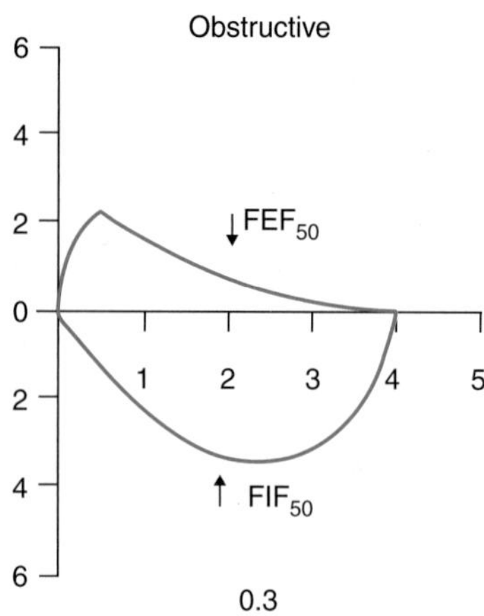

FIGURE 3-3. Obstructive lung disease flow-volume loop. (From Hyatt RE, Scanlon PD, Nakamura M. *Interpretation of Pulmonary Function Tests.* 4th ed. Philadelphia, PA: Lippincott Williams & Wilkins; 2014. © Mayo Foundation for Medical Education and Research.)

- Three forms of upper airway obstruction can be discerned:
  - Fixed obstruction
  - Variable intrathoracic obstruction
  - Variable extrathoracic obstruction

Fixed Upper Airway Obstruction

- When a central airway contains a fixed obstruction, the cross-sectional area of the obstructed airway does not change throughout the respiratory cycle (hence its characterization as *fixed*).
- The obstruction is present during both inspiration and expiration, and both limbs of the flow-volume loop are almost equally affected.
- There is characteristic truncation of both the inspiratory and expiratory limbs with the resulting "box" shape on the flow-volume loop (Fig. 3-4).[5]

Variable Upper Airway Obstruction

- When an airway contains a variable obstruction, manifestation of the obstruction is dependent on both the location of the obstruction (within or external to the thorax) and the phase of the respiratory cycle (inspiration or expiration).
- Changes in the cross-sectional area of the obstructed airway vary with both inspiration and expiration and intra- or extrathoracic location of the obstructing lesion.
  - In variable **intrathoracic** obstruction, the expiratory limb is primarily affected.
  - During forced expiration, pleural pressure exceeds the intrathoracic airway pressure. As a result, the airway narrows, and the obstruction worsens. During forced inspiration, the pressure relationships are reversed, and the obstruction is relieved. Thus, only the expiratory limb is truncated (Fig. 3-5).[5]
  - In variable **extrathoracic** obstruction, the inspiratory limb is primarily affected.

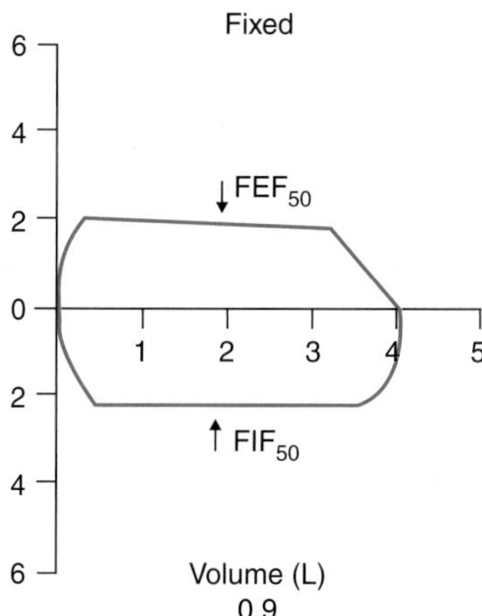

FIGURE 3-4. Fixed upper airway obstruction flow-volume loop. (From Hyatt RE, Scanlon PD, Nakamura M. *Interpretation of Pulmonary Function Tests*. 4th ed. Philadelphia, PA: Lippincott Williams & Wilkins; 2014. © Mayo Foundation for Medical Education and Research.)

- During forced inspiration, atmospheric pressure exceeds the extrathoracic tracheal pressure. As a result, the airway collapses, and the obstruction worsens. During forced expiration, the pressure relationships are reversed, and the obstruction is relieved. Thus, only the inspiratory limb is truncated (Fig. 3-6).[5]

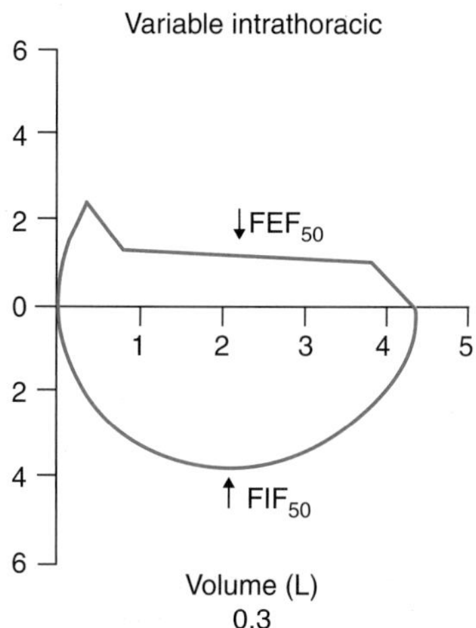

FIGURE 3-5. Variable intrathoracic obstruction flow-volume loop. (From Hyatt RE, Scanlon PD, Nakamura M. *Interpretation of Pulmonary Function Tests*. 4th ed. Philadelphia, PA: Lippincott Williams & Wilkins; 2014. © Mayo Foundation for Medical Education and Research.)

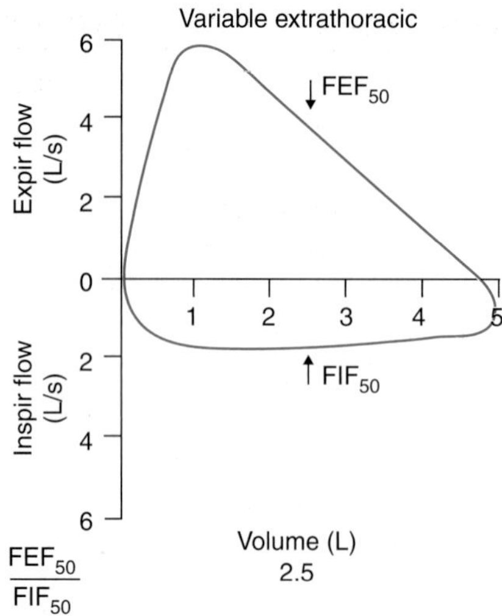

FIGURE 3-6. Variable extrathoracic obstruction flow-volume loop. (From Hyatt RE, Scanlon PD, Nakamura M. *Interpretation of Pulmonary Function Tests*. 4th ed. Philadelphia, PA: Lippincott Williams & Wilkins; 2014. © Mayo Foundation for Medical Education and Research.)

RESTRICTIVE VENTILATORY DEFECTS

- A restrictive ventilatory defect (RVD) exists when there is a reduction of maximum lung inflation, manifested by a reduction in TLC. Therefore, **a TLC <80% of predicted defines an RVD.**
- The presence of an RVD may be suspected using spirometry when the FVC is reduced in proportion to the reduction in FEV_1. In these cases, the FEV_1:FVC ratio will be either normal or increased.
- To diagnose an RVD definitively, however, lung volumes must be obtained to determine the TLC.
- An RVD is not specific for any specific disease. In interstitial pulmonary fibrosis, the restriction is the result of the fibrosis of the alveolar walls and "stiffening" of the lung parenchyma. In muscular dystrophy, weakened diaphragmatic and thoracic muscles are the etiologies.
- An RVD can also be caused by removal of lung tissue (lobectomy, pneumonectomy) as this results in a decrease in the total lung volume (hence TLC) compared to that predicted for the patient.
- Once the diagnosis of an RVD has been made, the defect needs to be quantified, which is done using the FEV_1 or the TLC percent predicted (Table 3-2).

The Flow-Volume Loop in Restrictive Ventilatory Defects

- The proportions of the flow-volume loop are essentially unchanged in RVDs.
- The curve is often narrowed and shifted to the right, reflecting the smaller lung volumes associated with RVDs (Fig. 3-7).[5]
- Although peak expiratory flow is decreased, note that at each measured lung volume, flow is often greater than in normal lungs.
- The features are only suggestive of an RVD; measurement of TLC must be performed to make the diagnosis.

TABLE 3-2 SEVERITY OF RESTRICTIVE VENTILATORY DEFECT

Severity	FEV_1	TLC
Mild	>70% of predicted	>70% of predicted
Moderate	60–69% of predicted	60–69% of predicted
Moderately severe	50–59% of predicted	50–59% of predicted
Severe	35–49% of predicted	35–49% of predicted
Very severe	<35% of predicted	<35% of predicted

DIFFUSING CAPACITY

- Diffusing capacity is often measured as part of a PFT. It is performed separately from spirometry and lung volume measurement.
- It is a measure of the integrity of the alveolar-capillary membrane across which gas exchange takes place.
- The diffusing capacity is a nonspecific measurement and provides only a physiologic assessment of the **efficiency of gas exchange.**
- Any disease affecting the pulmonary parenchyma or circulation can alter the diffusing capacity.
- The gas used to measure diffusing capacity is carbon monoxide, and the diffusing capacity is expressed as **diffusing capacity of the lung for carbon monoxide (DLCO).**
- The measured value is often adjusted to eliminate the effects of the hemoglobin concentration, which may artificially increase (high hemoglobin concentration) or reduce (low hemoglobin concentration) the DLCO.[8] The adjusted value is expressed as the **adjusted DLCO ($DLCO_{ADJ}$). The adjusted value for DLCO is sometimes called the corrected DLCO ($DLCO_C$).**

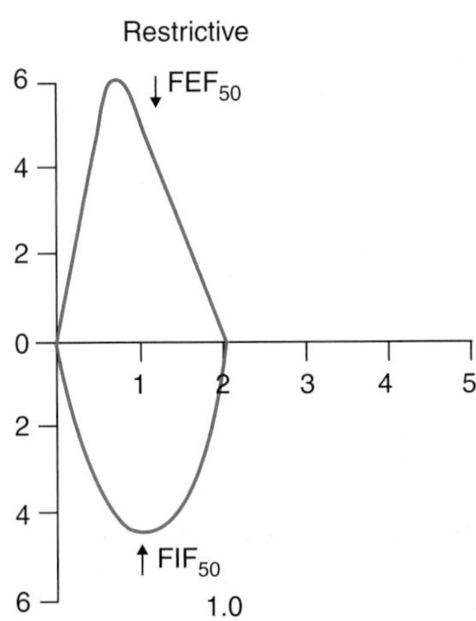

FIGURE 3-7. Restrictive lung disease flow-volume loop. (From Hyatt RE, Scanlon PD, Nakamura M. *Interpretation of Pulmonary Function Tests.* 4th ed. Philadelphia, PA: Lippincott Williams & Wilkins; 2014. © Mayo Foundation for Medical Education and Research.)

- Calculation of the $DLCO_{ADJ}$ is not mandatory but desirable.
- Measured values of DLCO and $DLCO_{ADJ}$ are compared to predicted values as a percent (the percentile method may also be used).
- Percent predicted values for **DLCO** between 70% and 120% are considered normal. Also percent predicted values for **$DLCO_{ADJ}$** between 70% and 120% are considered normal.
- The reason for the wide range in normal DLCO and $DLCO_{ADJ}$ is the large amount of variability between different measurements in the same individual at any given time. Of note the finding of normal PFTs with an isolated decrease in DLCO should raise a high index of suspicion for pulmonary vascular disease.

OTHER PULMONARY FUNCTION TESTS

Maximal Voluntary Ventilation

- Maximal voluntary ventilation (MVV), reported in liters per minute, is defined as the maximum amount of air that can be breathed in and out in 1 minute.
- For patient comfort, it is usually measured over 12 seconds and the value extrapolated to 1 minute.
- MVV is a very nonspecific measurement and can be reduced in either restrictive or obstructive disorders.
- MVV is often used to assess patient's respiratory musculature prior to surgery to help predict postoperative pulmonary complications.
- MVV is very effort dependent and requires good patient instruction.
- It is also a reflection of lung volume changes, lung–thorax compliance, and airway resistance. Therefore, MVV may be a less than accurate predictor of respiratory strength and endurance.
- Average values for males and females are 140–180 L/min and 80–120 L/min, respectively.
- However, interpretation is more complicated because MVV is proportional to FEV_1 and will decrease when FEV_1 is reduced.
- The following predictive equation is used to determine predicted MVV in the setting of a reduced FEV_1. **Predicted MVV = $FEV_1 \times 40$. Some sources use $FEV_1 \times 35$ to calculate predicted MVV. Other more complex formulas also exist.**
- In the setting of a reduced FEV_1, the predicted MVV may be reduced proportionately to the reduction in FEV_1, it may be reduced in excess of the reduced FEV_1, or it may be reduced to a lesser degree than predicted by the reduction in FEV_1.

Methacholine Challenge Testing

- Asthma is defined as a reversible obstructive airway disease. Therefore, in individuals suspected of having asthma, PFTs may appear normal, without evidence of obstruction.
- In individuals where PFTs are normal but asthma is strongly suspected, bronchial provocation testing is indicated to induce airway constriction and allow for the diagnosis (and further management) of asthma.
- Other individuals who should be considered for bronchial provocation testing include those with[9]:
    - **Chronic cough**
    - **Wheezing**
    - **Intermittent dyspnea**
    - **Workplace-related cough/wheezing/dyspnea**
    - **Exercise-associated cough/wheezing**
- The methacholine challenge test is a nonspecific test of airway responsiveness. It allows for a semiquantitative assessment of airway reactivity but gives no insight into the stimulus responsible for the reactivity in an individual.

TABLE 3-3 METHACHOLINE DILUTION SCHEDULE

Dose Number	Methacholine Concentration (mg/mL)
0	0 (baseline)
1	0.031
2	0.0625
3	0.125
4	0.025
5	0.5
6	1
7	2
8	4
9	8
10	16 (maximum)

- The advantage of the test is that it has good reproducibility.
- The disadvantage is that multiple factors can affect the test, including the following:
  - Medications (bronchodilators, steroids, antihistamines, β-agonists, calcium-channel blockers)
  - Respiratory infection
  - Exposure to sensitizers (allergens or chemicals)
- The test begins with the administration of a sterile saline aerosol followed by the measurement of the FEV_1 after 3–5 minutes (as a baseline).
- Increasing concentrations of methacholine diluted in sterile saline are then administered to the patient at 5-minute intervals, and the FEV_1 is measured 3–5 minutes after each increase in concentration.
- The concentrations range from 0.003 to 16 mg/mL of methacholine in sterile saline and are roughly doubled each time until either a positive response is obtained or a maximum concentration is achieved (Table 3-3).
- **A positive methacholine challenge is defined as a decrease in FEV_1 from baseline of >20% at a methacholine concentration of ≤8 mg/mL.**
- The methacholine concentration resulting in a positive challenge is reported as the PC20 (provocative concentration causing a 20% fall in FEV_1), for example, a decrease in FEV_1 from baseline occurring at a methacholine concentration of 0.5 mg/mL is reported as a PC20 = 0.5 mg/mL.
- **A negative methacholine challenge occurs if there is no change from baseline, or any decrease in FEV_1 from baseline is <20% and a concentration of >8 mg/mL has been reached.**
- When patients undergoing bronchial provocation testing are on inhaled corticosteroids, a decrease in FEV_1 from baseline of >20% at a methacholine concentration of 16 mg/mL may be considered a positive methacholine challenge test.[10]

REFERENCES

1. Roberts SD, Farber MO, Knox KS, et al. FEV1/FVC Ratio of 70% misclassifies patients with obstruction at the extremes of age. *Chest.* 2006;130:200–6.
2. Hardie JA, Buist AS, Vollmer WM, et al. Risk of over-diagnosis of COPD in asymptomatic elderly never-smokers. *Eur Respir J.* 2002;20:1117–22.
3. Lung function testing: selection of reference values and interpretative strategies. American Thoracic Society. *Am Rev Respir Dis.* 1991;144:1202–18.
4. Standardization of Spirometry, 1994 Update. American Thoracic Society. *Am J Respir Crit Care Med.* 1995;152:1107–36.

5. Hyatt RE, Scanlon PD, Nakamura M. *Interpretation of Pulmonary Function Tests.* 4th ed. Philadelphia, PA: Lippincott, Williams & Wilkins; 2014: 4–21.
6. Al Ashkar F, Mehra R, Mazzone PJ. Interpreting pulmonary function tests: recognize the pattern, and the diagnosis will follow. *Cleve Clin J Med.* 2003;70:866, 868, 871–3.
7. Pelligrino R, Viegi G, Brusasco V, et al. Interpretative strategies for lung function tests. *Eur Resp J.* 2005;26:948–68.
8. MacIntyre N, Crapo RO, Viegi G, et al. Standardization of the single-breath determination of carbon monoxide uptake in the lung. *Eur Respir J.* 2005;26:720–35.
9. Crapo RO, Casaburi R, Coates AL, et al. Guidelines for methacholine and exercise challenge testing—1999. This official statement of the American Thoracic Society was adopted by the ATS Board of Directors, July 1999. *Am J Respir Crit Care Med.* 2000;161:309–29.
10. Sumino K, Sugar EA, Irvin CG, et al. Methacholine challenge test: diagnostic characteristics in asthmatic patients receiving controller medications. *J Allergy Clin Immunol.* 2012;130(1):69–75.

Fiberoptic Bronchoscopy

4

Alexander C. Chen and Daniel J. Brown

GENERAL PRINCIPLES

- Fiberoptic bronchoscopy (FOB) was developed by Shigeto Ikeda in the 1960s.
- FOB has become a vital procedure for pulmonologists, with nearly 500,000 procedures performed in the United States every year.[1]
- The rise of the field of interventional pulmonology has increased the diagnostic and therapeutic range of the bronchoscope.
- As technology has improved, indications for FOB have increased (Table 4-1).
- Most contraindications are relative, and potential reward must merit the possible risk (Table 4-2). The major absolute contraindication is a significant increase in intracranial pressure (ICP), as coughing during the procedure can further increase ICP leading to brain herniation.

TABLE 4-1 INDICATIONS FOR FIBEROPTIC BRONCHOSCOPY

Inspection of	Evaluation, Diagnosis, or Management of		Other
Upper aerodigestive tract, larynx, vocal cords, and related structures	Chronic cough	Tracheoesophageal fistula	Assisting in intubation and extubation
	Wheezing	Tumor	Assisting percutaneous tracheostomy
	Pneumonia	Tracheobronchial stenosis	Brachytherapy
The major conductive airways	Persistent pulmonary infiltrates	Foreign body	Intralesional injection of drugs
	Disrupted bronchial tree secondary to trauma	Persistent atelectasis	Brachytherapy
	Thermal or chemical inhalational injury	Lymphadenopathy	Stent placement
	Anastomotic sites after lung transplantation	Pulmonary nodule	Surveillance for rejection after lung transplantation
	Position/patency of an ETT/tracheostomy tube		

TABLE 4-2 RELATIVE CONTRAINDICATIONS TO BRONCHOSCOPY

Relative Contraindication
Life-threatening arrhythmias
Severe hypoxemia
Recent myocardial infarction
Unstable angina
Uncorrected bleeding diathesis
Severe pulmonary hypertension
Thrombocytopenia
Superior vena cava syndrome
Unstable cervical spine

Prebronchoscopy Evaluation

- In an American College of Chest Physicians (ACCP) survey, a majority of operators obtain a preprocedure chest radiograph, coagulation studies, and complete blood count. Less than one-half obtain an EKG, arterial blood gas, electrolytes, or pulmonary function tests.[2] Routine preprocedure labs are not absolutely indicated unless specific concerns exist.
- Cardiac evaluation in patients with known coronary disease undergoing elective bronchoscopy can be considered, and guidelines have been published by the American College of Cardiology/American Heart Association.[3]

Procedural Medications

- Medications are commonly used before and during bronchoscopy to facilitate a safe, comfortable, and successful procedure.
- Antisialogogues are used with the intent of drying secretions and reducing the vasovagal response.
  - Atropine 0.4 mg IM is the antisialogogue most commonly used.
  - There are no convincing data that antisialogogues are efficacious, and because of the side effects, they are not recommended on a routine basis.[4]
- Benzodiazepines play a central role in providing amnesia and anxiolysis.
  - Midazolam given parenterally is often used for its fast onset of action and short half-life.[4]
  - Lorazepam has been used as a preprocedure medication with improved patient satisfaction at 24 hours versus placebo.
  - Flumazenil, a competitive inhibitor of the gamma-aminobutyric acid (GABA) receptor, can be used to reverse the sedative effects of benzodiazepines, though it should generally be avoided as it can precipitate withdrawal seizures.
- Opiates decrease the laryngeal reflexes and cough response, and provide some anxiolysis.
  - Fentanyl given parenterally is commonly used, again because of its short onset of action.[4]
  - Meperidine has been used pre- and intraprocedurally, but its use is increasingly discouraged because of its active metabolites, long half-life, and increased risk of seizures.
  - Naloxone reverses opiate sedation through direct competitive inhibition. It should only be used in cases of a significant narcotic overdose. Repeated doses or a continuous infusion may be required.
- Topical anesthesia to the upper aerodigestive tract, glottic area, and bronchial tree can be accomplished by the application of lidocaine, benzocaine, tetracaine, or historically, cocaine.
  - Lidocaine is the most commonly used topical anesthetic for FOB because of its fast onset of action and wide therapeutic window. It is applied in the glottic area, as well as directly on the tracheobronchial tree.[5]

  - Safety for lidocaine is well established at doses <7 mg/kg.[5]
  - Operators must be aware of the risk of methemoglobinemia when using topical anesthetics, even in small amounts. When it occurs, it can be reversed by administration of methylene blue.
- Propofol is a sedative-hypnotic drug with rapid onset and very short duration of action.[5] Recovery time after an infusion is only minutes.
  - Titration of propofol takes experience to avoid the most common side effect, hypotension.
  - Many institutions require anesthesia support for administration during procedures, and therefore it is often not used during routine bronchoscopies.

Monitoring

- The operator is ultimately responsible for the care and safety of the patient during the bronchoscopy.
- Additional assistance is required, including at least one respiratory therapist. A second assistant can be either a second respiratory therapist or a procedural nurse.
  - Assistants monitor the patient, record vital signs, administer and record medications, handle specimens, and assist with the bronchoscope and other equipment.
  - Special assistance is also needed when the patient is on a mechanical ventilator as insertion of a bronchoscope creates increased airway resistance.
- Equipment for monitoring and supporting the patient should include continuous pulse oximetry and EKG, vascular access, supplemental oxygen, suction, and an automated blood pressure cuff.
- Additional equipment that should be immediately available includes that needed for endotracheal intubation, cardiopulmonary resuscitation, vascular access, and needle decompression of pneumothorax.

Technique

- The most common patient position is supine, in bed, with the operator standing at the patient's head.
- A transoral approach is often used, sometimes with insertion of a laryngeal mask airway or endotracheal tube, and sometimes with no artificial airway. A transnasal or transtracheostomy approach may also be utilized.
- During insertion of the bronchoscope, the operator should note abnormalities of the upper airway, false and true vocal cords, and glottic area. After passage through the cords, the trachea and tracheobronchial tree are examined to at least the first subsegmental level.
- After examination of the airways, diagnostic or therapeutic procedures may be attempted.

Postprocedure

- After the procedure, the patient requires monitoring in a postprocedure area until they have recovered from sedation.
- A patient cannot drive home from the procedure, and should not operate machinery or perform other potentially dangerous activity after the procedure.
- Postprocedure chest radiograph is generally obtained if needle aspirations or biopsies have been performed.

DIAGNOSIS

- A list of diagnostic uses of bronchoscopy can be seen in Table 4-1.
- Airway inspection is the mainstay of FOB and is generally performed with each procedure.

- Tumors, cysts, source of hemoptysis, signs of infection, foreign bodies, and altered airway anatomy are some of the more common abnormalities encountered during inspection.
- Bronchoalveolar lavage (BAL) consists of wedging the end of the FOB in a distal airway, followed by instillation of sterile saline through the bronchoscope with subsequent aspiration back through the bronchoscope, in 50-mL aliquots.
  - BAL is most useful for obtaining microbiologic cultures in diagnosing typical and atypical infections.
  - Cytology can be sent to aid in diagnosis of infection, malignancy, and occasionally diffuse lung disease.
  - Cell count can show a preponderance of macrophages (normal), neutrophils, lymphocytes, eosinophils, or a fairly even mix of cell types, which are indicative of different disease states.
  - Successively bloodier BAL return aliquot is characteristic of diffuse alveolar hemorrhage.
- Transbronchial lung biopsy is performed by passing biopsy forceps through the bronchoscope and into the lung, with the goal of sampling the distal airways parenchyma.
  - Biopsies are examined by experienced pathologists and can diagnose a wide range of pulmonary pathology.
  - Transbronchial biopsies are generally performed using fluoroscopic guidance as the area being sampled is too distal for direct visualization, though this is not absolutely necessary.
- Endobronchial biopsy is performed by passing biopsy forceps through the bronchoscope and sampling airways lesions in the larger airways under direct visualization.
- Transbronchial needle aspirations (TBNA) are used to take cytologic samples from enlarged mediastinal lymph nodes and mediastinal masses.
- Endobronchial ultrasound has led to a marked increase in the range of diagnostic uses of FOB.
  - Endobronchial ultrasound using a linear array ultrasound is becoming the standard of care for diagnosis of mediastinal lymphadenopathy and masses, replacing traditional TBNA, and can also be used for sampling masses within 3–4 cm of the large airways in experienced hands. It is also superior to other modalities for imaging the structure of the trachea and mainstem bronchi.
  - Radial endobronchial ultrasound consists of a small, high-frequency ultrasound probe that can be guided through the bronchoscope into the distal airways, and advanced under fluoroscopic guidance with the goal of obtaining a real-time ultrasound image of a distal pulmonary nodule, allowing for biopsy and needle aspiration.
- Along with radial endobronchial ultrasound, 3D navigational systems have been developed that are being increasingly used to sample pulmonary nodules.

TREATMENT

- A list of therapeutic uses of bronchoscopy is seen in Table 4-1.
- Advances in the field of interventional pulmonology have led to a large increase in the therapeutic uses of FOB, several of which are listed below. Some of these procedures are performed solely by these bronchoscopic specialists, while some are also performed by general pulmonologists.
  - Tracheobronchial narrowing from malignancy, strictures, or other pathology can be alleviated by stent placement or balloon dilatation, though the latter's effects are much less permanent.
  - Cryotherapy can remove malignancies or other airway obstructions. During cryotherapy, a probe is placed on the obstruction at extremely low temperatures, in essence freezing the obstruction to the probe and allowing for extrication.[6]

- ◦ Argon plasma coagulation can be used to stop focal bleeding or obliterate obstructive airway lesions, neodymium:yttrium aluminium garnet (Nd:YAG) lasers may also do the latter.
- ◦ Foreign body removals are usually performed using biopsy forceps and sometimes occur under fluoroscopic guidance depending on the density of the foreign body.
- ◦ Therapeutic aspiration of secretions is sometimes performed in the presence of atelectasis with respiratory failure.[6]
- ◦ Management of anastomotic stricture or dehiscence after lung transplantation can generally be managed by debridement or stenting.
- ◦ Placement of one-way endobronchial valves will lead to collapse of selective subsegments of the lung and is being increasingly used in management of refractory, localized bronchopleural fistulas.

COMPLICATIONS

- FOB is overall very safe, with a reported mortality of 0–0.013%.[7,8]
- Major complications (pneumothorax, pulmonary hemorrhage, or respiratory failure) occur in <1% of procedures.[7]
- After bronchoscopy, the patient may experience low-grade fever, cough, hypoxemia, sore throat, hoarseness, or low-grade hemoptysis.
- Pneumothorax occurs in ~4% of patients after transbronchial lung biopsy,[8] and is usually detected by postprocedure chest radiograph.

REFERENCES

1. Ernst A, Silvestri GA, Johnstone D. Interventional pulmonary procedures: guidelines from the American College of Chest Physicians. *Chest.* 2003;123(5):1693–717.
2. Prakash UB, Offord KP, Stubbs SE. Bronchoscopy in North America: the ACCP Survey. *Chest.* 1991;100(6):1668–75.
3. Eagle KA, Brundage B, Chaitman B, et al. Guidelines for perioperative cardiovascular evaluation for noncardiac surgery. *Circulation.* 1996;93(6):1278–317.
4. Wahidi MM, Jain P, Jantz M, et al. American College of Chest Physicians consensus statement on the use of topical anesthesia, analgesia, and sedation during flexible bronchoscopy in adult patients. *Chest.* 2011;140(5):1342–50.
5. Matot I, Kramer MR. Sedation in outpatient bronchoscopy. *Respir Med.* 2000;94(12):1145–53.
6. Mehishi S, Raoof S, Mehta AC. Therapeutic flexible bronchoscopy. *Chest Surg Clin N Am.* 2001;11(4):657–90.
7. Jin F, Mu D, Chu D, et al. Severe complications of bronchoscopy. *Respiration.* 2008;76(4):429–33.
8. Pue CA, Pacht ER. Complications of fiberoptic bronchoscopy at a university hospital. *Chest.* 1995;107(2):430–2.

Hypoxic Respiratory Failure

5

Brad Bemiss, Adrian Shifren,
and James Bosanquet

GENERAL PRINCIPLES

Definition

Respiratory failure describes a set of conditions impairing delivery of oxygen to the tissues or removal of carbon dioxide from the tissues.

Classification

- Respiratory failure can be classified under many different schemas, each having its advantages.
- Classification by timing of onset, underlying etiology and/or anatomic area is useful when determining a differential diagnosis.
- Understanding the pathophysiology of respiratory failure and applying physiologic principles can guide the physician in developing a differential diagnosis and administering timely treatment to the patient.
- On the basis of pathophysiologic abnormalities, there are four types of respiratory failure.
  - Type 1: hypoxic respiratory failure.
  - Type 2: hypercapnic respiratory failure (see Chapters 6, 10, and 24).
  - Type 3: postoperative or atelectatic respiratory failure.
  - Type 4: circulatory shock-associated respiratory failure associated with hypoperfusion of respiratory muscles.

Etiology

- Causes of hypoxemic respiratory failure are shown in Figure 5-1.[1]
- The primary derangement in acute hypoxic respiratory failure is an inability of the cardiopulmonary system to deliver adequate oxygen supply to the tissues.
- Clinically, this can be further defined as the partial pressure of arterial oxygen (PaO_2) <60 mm Hg.
- It is also important to differentiate hypoxia from hypoxemia.
- **Hypoxia** occurs when tissues are not adequately supplied with sufficient oxygen to accomplish cellular respiration.
- **Hypoxemia** is characterized by a decrease in the content of oxygen in arterial blood. This includes both oxygen bound to hemoglobin and oxygen dissolved in the blood.
- Hypoxemia is, therefore, a form of hypoxia.
- There are four basic **classes of hypoxia:**
  - Hypoxemic hypoxia: low arterial oxygen content with impaired oxygen delivery.
  - Anemic hypoxia: low circulating hemoglobin concentration with impaired oxygen delivery.
  - Circulatory hypoxia: low cardiac output with impaired oxygen delivery.
  - Cytotoxic hypoxia: poisoning with cyanide where oxygen is delivered to the tissues but cannot be used.

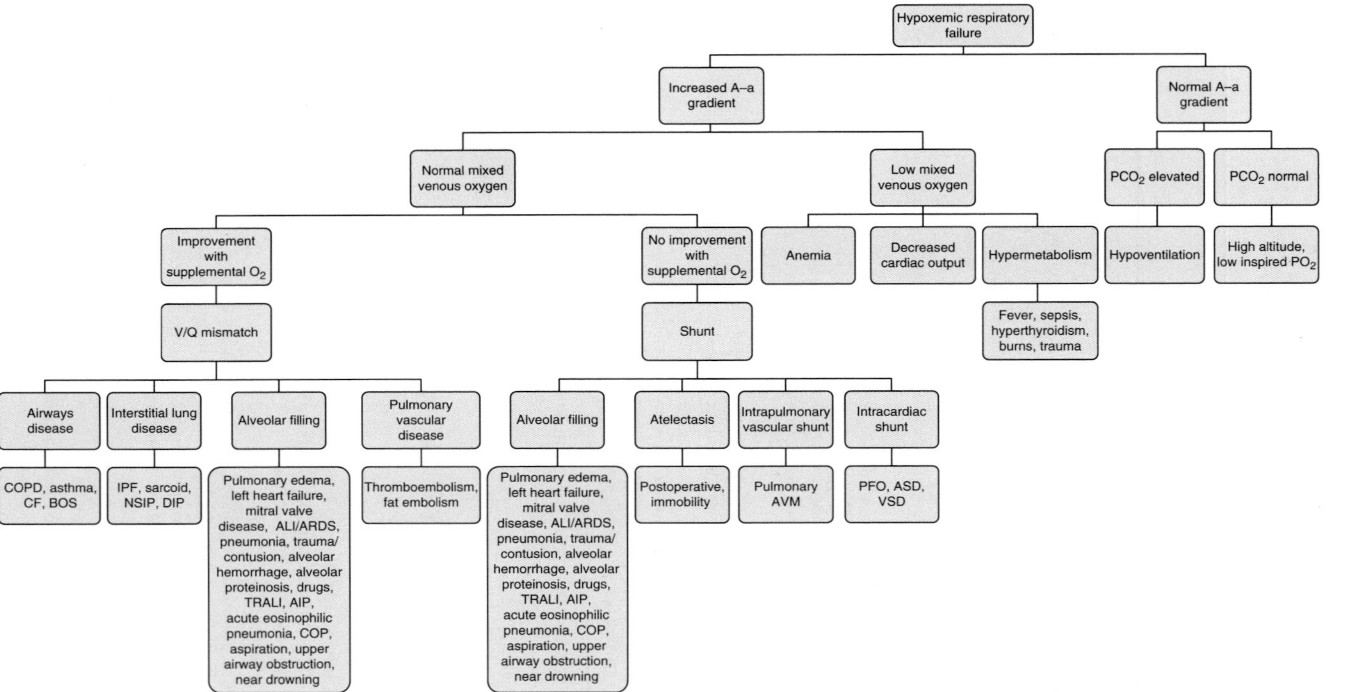

FIGURE 5-1. Etiology and approach to hypoxemic respiratory failure. (From Kollef M, Isakow W. *The Washington Manual of Critical Care*. 2nd ed. Philadelphia, PA: Lippincott Williams & Wilkins; 2012:42.)

Pathophysiology

- **Hypoxemia** results from one of six basic pathophysiologic mechanisms.
  - Decreased inspired oxygen pressure
  - Hypoventilation
  - Impaired diffusion
  - Ventilation/perfusion mismatch
  - Shunt
  - Low mixed venous oxygen content
- Multiple pathophysiologic mechanisms may be at play in a single hypoxemic patient at any given time.
- However, while all six mechanisms can contribute, typically, the only clinically significant mechanisms are ventilation/perfusion mismatch (V/Q mismatch), right-to-left shunting (shunt), and low mixed venous oxygen content.

Decreased Inspired Oxygen Pressure

- In conditions of low atmospheric pressure (P_{atm}), a decreased partial pressure of inspired oxygen (PiO_2) occurs.
- PiO_2 is calculated as: $PiO_2 = FiO_2 (P_{atm} - P_{H_2O})$
- Therefore, while the FiO_2 (fraction of inspired oxygen) in the atmosphere is a constant 21%, the PiO_2, and thus the driving pressure for oxygen diffusion across the alveolar membrane, is reduced in circumstances where atmospheric pressure is decreased (i.e., at altitude).

Hypoventilation

- With a reduction in alveolar ventilation, partial pressure of arterial carbon dioxide ($PaCO_2$) will increase.
- Using the alveolar gas equation we can predict that with the increased CO_2 resulting from hypoventilation, the partial pressure of alveolar oxygen (PAO_2) will decrease:
  - $PAO_2 = (FiO_2 \times [P_{atm} - P_{H_2O}]) - (PaCO_2/0.8)$
- Hypoxemia related to hypoventilation can be reversed by an increase in FiO_2 using supplementary oxygen, or an increase in alveolar ventilation.

Impaired Diffusion

- Diffusion of oxygen across the alveolar–capillary membrane is rarely the sole reason for hypoxemia.
- Diffusion of gas across a membrane is governed by Fick Law: $V_{gas} + (A \times D \times [P1 - P2])/T$
  - V_{gas} = volume of gas diffusing
  - A = surface area available for diffusion
  - D = diffusion coefficient of the gas
  - P1 – P2 = difference in partial pressures of the gas across the membrane
  - T = thickness of the membrane
- In healthy subjects at rest, a single red blood cell will spend ~0.75 seconds moving through a pulmonary capillary in contact with an alveolus.
- Oxygen is a perfusion-limited gas. Therefore, the partial pressure of oxygen in the alveolus equilibrates quickly with that in the capillary. This takes ~0.25 seconds.
- Thus, there is considerable diffusion reserve if other variables in Fick Law are compromised.
- However, in conditions where cardiac output is increased (i.e., exercise) the red blood cell spends significantly less time in contact with the alveolus. In these instances, impaired diffusion may contribute to the development of hypoxemia (e.g., interstitial lung disease).
- Impaired diffusion is characterized by a widened Alveolar–arterial (A–a) gradient and will correct with supplemental oxygen.

Ventilation/Perfusion Mismatch

- V/Q mismatch is the most common cause of hypoxemic respiratory failure, owing to the wide variety of clinical conditions in which it occurs.
- Ideally, ventilation of alveoli would perfectly match the perfusion of blood to those alveoli resulting in a V/Q ratio of 1.
- However, even in healthy subjects, differential ventilation and perfusion of the lung from apex to base is not perfectly matched. Normally, the ventilation to perfusion ratio of the entire lung is around 0.8, accounting for the physiologic A–a gradient.
- In certain disease states (see Fig. 5-1) this ratio can be altered leading to hypoxemia.[1]
- V/Q mismatch can vary widely depending on the disease state.
- A V/Q ratio of infinity, where alveoli are fully ventilated but have no perfusion, is referred to as **dead space.**
- A V/Q ratio of 0, where alveoli are perfused but have no ventilation is referred to as a **shunt.**
- These two extremes of V/Q mismatch are at opposite ends of a continuous spectrum that may result in hypoxemia, hypercapnia, or both.
- V/Q mismatch is characterized by a widened A–a gradient and will correct with supplemental oxygen.

Shunt

- As discussed above, a right-to-left shunt is a specific type of V/Q mismatch with a V/Q ratio of 0.
- In true shunt physiology, deoxygenated mixed venous blood will return to systemic circulation after bypassing unventilated alveoli.
- Shunts can be **congenital**, as occurs in developmental abnormalities of the heart and great vessels, or **acquired**, as occurs in diseases affecting the lungs (see Fig. 5-1).[1]
- Shunt is characterized by a widened A–a gradient and **inability to correct with supplemental oxygen** when the shunt fraction is >30%.

Low Mixed Venous Oxygen Content

- Typically, the mixed venous oxygen content of blood returning to the right side of the heart does not affect the PaO_2 significantly.
- However, in the setting of shunt or V/Q mismatch, subjects may become hypoxemic secondary to low mixed venous oxygen.
- Disease states that lower mixed venous oxygen are shown in Figure 5-1.[1]

DIAGNOSIS

Clinical Presentation

History

- Although hypoxemia can be asymptomatic, the most frequent presenting sign of profound hypoxemia is dyspnea.
- Copious airway secretions and abundant expectoration (among other clinical signs) can occur in pulmonary edema.
- Cough and purulent sputum (among other clinical signs) can occur in pneumonia.

Physical Examination

Manifestations of hypoxemia include cyanosis, restlessness, confusion, anxiety, delirium, tachypnea, tachycardia, hypertension, cardiac arrhythmias, and tremor.

- All of these clinical signs are both insensitive and nonspecific.

Diagnostic Criteria

Hypoxemia is defined as: PaO_2 <60 mm Hg and/or (arterial oxygen saturation) SaO_2 <90%.

Diagnostic Testing

- Initial diagnostic testing will likely include pulse oximetry, CXR, and arterial blood gas (ABG).
- Further diagnostic testing will depend on the differential diagnosis.

Laboratories

- A standard complete blood count (CBC) should be obtained as changes in hemoglobin can alter oxygen delivery.
- A drug screen (serum or urine) can assist in some cases of hypoventilation.
- If that patient is believed to have acute respiratory distress syndrome (ARDS), it is prudent to obtain more specific labs to diagnose the cause.
- Cultures (blood, sputum, and urine) should always be obtained if the possibility of infection is entertained.
- If diffuse alveolar hemorrhage is suspected, a vasculitis work-up would consist of anti-neutrophil cytoplasmic antibody (ANCA), antinuclear antibody (ANA), antiglomerular basement membrane (anti-GBM), rheumatoid factor (RF), complement levels, cryoglobulins, creatine phosphokinase (CPK), and other pertinent testing.

Imaging

- **CXR**: a standard two-view posterior–anterior (PA) and lateral CXR is always preferred to a portable CXR and is more sensitive for detecting and characterizing underlying lung pathology. However, the clinical situation must be taken into account.
- **CT chest**: depending on the clinical situation, a CT of the chest can help narrow the differential diagnosis for hypoxemic respiratory failure. A noncontrast CT scan almost always suffices, with the exception of suspicion for pulmonary embolus in which case a CT pulmonary angiogram is indicated.

Diagnostic Procedures

Echocardiogram: a cardiac echo may assist in evaluation of some causes of hypoxemia (e.g., heart failure, intracardiac right-to-left shunting, and valvular or pericardial disease).

TREATMENT

- Treatment of acute respiratory failure involves treatment of the underlying cause as well as general and respiratory supportive care.
- The therapeutic goal is to ensure adequate oxygenation of vital organs.
- For conscious, spontaneously breathing patients, supplemental oxygen is one of the most important initial treatments for acute hypoxic respiratory failure.
- The inspired oxygen concentration should be the lowest amount of supplemental oxygen that results in a **PaO_2 ≥60 mm Hg** or a **SaO_2 ≥92%**. Higher arterial oxygen tensions are of no proven benefit.
    - An important distinction must be made between adequate blood oxygenation and tissue oxygenation.
    - There is poor correlation between arterial hypoxemia and tissue hypoxia.
    - Improvement in arterial oxygenation may not provide a subsequent or adequate improvement in tissue oxygen availability owing to a drop in cardiac output or systemic vasoconstriction.

  - Obtaining a mixed venous oxygen saturation (SvO_2) or central venous oxygen saturation ($ScvO_2$) can assist with further management.
  - A profound decrease in tissue oxygenation is defined as shock.
- Appropriate oxygen delivery generally involves slowly increasing the inspired oxygen concentration (FiO_2) with monitoring of both PaO_2 and $PaCO_2$.
- The FiO_2 should slowly be increased to a goal PaO_2 of 60–70 mm Hg or a SaO_2 of ≥92%.
- It is important to realize that in some patients with chronic obstructive pulmonary disease (COPD) with acute-on-chronic respiratory failure there exists a compensated chronic respiratory acidosis with a small derangement of arterial pH.
- Although there is concern for CO_2 retention (and resultant worsening respiratory acidosis) in COPD patients when oxygen is administered, these patients are at greater risk from acute hypoxemia than hypercapnia.
- Therefore, the goals of oxygen therapy in COPD patients are the same as for other subjects, although some sources advocate for using a SaO_2 of ≥88% in these cases.

Oxygen Delivery Devices

- The selection of the appropriate noninvasive delivery system depends on the stability of the patient, availability of devices, and level of respiratory support required.
- For the critically ill or unstable patient, a planned, controlled intubation is always more desirable than emergent intubation. Predefined criteria for intubation and mechanical ventilation are broad and nonspecific, and are not covered in this chapter.
- Oxygen delivery devices for hypoxic respiratory failure can broadly be divided into two classes.
  - **Low-flow devices**, for example, nasal cannulas and face masks
  - **High-flow devices**, for example, Venturi masks and high-flow nasal cannulas

Low-Flow Oxygen Delivery Devices

Low-flow oxygen delivery devices provide a variable FiO_2 based on the size of the oxygen reservoir, the rate at which the reservoir is filled, and the ventilatory pattern of the patient.

Nasal Cannulas

- These low-flow systems provide insufficient gas to replace an entire inspired tidal volume (V_t). As a result, a large part of each inhaled breath is composed of ambient (room air) gas.
- Nasal cannulas are appropriate in patients with minimal or no respiratory distress, or those who are unable to tolerate a facemask.
- The benefits include allowing the patient to eat, drink, and speak.
- Their main disadvantage is that the exact FiO_2 is unknown. This is because the oxygen flow rate, the patient's inspiratory flow rate, and the inhaled V_t all influence the final FiO_2.
- As a general rule, for every liter per minute delivered, the oxygen concentration increases by ~3%. Therefore, with a normal V_t, the commonly utilized nasal cannula flow rates of 1–6 L/min provide an FiO_2 of 24–40%.
- Routine humidification of oxygen may provide little or no benefit in reducing the drying effects of nasal cannula oxygen on the nose and throat, especially with flow rates >5 L/min.
- At rates >6 L/min, flows become turbulent and the oxygen being delivered is no more effective than that delivered at 6 L/min.

Reservoir Nasal Cannulas

- Reservoir nasal cannulas are also called oxymizers.
- These low-flow systems can either increase the percentage of oxygen delivered compared to nasal cannulas, or act as oxygen-conserving devices.

- There are two types of reservoir cannulas commonly available: a nasal cannula with a reservoir situated below the nose (mustache-type), and a nasal cannula with a pendant reservoir situated on the patient's chest (pendant-type).
- The reservoirs facilitate conservation of oxygen by storing oxygen from exhalation for delivery during subsequent inhalation.
- The reservoirs trap the initial portion of expired gas from the large conducting airways that contain a high percentage of oxygen (i.e., dead-space gas that did not participate in gas exchange in the alveoli).
- The reservoirs also receive a continuous flow of oxygen from the oxygen source.
- The combination of oxygen from the source and the reservoir results in a higher FiO_2 during the subsequent inspiration and allows for total flow rates to be reduced.

Simple Facemasks

- These low-flow systems also provide a means of delivering a higher FiO_2 than can be achieved via nasal cannula.
- Two types of facemask exist: those with and those without an oxygen reservoir.
- To avoid accumulation of expired air within the mask, and subsequent retention of CO_2, the oxygen flow rates should be >5–6 L/min.
- Simple facemasks generally provide a FiO_2 of 35–60%.

High-Flow Oxygen Delivery Devices

High-flow oxygen delivery devices provide a constant FiO_2 by delivering either a higher-flow rate of oxygen than the patient's peak inspiratory flow rate, and/or by providing an oxygen flow admixed with a fixed proportion of room air.

High-Flow Nasal Cannulas

- **These high-flow systems** (e.g., Optiflo) allow oxygen to be delivered at rates that exceed a patient's inspiratory flow rate.
- Using special tubing, along with warming and humidification, allows for nasal delivery of oxygen flows of >60 L/min.
- This allows for the elimination of room air during inspiration so that a patient can breathe high fractions of oxygen without dilution by ambient air. Fractions of oxygen of up to 100% can be effectively delivered.
- In addition, the high flows used result in positive airway pressures of between 3 and 7 cm H_2O that assists in preventing atelectasis.
- The main benefit of the high-flow nasal cannula over other high-flow systems is patient comfort.

Venturi Masks

- These high-flow systems deliver precise oxygen concentrations.
- Oxygen passes through a narrow orifice under pressure into a larger tube, creating a subatmospheric pressure. This drop in pressure results in a shearing force that draws room air into the delivery system through a number of openings (entrainment ports) in the tube.
- Oxygen concentration is adjusted by changing both the size of the entrainment ports and the oxygen flow.
- The maximum FiO_2 achievable is 50%.
- This type of mask provides a constant FiO_2 independent of changes in inspiratory flow rate.
- It allows for easy step-wise increases or decreases in FiO_2 as oxygen delivery is titrated to PaO_2 or SaO_2.

- The main disadvantage is that the FiO_2 provided by these masks is limited and may be insufficient to maintain appropriate oxygen saturations in sicker patients.

Nonrebreather Facemasks

- These high-flow systems consist of a facemask that provides a constant flow of oxygen into an attached reservoir bag, resulting in a FiO_2 of >60% at 6 L/min oxygen flow.
- Each liter per minute of flow over 6 L/min increases the inspired oxygen concentration by around 10%.
- Placed correctly, the oxygen concentration can reach almost 100%.
- This type of mask is most appropriate for spontaneously breathing patients who require the highest possible oxygen concentration.
- The disadvantages of nonrebreather facemasks include oxygen toxicity, inability to feed patients owing to the tight seal required, limitation of speech, patient discomfort, and inability to provide aerosolized treatments.

Partial Rebreather Facemasks

- These high-flow systems are similar to nonrebreather facemasks.
- They differ in that they allow exhaled air to enter the reservoir, although this air is mainly from the large conducting airways and is therefore high in oxygen.
- Using the masks, a FiO_2 of between 40% and 70% is achievable.

Other Therapies

- **Incentive spirometry** assists patients with deep breathing.
- The deep inspiration is believed to help prevent the development of significant atelectasis.
- In the setting of elective surgery, it should be started prior to the operative procedure.
- The incentive spirometer should be used >10× per hour.
- **Mobilization** and **ambulation**, through both maintenance of an upright position and exercise, may help prevent atelectasis.

MONITORING, PATIENT EDUCATION, AND FOLLOW-UP

- Oxygen should continually be weaned to a goal PaO_2 of 60–70 mm Hg or a goal SaO_2 of ≥92% while the patient is hospitalized and treated for their underlying ailment.
- Patients should be educated on their specific disease and what to expect in relation to long-term oxygen therapy if needed.
- Long-term oxygen therapy is indicated in patients with a PaO_2 ≤55 mm Hg or SaO_2 ≤88%. However, this recommendation is based on patients with COPD and may not apply to all patients with hypoxemic respiratory failure.
- Prior to discharge, a patient should be assessed for a requirement for long-term oxygen therapy both at rest and with exertion since these requirements often differ.
- A 6-minute walk can provide this information by allowing for titration of oxygen at rest and with exercise. Oxygen can then be prescribed as needed.
- If chronic oxygen needs to be administered as an outpatient, patients should be educated on the use of long-term oxygen, and the dangers associated with oxygen administration (specifically the harms of smoking or cooking with open flames when oxygen is present).
- Concentrated sources of oxygen promote rapid combustion, and when exposed to open flames highly concentrated oxygen can result in explosions.

- The amount of oxygen required to maintain oxygen saturations ≥88% can vary over time.
- Patients discharged on oxygen should be followed in the outpatient setting within 2–6 weeks depending on the etiology of their hypoxemic respiratory failure and their oxygen requirements on discharge.
- In patients requiring ongoing oxygen therapy, a 6-minute walk should be performed at least yearly to ensure an adequate oxygen prescription.
- In certain cases an ABG may be clinically indicated at follow-up.

REFERENCE

1. Kollef M, Isakow W: *The Washington Manual of Critical Care.* 2nd ed. Philadelphia, PA: Lippincott Williams & Wilkins; 2012.

Noninvasive Ventilation

6

Warren Isakow

GENERAL PRINCIPLES

- **Noninvasive ventilation** (NIV) or **noninvasive positive pressure ventilation** refers to the use of a mask or similar device to provide ventilatory support.
- This definition is broad and could include external negative pressure devices (e.g., the "iron lung," historically used for ventilation of patients suffering from poliomyelitis-induced paralysis), cuirass ventilation (external shell with applied negative pressure), and rocking beds—an effective means to ventilate a patient with bilateral diaphragmatic paralysis.
- NIV by definition excludes any modality that bypasses the upper airway, such as laryngeal masks, endotracheal intubation, or tracheostomy.
- For the purposes of this chapter, NIV refers to mechanical ventilatory support delivered through a face mask, nasal mask, or similar device.

CLASSIFICATION

- Invasive mechanical ventilation and NIV have similar physiologic principles.
- The modes of ventilatory support (i.e., the way in which the ventilator triggers, delivers, and ends the breath) are similar to invasive mechanical ventilation. However, there is no standardization between manufacturers regarding mode terminology.
- Two of the most commonly encountered modes include continuous positive airway pressure (CPAP) and bilevel positive airway pressure (BiPAP).

Continuous Positive Airway Pressure

- CPAP maintains a set positive pressure throughout the respiratory cycle (inhalation and exhalation) and is not ventilatory support in a strict physiologic sense.
- CPAP "stents open" the upper airway with continuous pressure. This concept helps explain the utility of CPAP in disorders such as obstructive sleep apnea but does not explain why a treatment that does not provide ventilatory support can be of use in the patient who is suffering from hypoxemic or hypercapnic respiratory failure.
- Clinical applications include:
  - **Hypoxemic respiratory failure**
    - **Increases partial pressure of oxygen in the alveoli.** In the alveolar gas equation, $PAO_2 = FiO_2 (P_B - 47) - 1.2 (PaCO_2)$, if P_B is barometric pressure (or in our case, the pressure delivered from the ventilator through the mask), an increase in the mean airway pressure throughout the respiratory cycle for a given fraction of inspired oxygen (FiO_2) will increase the partial pressure of inspiratory oxygen and therefore oxygen tension in the alveoli (PAO_2).
    - **Provides extrinsic positive end-expiratory pressure (PEEP).** It recruits the underventilated or collapsed lung, probably by preventing alveolar collapse during exhalation.
  - **Hypercapnic respiratory failure** can decrease the work of breathing, by overcoming intrinsic PEEP in patients with chronic obstructive airway disease.

- In advanced chronic obstructive pulmonary disease (COPD) with hyperinflation, airflow obstruction and decreased elastic recoil lead to a prolonged expiratory phase. In respiratory distress, inspiration may occur before expiration is completed, leading to dynamic hyperinflation.
- Ineffective ventilation and increasing work of breathing cause the buildup of carbon dioxide and worsening respiratory acidosis. The positive elastic recoil pressure left behind in this hyperinflated patient at the end of expiration is termed intrinsic PEEP.
- Delivering PEEP via CPAP lessens the work of breathing by overcoming intrinsic PEEP. In intubated patients with acute respiratory failure, extrinsic PEEP ($PEEP_e$) has been demonstrated to reduce the work of breathing by 50%. The same principle applies to the noninvasively ventilated patient.

Bilevel Positive Airway Pressure

- **BiPAP** is CPAP with a second level of pressure support during inspiration, akin to pressure support ventilation for mechanically ventilated patients.
- In practical terms, BiPAP requires the operator to set two variables, inspiratory positive airway pressure (IPAP) and expiratory positive airway pressure (EPAP), that are measured in cm H_2O.
  - IPAP is the ventilatory pressure support the patient receives when either the machine or the patient initiates a breath.
  - EPAP is the pressure against which the patient exhales at the termination of inhalation.
  - "Initial settings" are often referred to by the IPAP followed by the EPAP (e.g., 12 cm H_2O and 5 cm H_2O).
    - The greater the difference between the IPAP and the EPAP, the greater the theoretical ventilatory support the patient receives.
    - However, progressively higher levels of EPAP and IPAP are not usually well tolerated by the patient, and as with any initiation of NIV, the patient should be observed closely to see if effective patient–ventilator synchrony occurs.

SPECIFIC DISEASE INDICATIONS FOR NONINVASIVE VENTILATION

- NIV may improve outcomes by avoiding intubation and the attendant risks of secondary infections in this patient population.
- In general, NIV is most effective in patients with cardiogenic pulmonary edema, patients with hypercapnic respiratory failure, and in weaning patients from invasive mechanical ventilation.

Cardiogenic Pulmonary Edema

- NIV helps to unload the respiratory muscles in respiratory failure caused by heart failure and pulmonary edema and improves cardiac performance by reducing right and left ventricular preload and mean transmural filling pressures.
- CPAP is recommended for hypoxemic patients with cardiogenic pulmonary edema who remain hypoxemic despite maximal medical therapy.
- A recent meta-analysis pooled the results of 34 trials in patients with acute cardiogenic pulmonary edema confirmed an overall mortality benefit utilizing NIV (both CPAP or bilevel modes), as well as a reduction in the risk of intubation.[1]
- Noninvasive methods of respiratory support **should not** be used in hemodynamically unstable patients or in those with ongoing cardiac ischemia.

Chronic Obstructive Pulmonary Disease

- NIV can be an effective initial respiratory support modality in the setting of acute COPD exacerbation. Studies have shown improvements in pH, PCO_2, and respiratory rate, and lower intubation rates and lower mortality when compared to standard therapy.[2,3]
  - NIV should be considered in patients with acute exacerbations of COPD in whom a respiratory acidosis persists (pH <7.35) despite maximum medical therapy. In a multicenter randomized controlled trial of BiPAP via nasal or face mask with standard therapy ($n = 236$ patients), NIV reduced the need for intubation and rate of in-hospital mortality was significantly reduced compared to the standard therapy group.
  - NIV helps to decrease the need for invasive mechanical ventilation. Between 1998 and 2008 in the United States, NIV use increased from about 1% to 4.5% of all patients admitted with COPD exacerbations, and invasive ventilation dropped from 6% to 3.5% accordingly. Similarly, patients who fail NIV and require intubation have a much higher mortality.[4]
- NIV can also facilitate weaning and extubation of COPD patients from invasive mechanical ventilation. Randomized trials in this population of patients have shown shorter durations of intubation, lower rates of nosocomial pneumonia, shorter hospital stays, and improved survival.[5]

Postextubation Respiratory Failure

- Most of the benefit of NIV in postextubation respiratory failure applies to hypercapnic patients who may benefit from a trial of NIV and close monitoring.
- In most cases, reintubation is more prudent and helps to prevent situations of emergent reintubation from a failure of trial of NIV.

Chest Wall Deformity and Neuromuscular Disease

- NIV can be an appropriate first-line choice in patients with acute and acute-on-chronic respiratory failure.
- In our experience at Washington University, these patients often do better in the long term with NIV that delivers a fixed tidal volume using laptop ventilators in assist control (AC), synchronized intermittent mandatory ventilation (SIMV), or even newer modes of average volume assured pressure support (AVAPS).
  - With bilevel pressure ventilation, tidal volume and minute ventilation may decrease with disease progression.
  - Similarly, acute changes in lung compliance due to alveolar consolidation due to pneumonia may render pressure-based NIV inadequate.

Trauma Patients

- CPAP can be considered in patients with chest wall trauma who remain hypoxemic despite regional anesthesia.
- Several small randomized, controlled trials support using CPAP for patients with isolated chest trauma, rib fractures, and hypoxemia.[6,7]
- Standard mechanical ventilation should still be used in patients with greater than moderate lung injury (defined by a PaO_2 of <60 mm Hg on an FiO_2 of ≥40%), as these patients were excluded from the study. Furthermore, the injury severity score was higher in the intubated group.[6]

Acute Hypoxemic Respiratory Failure and Pneumonia

- The use of NIV in hypoxemic respiratory failure is less clear than in the above disorders and depends on the severity of disease.
- The current recommendation is that NIV can be used as an alternative to endotracheal intubation in carefully selected patients with acute hypoxemic respiratory failure with

recognition that many of these patients may require intubation and if NIV is chosen, the patient should be intubated if not improving within 1–2 hours of initiation.

Asthma

- Routine use of NIV is not recommended.
- Severe respiratory acidosis in the setting of an acute asthma exacerbation should be treated with intubation and invasive ventilation.

Palliative Noninvasive Ventilation

- NIV has the potential to alleviate dyspnea in end-of-life circumstances.[8]
- Use of NIV should be weighed with issues of discomfort and claustrophobia from face–mask ventilation. Effective communication and clarification of the goals of care need to occur and managed on a case-by-case basis.

INITIATION OF NONINVASIVE VENTILATION

- NIV is best used for patients with:
  - High $PaCO_2$ (pH range of 7.25–7.35)
  - Low alveolar–arterial oxygen gradient
  - A good level of consciousness and cooperation
- NIV should only be initiated in locations with experienced staff, including respiratory therapists who are immediately available. In practice, this tends to restrict NIV to intensive care units (ICUs) or a designated respiratory ward.
- For initial settings see Table 6-1.[9]
  - IPAP
  - EPAP
  - FiO_2: this may be from a flow rate of O_2 L/min or from direct FiO_2 setting.
    - In some models, high flow rates may become uncomfortable and can lead to ventilator dyssynchrony.
    - Newer ventilators use an oxygen mixer that allows for titration of FiO_2 before its entry into the circuit without adjusting the flow rate. This setup is subsequently more comfortable for the patient and more beneficial for ventilation.

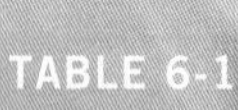

TYPICAL INITIAL VENTILATOR SETTINGS FOR BILEVEL POSITIVE AIRWAY PRESSURE IN A PATIENT WITH ACUTE HYPERCAPNIC RESPIRATORY FAILURE DUE TO COPD

Mode	Spontaneous/Timed
Expiratory positive airway pressure	4–5 cm H_2O
Inspiratory positive airway pressure	12–15 cm H_2O (to be increased as tolerated to 20 cm H_2O)
Triggers	Maximum sensitivity
Back up rate	15 breaths/min
Back up inspiration:expiration ratio	1:3

Adapted from British Thoracic Society Standards of Care Committee. Non-invasive ventilation in acute respiratory failure. *Thorax*. 2002;57:192–211.

TABLE 6-2 CONTRAINDICATIONS TO NONINVASIVE VENTILATION

Cardiac or respiratory arrest
Nonrespiratory organ failure (e.g., hemodynamic instability, unstable angina, severe GI bleeding, severe encephalopathy)
Life-threatening hypoxemia
Facial surgery or trauma/burns
Fixed upper-airway obstruction
Inability to protect the airway and/or high risk of aspiration (e.g., severe encephalopathy, upper gastrointestinal hemorrhage, vomiting)
Inability to clear secretions
Undrained pneumothorax

Adapted from Vianello A, Bevilacqua M, Arcaro G, et al. Non-invasive ventilatory approach to treatment of acute respiratory failure in neuromuscular disorders. A comparison with endotracheal intubation. *Intensive Care Med.* 2000;26:384–90; and Mehta S, Hill NS. Noninvasive ventilation. *Am J Respir Crit Care Med.* 2001;163:540–77.

CONTRAINDICATIONS FOR NONINVASIVE VENTILATION

- Absolute and relative contraindications are listed in Table 6-2.[10,11]
- Certain situations such as severe acidosis (pH <7.30) or a lack of improvement in clinical state and blood gas values make the immediate availability of intubation and critical care a necessity.

SPECIAL CONSIDERATIONS AND MONITORING

- Check arterial blood gas (ABG) within the first hour after initiation. ABG values usually improve within the first 1–2 hours if NIV is going to succeed.
- Clinical stabilization and improvement should occur within the first 4–6 hours.
- Optimize patient–ventilator synchrony and minute ventilation by fine-tuning flow rate, IPAP, EPAP, and FiO_2.
- Do not hesitate to intubate the patient if NIV is failing. Delay in intubation is a significant cause of rapid clinical deterioration and significant morbidity and mortality.

REFERENCES

1. Mariani J, Macchia A, Belziti C, et al. Noninvasive ventilation in acute cardiogenic pulmonary edema: a meta-analysis of randomized controlled trials. *J Card Fail.* 2011;17(10):850–9.
2. Brochard L, Mancebo J, Wysocki M, et al. Noninvasive ventilation for acute exacerbations of chronic obstructive pulmonary disease. *N Engl J Med.* 1995;333:817–22.
3. Celikel T, Sungur M, Ceyhan B, et al. Comparison of non-invasive positive pressure ventilation with standard medical therapy in hypercapnic acute respiratory failure. *Chest.* 1998;114:1636–42.
4. Chandra D, Stamm JA, Taylor B, et al. Outcomes of noninvasive ventilation for acute exacerbations of chronic obstructive pulmonary disease in the United States, 1998–2008. *Am J Respir Crit Care Med.* 2012;185(2):152–9.
5. Nava S, Amrosini N, Clini E, et al. Non-invasive mechanical ventilation in the weaning of patients with respiratory failure due to chronic obstructive pulmonary disease: a randomized study. *Ann Intern Med.* 1998;128:721–8.
6. Bollinger CT, Van Eeden SF. Treatment of multiple rib fractures. Randomized controlled trial comparing ventilatory with nonventilatory management. Chest. 1990;97(4):943–8.

7. Hernandez G, Fernandez R, Lopez-Reina P, et al. Noninvasive ventilation reduces intubation in chest trauma-related hypoxemia: a randomized clinical trial. *Chest.* 2010;137(1):74–80.
8. Azoulay E, Demoule A, Jaber S, et al. Palliative noninvasive ventilation in patients with acute respiratory failure. *Intensive Care Med.* 2011;37(8):1250–7.
9. British Thoracic Society Standards of Care Committee. Non-invasive ventilation in acute respiratory failure. *Thorax.* 2002;57(3):192–211.
10. Vianello A, Bevilacqua M, Arcaro G, et al. Non-invasive ventilatory approach to treatment of acute respiratory failure in neuromuscular disorders. A comparison with endotracheal intubation. *Intensive Care Med.* 2000;26(4):384–90.
11. Mehta S, Hill NS. Noninvasive ventilation. *Am J Respir Crit Care Med.* 2001;163(2):540–77.

Singultus

7

Sandeep Sodhi

GENERAL PRINCIPLES

- **Singultus**, more commonly known as **hiccups**, is a pervasive problem affecting almost everyone in his or her lifetime.
- Hiccups spare no population and have been observed in human beings from preterm infants to adults.
- Hiccups appear to serve no particular function and may be remnants of a primitive reflex. In utero hiccups may be a programmed isometric contraction of the inspiratory muscles.
- Singultus is derived from the Latin **singult**, meaning "a gasp."
- A hiccup is an involuntary and intermittent contraction or spasm of the diaphragm and intercostal muscles.
- Hiccups are divided into three categories, classified by the duration of the episodes.
    - **Hiccup bouts** are acute episodes that terminate within 48 hours.
    - Hiccups lasting >48 hours but <1 month are identified as **persistent hiccups**.
    - Those afflicted with hiccups for >1 month are identified as having **intractable hiccups**.
- Transient hiccups tend to occur at night.
- Although the majority of hiccups are benign, chronic hiccups may portend more ominous pathology, such as infection or structural abnormalities.

ETIOLOGY

- **Benign transient hiccups** are believed to arise from such common occurrences as gastric distention from overeating or aerophagia, tobacco use, sudden excitement or stress, or sudden changes in environmental or internal temperatures.
- **Chronic hiccups** are often pathologic in nature and can be broadly classified into organic, psychogenic, medication-induced, and miscellaneous origins.
    - Central processes include any disruption of the brainstem or midbrain areas.
    - Peripheral nervous system etiologies include those that irritate the vagus or phrenic nerves anywhere along their courses, including their cranial (vagus), cervical, thoracic, or abdominal portions.

PATHOPHYSIOLOGY

- Hiccups are believed to result from the stimulation of a **hiccup reflex arc** that involves both central and peripheral components.
- The afferent limb is composed of the phrenic nerve, vagus nerve, and sympathetic chain from T6 to T12.
- The efferent limb includes multiple brainstem and midbrain areas interacting with the motor fibers of the phrenic nerve.
- Previously, it was thought that a central connection between afferent and efferent limbs existed in the spinal cord between C3 and C5.
- It is now believed that this central connection involves an interaction among the medulla oblongata and reticular formation of the brainstem, phrenic nerve nuclei, and

the hypothalamus. These interactions then manifest as repetitive, involuntary contractions of intercostal and diaphragmatic muscles with glottic closure resulting in the familiar "hic" sound.

- Irritation in any component of this reflex arc may result in hiccups.
- Hiccups more commonly (in ~80% of cases) involve unilateral contraction of the left hemidiaphragm.
- The frequency of hiccups ranges between 4 and 60 per minute.
- Increased frequency is noted with decreased $PaCO_2$.

DIAGNOSIS

Clinical Presentation

History

- The onset, severity, and duration of hiccups are useful details. For example, hiccups occurring during sleep often point to an organic rather than a psychogenic cause.
- A careful review of systems allows further assessment of the clinical impact of hiccups.
- Chronic persistent hiccups have been associated with such complications as malnutrition, fatigue, dehydration, cardiac arrhythmias, and insomnia.
- Social history also provides helpful diagnostic clues, as excessive alcohol and tobacco use can cause hiccups.
- Medications need to be discussed, as a number of medicines are known to precipitate hiccups (Table 7-1).[1,2]

Physical Examination

- A thorough examination of the head and neck should be performed to evaluate for masses, foreign bodies, or evidence of infection—all of which may be culprits in inducing hiccups.
- Lymphadenopathy may cause compression of neural structures and merit more intensive investigation for underlying pathologies.
- Given the extensive number of thoracic causes of hiccups, the chest examination is crucial to identifying the underlying diagnosis and can shed light on underlying processes such as pneumonia or asthma.
- The physical examination should also include a careful neurologic assessment because strokes and various neurologic disorders such as multiple sclerosis can often manifest with hiccups.[3]

Diagnostic Testing

- No single laboratory study can diagnose hiccups. However, based on suspected etiologies from the history and physical examination, specific laboratory studies may be helpful.
- Specific tests such as serum alcohol or electrolyte levels can exclude metabolic and toxic causes of persistent hiccups.
- The CXR and/or chest CT can be helpful for ruling out cardiac, pulmonary, and mediastinal sources of peripheral nerve irritation.
- More specialized tests such as electroencephalogram (EEG), MRI, lumbar puncture (LP), bronchoscopy, and endoscopy may be performed based on clinical findings/necessity.[3]

TREATMENT

- Few controlled trials have been conducted to guide the approach to hiccup therapy.
- The literature consists primarily of case reports and series that do not directly compare treatment options.

TABLE 7-1 CAUSES OF HICCUPS

Organic
- Central
  - Vascular: ischemic/hemorrhagic strokes, arteriovenous malformations, head trauma lesions, vasculitis
  - Infections: encephalitis/meningitis, brain abscess, neurosyphilis
  - Structural: mass lesions
- Peripheral
  - Meningeal/pharyngeal afferents: meningitis/laryngitis/abscess, goiters/cysts/tumors
  - Auricular afferents: foreign body
  - Thoracic afferents: chest trauma, neoplasm of lung, lymphadenopathy, myocardial infarction, pulmonary edema, pericarditis/pleuritis/esophagitis, aortic aneurysm, asthma/bronchitis/pneumonia, esophagitis/stricture/hernia, achalasia
  - Abdominal afferents: gastric distention, gastritis/hepatitis, peptic ulcers, pancreatic/biliary disease, bowel obstruction, appendicitis, inflammatory bowel disease, intra-abdominal surgery, genitourinary disorders, direct diaphragmatic irritation

Psychogenic: stress/excitement, conversion/grief reactions, anorexia nervosa, malingering

Medications: corticosteroids, barbiturates, benzodiazepines, α-blockers, dopaminergic agonists, antibiotics, nonsteroidal anti-inflammatories, general anesthetics

Miscellaneous: idiopathic, toxic/metabolic causes, alcohol, tobacco, sepsis, electrolyte abnormalities (sodium/calcium/potassium), uremia, diabetes mellitus, intubation (with glottic stimulation)

- Nonetheless, when persistent hiccups adversely affect a patient's quality of life, treatment is indicated.
- Given the numerous etiologies of hiccups, treatment should first be directed at rectifying the specific cause as determined by history, physical examination, and testing.
- If a cause for hiccups cannot be found nonpharmacologic therapies should be first-line treatment.

Medications

- Targeted pharmacologic therapy is aimed at inhibition of stimulated points in the hiccup reflex arc, largely effecting blockade through inhibitory neurotransmitters.
- Again, most pharmacologic therapies have been evaluated in case studies rather than in controlled clinical trials, and should be used only after physical maneuvers have failed.
- Idiopathic chronic hiccups have been treated with such pharmacologic agents as gamma-aminobutyric acid (GABA) and dopamine antagonists (baclofen, chlorpromazine, haloperidol, metoclopramide); anticonvulsants (valproic acid, carbamazepine, phenytoin); and numerous miscellaneous agents (nifedipine, sertraline, anesthetics, gastric acid suppressors).[4]
- To date, chlorpromazine has been one of the most commonly used medications in the treatment of hiccups. It has been shown to have good efficacy and is well tolerated at low doses.[5]
- In a small number of case studies, gabapentin has been reported as successful therapy in refractory hiccups.[6]

- Hiccups usually respond rapidly to therapy if the therapy is to be effective. However, multiple agents may be initiated before a successful drug is found.
- If hiccups subside following treatment, medical therapy can generally be discontinued 24 hours after the resolution of symptoms.
- Most drug therapies for hiccups can be used for 7–10 days.

Other Nonpharmacologic Therapies

- Such ancient remedies include sneezing, inducing unexpected fright, swallowing granulated sugar, carotid massage, Valsalva maneuvers, supraorbital pressure, and holding one's breath.[4]
- These maneuvers carry a low risk of complications, but their efficacy has not been confirmed.

Surgical Management

In cases refractory to both conservative (nonpharmacologic) and pharmacologic therapy, surgical manipulation of either the phrenic or vagal nerves may be considered.

REFERENCES

1. Hansen BJ, Rosenberg J. Persistent postoperative hiccups: a review. *Acta Anaesthesiol Scand.* 1993; 37(7):643–6.
2. Thompson DF, Landry JP. Drug-induced hiccups. *Ann Pharmacother.* 1997;31(3):367–9.
3. Kolodzik PW, Eilers MA. Hiccups (singultus): review and approach to management. *Ann Emerg Med.* 1991;20(5):565–73.
4. Friedman NL. Hiccups: a treatment review. *Pharmacotherapy.* 1996;16(6):986–95.
5. Friedgood CE, Ripstein CB. Chlorpromazine in the treatment of intractable hiccups. *J Am Med Assoc.* 1955;157(4):309–10.
6. Hernandez JL, Pajaron M, Garcia-Regata O, et al. Gabapentin for intractable hiccup. *Am J Med.* 2004;117(4):279–81.

Cough

8

David Picker and Praveen R. Chenna

GENERAL PRINCIPLES

- Cough is a common symptom and a substantial driver of outpatient care visits.
- Cough accounts for nearly 30 million physician visits per year. Estimated costs for treatment may reach $1 billion annually, not including the cost of diagnostic testing and complications such as headache, hoarseness, urinary incontinence, musculoskeletal pain, and exhaustion.
- Due to the adverse effects on the quality of patients' lives, a systematic approach is necessary for the diagnosis and management of cough in the adult patient.

CLASSIFICATION

Cough is classified based on the duration of symptoms, which can help provide a framework for diagnosis.[1]

- **Acute** cough is defined as <3 weeks.
- **Subacute** cough is defined as >3 weeks, and <8 weeks.
- **Chronic** cough is defined as >8 weeks.

Acute Cough

Acute cough can be divided into three main categories; infectious, exacerbation of underlying disease process, and exposure-related.

- **Infectious**
  - Viral infections of the upper respiratory tract are the most common cause of acute cough. Rhinovirus, coronavirus, and respiratory syncytial virus are the pathogens most frequently associated with common cold symptoms. Less frequent causes include influenza, parainfluenza, and adenovirus.
  - Clinical features of the common cold include rhinorrhea, sneezing, irritation of the throat, lacrimation, and nasal obstruction. Fever may or may not be a presenting symptom. Coughing usually presents on day 4 or 5 after infection.
  - Chest radiograph is usually negative and therefore of low yield in the general population. However, certain exceptions should be considered in the elderly and immunocompromised to rule out potential pneumonia, or other insidious infection.
  - **Viral or bacterial rhinosinusitis** can also result in postnasal drainage and acute cough.
    - Viral rhinosinusitis may be difficult to distinguish from bacterial sinusitis.
    - Viral rhinosinusitis can be symptomatically managed with antihistamines and nasal decongestants.
  - *Bordetella pertussis* infection is common cause of acute cough in adults. Symptoms may include a barking cough and post-tussive emesis. Diagnosis may be confirmed by sputum culture or *B. pertussis* PCR testing.

- **Exacerbation of underlying disease process**
  - **Allergic rhinitis** is an IgE-mediated syndrome characterized by paroxysms of sneezing, nasal congestion, and irritation of the eyes and nose.
    - Postnasal drainage is probably the mechanism leading to acute exacerbation and may be a prominent symptom when cough is severe.
    - Symptoms are often improved by using nonsedating antihistamines and avoiding offending allergens.
  - **COPD exacerbation** may result from smoking, air pollutants, allergens, and infections.
    - *Streptococcus pneumoniae, Haemophilus influenza,* and *Moraxella catarrhalis* are among the most common bacterial pathogens isolated in COPD exacerbations.
    - Antibiotics may be prescribed if the acute cough is accompanied by worsening shortness of breath, increased oxygen requirements, increased sputum production, or change in the character of sputum.
- **Exposure**

Occupation or environmental exposures may also be contributors to cough. A thorough history, including workplace exposures, household exposures (including pets or new carpeting), and change in medications will help to pinpoint the diagnosis.

Chronic Cough

Cough >3 weeks is often attributable to one of a handful of diagnoses in nonsmokers. These include upper airway cough syndrome (UACS) which was previously referred to as postnasal drip syndrome, asthma, and gastroesophageal reflux disease (GERD).[2]

- **Upper airway cough syndrome**
  - The most common cause of persistent cough in nonsmokers.
  - Symptoms may include nasal discharge, frequent throat clearing, and a sensation of nasal discharge dripping into the back of the throat.
  - Physical examination may show secretions in the nasopharynx, and presence of cobblestoning.
    - However, postnasal drip may be silent, leaving the practitioner with nonspecific symptoms to help guide treatment.
    - Therefore, when there is a lack of alternative cause of a patient's cough, empiric therapy for postnasal drip should be attempted before other extensive workups for alternate cough etiologies.
- **Asthma**
  - The leading cause of chronic cough in children and second most common cause of chronic cough in the adult population.
  - The clinical spectrum of symptoms includes recurrent episodic wheezing, chest tightness, breathlessness, and cough, particularly at nighttime and/or in the early morning.
  - **Cough-variant asthma** will often present with cough and may progress to encompass other common asthma symptoms.
- **Gastroesophageal reflux**
  - GERD is the third most common cause of chronic cough.
  - Symptoms include heartburn or a sour taste in the mouth, but some patients may also lack these symptoms.
  - Prolonged esophageal pH monitoring is generally considered the gold standard for confirmation of GERD.
- **Chronic bronchitis**
  - The most common cause of chronic cough in smokers.
  - Defined as cough productive of sputum ≥3 month's duration in at least 2 consecutive years in the absence of other lung diseases that may cause cough.

  - Usually found with extensive smoking history, often >1 pack per day for more than 20 years.
  - An acute change of cough, or caliber of sputum is what may lead to initial presentation. It is important to remember these patients are at higher risk of developing neoplasm secondary to underlying smoking history.
- **Angiotensin-converting enzyme inhibitors**
  - Angiotensin-converting enzyme (ACE) inhibitors have been associated with cough in up to 15% of patients taking this class of medication.
  - Usually begins within 1 week of starting treatment but can be seen up to 6 months later.
  - Patients often report a "tickling" or "scratching" sensation in their throat, and the symptoms usually resolve within 1 week of discontinuing therapy (although it may take longer in some patients).
  - Mechanism is not entirely clear, but it is believed that accumulation of bradykinin may stimulate afferent nerve fibers in the airway. This is supported by data in patients who take angiotensin II receptor blockers (this class of medication does not affect kinin levels) and are not at increased risk of cough.
- **Bronchiectasis**
  - Bronchiectasis occurs less frequently.
  - Some studies show bronchiectasis is responsible for chronic cough in ~4% of patients in the United States.
  - Bronchiectasis is the result of repeated damage from chronic infections and airway inflammation in the bronchial tree that leads to irreversible dilatation of the affected airways. This anatomical alteration can lead to easily collapsible airways, poor mucus excretion, and chronic infection.
  - Most patients will produce chronic mucopurulent sputum at baseline that becomes more purulent during acute infectious processes.
- **Other etiologies of chronic cough**
  - **Eosinophilic bronchitis** is increasingly being recognized as a cause of chronic cough.
    - Patients often have atopic sensitivities, elevated sputum eosinophils, and airway inflammation.
    - Although similar characteristics can be seen in patients with cough-variant asthma, patients with eosinophilic bronchitis do not demonstrate airway hyperresponsiveness.
  - Other causes include interstitial lung diseases, lung cancers, and lesions that compromise the upper airway, including arteriovenous malformations, retrotracheal masses, and broncholiths.
  - Although practitioners are frequently concerned about missing lung cancer as a cause of chronic cough, cough is an infrequent presentation of occult bronchogenic carcinoma.
  - Rare causes include tracheobronchomalacia, TB, tracheal diverticuli, occult cystic fibrosis, recurrent aspiration, hyperthyroidism, carcinoid syndrome, and psychogenic cough.
  - Psychogenic cough is always a diagnosis of exclusion, and occurs less frequently in adults than in children.
    - Many patients with this condition do not cough during sleep, are not awakened by cough, and do not cough when otherwise occupied (working or playing).

PATHOPHYSIOLOGY

- Cough receptors exist in the epithelium of the upper and lower respiratory tracts, pericardium, stomach, esophagus, and diaphragm.
  - Afferent receptors are located within the sensory distribution of the trigeminal, glossopharyngeal, superior laryngeal, and vagus nerves.
  - Efferent receptors located in the recurrent laryngeal and spinal nerves respond to signals from a cough center in the medulla.

- Irritation of the cough receptors by smoke, dust, or fumes leads to stimulation of a complex reflex arc.
  - Once stimulated, an impulse is sent to the cough center.
  - After a series of muscle contractions, an increase in intrathoracic pressure develops, leading to increased airflow through the trachea.
  - These shearing forces help to eliminate mucus and foreign materials.

DIAGNOSIS

The diagnosis can be narrowed down by a careful review of the patient's history and physical examination. Focusing on the three most common causes of chronic cough—UACS, GERD, and asthma—is helpful in limiting the need for extensive evaluation.

Clinical Presentation

History

- Important clues include the onset, frequency, severity of the cough, as well as coexisting symptoms (fever, weight loss, dyspnea, night sweats).
- Patients should be questioned about medications, especially β-blockers and ACE inhibitors, environmental exposures, and recent respiratory tract infections within the past 3 months.
- Sputum production is an important consideration.
  - For patients with chronic bronchitis, sputum production is usually insidious.
  - It is often worse in the morning, and the appearance is whitish to gray.
  - During exacerbations, the sputum may become more profuse and more purulent.
  - Cigarette smokers are often used to their baseline productive cough, and are less likely to present to their physician unless there is a change in their respiratory status or the character of their sputum.
- It is also important to establish TB risk factors, and when appropriate, to determine when the last PPD skin test was completed.
- The medical history should focus on any underlying conditions that may predispose a patient to aspiration, congestive heart failure, and interstitial lung disease.
- Social history should include a detailed history of tobacco and alcohol use. A detailed occupational history should be obtained, including past and present exposure to asbestos, silica, coal dust, and fumes.
- Family history should include information regarding asthma and cystic fibrosis.

Physical Examination

- The patient should be observed for any signs of labored breathing.
- Frontal and maxillary sinuses should be palpated for tenderness.
- It is also important to evaluate the auditory canal and tympanic membranes, as irritation of the external canal by impacted foreign bodies or cerumen can lead to a chronic dry cough.
- The nose should be examined with attention to boggy turbinates, mucopurulent secretions, and polyps.
- Cobblestone appearance of the oropharynx suggests postnasal drip.
- Lung auscultation is a key component of the examination, and one must pay special attention to breath sounds, wheezes, and crackles.
- Remember to inspect the extremities for clubbing and peripheral edema. Clubbing may occur with interstitial lung disease, cystic fibrosis, and lung cancer.

Differential Diagnosis

- **Upper airway cough syndrome**
  - Absence of symptoms does not exclude the diagnosis of postnasal drip.

- Patients may have silent postnasal drip and still have a favorable response to combination therapy with an antihistamine, nasal decongestant, and/or nasal steroids.

- **Gastroesophageal reflux disease**
  - The patient may complain of heartburn, regurgitation, or dysphagia.
  - Although these symptoms are seen in the majority of patients, they may be absent in up to 75% of cases.
- **Asthma**
  - The classic triad of cough, shortness of breath, and wheezing does not occur in every patient.
  - Chronic cough may be the sole presenting symptom in up to nearly 25% of all cases.

Diagnostic Testing

- **CXR**
  - CXR can be helpful in establishing an initial diagnosis in chronic cough cases for which there is low clinical suspicion of postnasal drip, asthma, or GERD.
  - A normal radiograph in an immunocompetent host makes a diagnosis such as sarcoidosis, TB, or bronchiectasis less likely.
  - Recent data suggest that a normal CXR is not the best way to screen for malignancy in the lung. If suspicion is high, CT scan is the preferred method.[3]
- **Sinus CT scan**
  - Limited sinus CT is the usual test of choice in selected cases with suspected sinus disease.
  - Plain films of the sinuses are not generally recommended.
  - A CT scan should be obtained if a patient has not responded to one or two courses of appropriate antibiotic therapy for sinusitis, which occurs in ~10% of treated patients.
  - Nasal endoscopy is generally not indicated except in cases in which resistant or unusual organisms are suspected.
- **Pulmonary function tests**
  - **Methacholine challenge testing** should be performed in patients with a history and physical examination suggestive of asthma.
  - A negative test result essentially eliminates cough-variant asthma as the cause of chronic cough.
  - In patients with a positive response to methacholine challenge, a lack of improvement with bronchodilators may indicate a false positive test, and further workup should be initiated.
- **Gastrointestinal evaluation**
  - Diagnostic testing for suspected gastroesophageal disease is not routinely recommended.
  - An abnormal barium swallow may demonstrate cough induced by gastroesophageal reflux. However, this study is negative in the majority of patients.
  - Twenty-four–hour esophageal pH monitoring is the single most sensitive and specific test for reflux disease, but it is inconvenient and may not be readily available in some practices.
  - When postnasal drip and asthma have been ruled out, a 4-week trial of antireflux therapy can be initiated.
  - In the face of an inadequate response to a proton pump inhibitor, pH monitoring may be performed. The study should be performed while the patient is on the antireflux therapy to document the efficacy of the medication.
- **Additional testing**
  - If the history, physical examination, laboratory tests, and x-ray data do not provide a diagnosis, referral to a specialist should be considered.
  - A high-resolution chest CT can be performed to rule out rare causes of chronic cough such as bronchiectasis or interstitial lung disease. If the high-resolution CT scan is negative, then more invasive studies can be considered.

- A bronchoscopy with or without biopsy may be indicated.
- Echocardiography can be performed to rule out left ventricular dysfunction.
- Other tests that may be performed include a sweat chloride test for cystic fibrosis and quantitative immunoglobulin's to evaluate for rare immunodeficiencies.

TREATMENT

The first step is establishing the underlying etiology. A systematic approach to the evaluation of persistent cough and treatment aimed at the underlying disorder is successful in >95% of cases.

- **Chronic bronchitis**
  - Chronic bronchitis is managed with smoking cessation and bronchodilator therapy (see Chapter 10).
  - Cough will improve in ~95% of patients with cessation of smoking.
  - In patients who continue to smoke, medical therapy may still be helpful.
- **Postnasal drip**
  - Postnasal drip may be due to allergic, perennial nonallergic, or vasomotor rhinitis.
  - Removal of the offending environmental precipitant (if possible) is the treatment of choice.
  - Nasal steroids (i.e., fluticasone nasal spray, 2 sprays per nostril daily) can also be helpful.
  - Nonspecific therapy for any form of rhinitis includes antihistamines and topical decongestants in combination, and ipratropium nasal spray (0.03% nasal solution, 2 sprays each nostril 2–3 times daily).
  - First-generation antihistamines have been shown to be more effective in the treatment of cough than the newer, nonsedating agents.
  - Improvement can be expected within 7 days.
- **Asthma**
  - The treatment of cough-variant asthma is identical to that of atopic asthma.
  - Inhaled bronchodilators and/or inhaled corticosteroids (see Chapter 9) are the mainstays of therapy.
  - Short-course oral prednisone (0.5 mg/kg/d for 1–2 weeks) may be used with the initiation of inhaled therapy to decrease airway hyperreactivity.
- **Gastroesophageal reflux disease**
  - GERD is treated with both behavioral modification and medication.
  - Patients should avoid eating for 3 hours before bedtime, and specifically, avoid reflux-inducing foods (i.e., fatty foods, chocolate, and alcohol).
  - Patients should elevate the head of their bed with foam wedges or use a mechanized bed.
  - Treatment with a proton pump inhibitor should be instituted, especially in patients who do not respond to behavioral therapy, or in those patients with severe symptoms.
- **Sinusitis**
  - Most mild cases of mild sinusitis respond to topical or oral decongestants.
  - In more severe cases, or in recurrent infections, an antihistamine in combination with a decongestant may be more effective.
  - Bacterial sinusitis can be treated with an appropriate antibiotic (amoxicillin–clavulanate, 500 mg by mouth tid, or clarithromycin, 500 mg by mouth bid) for a 10–14-day course.
- **Medication-induced cough**
  - Discontinuation of the offending ACE inhibitors of β-blockers often results in relief of symptoms within 1–4 days, but may take up to 4 weeks.
  - Substitutions of alternate drugs within the same class are unlikely to be effective, although alternatives such as angiotensin II receptor blockers may be useful substitutes.

   - When a patient's condition necessitates an ACE inhibitor, oral sulindac, indomethacin, or inhaled cromolyn sodium may provide relief.
- **Eosinophilic bronchitis**
   - Eosinophilic bronchitis is most often treated with a trial of inhaled corticosteroids.
   - In one study, inhaled budesonide, 400 μg bid for 4 weeks, markedly improved airway inflammation and cough sensitivity in patients with eosinophilic bronchitis.[4]
   - Optimal duration of therapy is not clear.
- **Bronchiectasis**
   - Antibiotics directed against the most frequently encountered pathogens (*H. influenza, Pseudomonas aeruginosa, and S. pneumonia*) help to reduce cough and sputum production.
   - Patients generally require a minimum of 7 days of therapy.
- **Interstitial lung disease**
  Treatment is directed at the underlying lung disease.
- **Lung cancer**
   - For non–small-cell lung cancer, resection, if possible, is the treatment of choice.
   - Treatment for nonresectable malignancy involves chemotherapy and/or radiation therapy.
- **Congestive heart failure**
  Treatment is directed at the underlying disorder.
- **Psychogenic cough**
   - Removal of psychological stressors and behavioral modification therapy are probably the best treatment modalities for psychogenic cough.
   - Antitussives have little or no proven role in the therapy of psychogenic cough.
- **Cough of unknown etiology**
   - Nonspecific therapy may be useful in those circumstances in which no cause of cough can be found.
   - Several therapies are believed to suppress cough through action on the central medullary cough center.
      - Codeine (codeine sulfate, 10–20 mg PO q4–6h) is the traditional narcotic agent used for cough suppression.
      - Dextromethorphan is the most common nonnarcotic agent used for treating cough.
      - Studies comparing these two agents have been limited and have yielded variable results with respect to efficacy.

REFERENCES

1. Irwin RS, Baumann MH, Bolser DC, et al. Diagnosis and management of cough executive summary: ACCP evidence based clinical practice guidelines. *Chest.* 2006;129:1S–23S.
2. Pratter MR. Overview of common causes of chronic cough: ACCP evidence-based clinical practice guidelines. *Chest.* 2006;129:59S–62S.
3. The National Lung Screening Trial Research Team; Aberle DR, Adams AM, Berg CD, et al. Reduced lung-cancer mortality with low-dose computed tomographic screening. *N Engl J Med.* 2011;365:395–409.
4. Brightling CE, Ward R, Wardlaw AJ, et al. Airway inflammation, airway responsiveness and cough before and after inhaled budesonide in patients with eosinophilic bronchitis. *Eur Respir J.* 2000;15:682–6.

Asthma

9

Chad A. Witt and Mario Castro

GENERAL PRINCIPLES

- Asthma is a disease of the airways characterized by airway inflammation and increased responsiveness (hyperreactivity) to a wide variety of stimuli (triggers).
- Hyperreactivity leads to obstruction of the airways, the severity of which may be widely variable in the same individual.
- As a consequence, patients have paroxysms of cough, dyspnea, chest tightness, and wheezing.
- Other conditions may present with wheezing and must be considered, especially in patients who are unresponsive to therapy, see Table 9-1.
- Asthma is an episodic disease, with acute exacerbations and attacks often interspersed with symptom-free periods.
  - Asthma exacerbations occur when airway reactivity is increased and lung function becomes unstable.
  - During an exacerbation, attacks occur more easily and are more severe and persistent.
  - Asthma attacks are episodes of shortness of breath or wheezing lasting minutes to hours.
  - Patients may be completely symptom-free between attacks.
  - Typically, attacks are triggered by acute exposure to irritants (e.g., smoke) or allergens.
  - Exacerbations are associated with factors that increase airway hyperreactivity, such as viral infections, allergens, and occupational exposures.

DIAGNOSIS

Clinical Presentation

History

- **Acute asthma exacerbation**
  - Patients with an acute asthma exacerbation present with worsening shortness of breath, wheezing, and/or cough.
  - Risk factors for severe exacerbations include
    - Previous history of mechanical ventilation

TABLE 9-1 CONDITIONS THAT MAY MIMIC ASTHMA

Upper Airway Obstruction	Adverse Drug Reaction	Other	
Tumor	Aspirin	Tracheomalacia	Foreign body
Epiglottitis	β-adrenergic antagonist	Endobronchial lesion	Congestive heart failure
Vocal cord dysfunction	ACE inhibitors	Allergic bronchopulmonary aspergillosis	Gastroesophageal reflux
Obstructive sleep apnea	Inhaled pentamidine	Sinusitis	Hyperventilation with panic attacks

    - Recurrent need for oral corticosteroids
    - Hospitalization within the past year
    - Use of more than two canisters per month of inhaled short-acting bronchodilator
    - Seizures related to asthma attacks
- **Chronic asthma**
  - Patients with chronic asthma present with episodic shortness of breath and/or cough, frequently accompanied by wheezing.
  - Patients often report worsening symptoms with specific exposures (e.g., smoke, volatile cleaning products, gasoline fumes, allergens, dust, etc.).

Physical Examination

- **Acute asthma exacerbation**
  - Initial rapid assessment to identify patients who need immediate intervention is required.
  - Decreased breath sounds may be noted during severe exacerbations because there is not enough air flow to generate wheeze, thus wheezing is an unreliable indicator of severity of an attack.
  - Severe airflow obstruction is indicated by:
    - Pulsus paradoxus >25 mm Hg
    - Accessory respiratory muscle use
    - Nasal alar flaring
    - Inability to speak in full sentences
    - Tachycardia >110 beats/min
    - Tachypnea >28 breaths/min
  - Patients with decreased mental status require intubation.
  - SC emphysema should alert the examiner to the presence of a pneumothorax and/or pneumomediastinum.
  - Impending respiratory muscle fatigue may lead to depressed respiratory effort and paradoxical diaphragmatic movement.
  - Up to 50% of patients with severe airflow obstruction do not manifest any of the above findings.
- **Chronic asthma**
  - Physical examination is frequently normal during symptom-free periods.
  - Auscultation of the lungs may reveal wheezing when asthma is symptomatic.

Diagnostic Testing

- **Acute asthma exacerbation**
  - **Peak expiratory flow** (PEF) assessment:
    - Best method for assessment of severity of asthma attack
    - Normal values vary with size and age
    - PEF rate <200 L/min indicates severe obstruction for most adults
    - Serial PEF measurements are effective tools in assessment of patient's response to therapy
  - **Transcutaneous pulse oximetry**:
    - PEF is a poor predictor of hypoxemia and thus transcutaneous pulse oximetry may be necessary
    - Supplemental oxygen is administered to maintain oxygen saturations >90%
  - **Arterial blood gas** (ABG):
    - PEF is a useful screening tool for the presence of hypercapnia
    - Hypercapnia typically develops when PEF <25% of normal

        - ABG is indicated with PEF remains <25% predicted after initial treatment
        - Most patients initially have a low $PaCO_2$ secondary to hyperventilation
        - Normal or elevated $PaCO_2$ indicates inability of the respiratory system to increase ventilation as needed because of severe airway obstruction, increased dead space ventilation, and/or respiratory muscle fatigue
        - Rising $PaCO_2$ is concerning for impending respiratory failure
    - **Imaging**
        - CXR can be obtained and most frequently reveals hyperinflation.
        - Obtaining CXRs in the setting of asthma exacerbation should be limited to patients with suspected complications or significant comorbidities.[1]
        - Pneumothorax, pneumomediastinum, pneumonia, and atelectasis are sometimes found on CXRs obtained from patients presenting to ER with an asthma exacerbation.
- **Chronic asthma**
    - **Pulmonary function tests** (PFTs) are essential for diagnosing asthma.
        - PFTs demonstrate an obstructive pattern, the hallmark of which is a decrease in expiratory flow rates.
        - Reduction in the forced expiratory volume over 1 second (FEV_1) and a proportionally smaller reduction in the forced vital capacity (FVC), result in a decreased FEV_1/FVC ratio (generally <0.70).
        - With mild obstructive disease that involves only the small airways, the FEV_1/FVC ratio may be normal, and the only abnormality may be a decrease in airflow at mid-lung volumes (forced expiratory flow, 25–75%).
        - Lung hyperinflation causes an increased residual volume and increased residual volume–total lung capacity ratio.
        - The flow–volume loop demonstrates a decreased flow rate for any lung volume and is useful to rule out other causes of dyspnea, such as upper airway obstruction or restrictive lung disease.
        - The diagnosis of asthma is supported by an obstructive pattern that improves after bronchodilator therapy, defined as an increase in FEV_1 of >12% and 200 mL after 2–4 puffs of a short-acting bronchodilator.
            - In patients with chronic, severe asthma with airway remodeling, the airflow obstruction may no longer be completely reversible.
            - An alternative method of establishing the maximal degree of airway reversibility is to repeat the spirometry after a course of oral corticosteroids (usually prednisone 40 mg/d PO in adults for 10 days).
        - Lack of demonstrable airway obstruction or bronchodilator reversibility does not rule out a diagnosis of asthma.
        - When the spirometry is normal, demonstrating heightened airway responsiveness to a methacholine or exercise bronchoprovocation challenge can substantiate the diagnosis of asthma.
    - **Imaging:** A CXR should be obtained to rule out other causes of dyspnea, cough, or wheezing in patients being evaluated for asthma.

TREATMENT

Acute Exacerbations

Indications for hospitalization and level of care:

- Patient response to initial treatment (60–90 minutes after three treatments with short-acting bronchodilator) is a better predictor of need for hospitalization than initial severity of attack.

- Prompt resolution of symptoms and PEF >70% of predicted can be discharged from the ER. Because bronchospasm can recur within 72 hours, education and an asthma action plan are essential.
- Admission to the hospital is recommended when PEF <50% of predicted.
- Recent hospitalization, failure of aggressive outpatient management (using oral corticosteroids), and history of life-threatening exacerbation should all prompt consideration for admission.
- Admission to the ICU should be considered in patients with fatigue, drowsiness, confusion, use of accessory muscles of respiration, hypercapnia, marked hypoxemia, or PEF <150 L/min.

Medications

First Line

- **Inhaled short-acting β-adrenergic agonists (SABAs) are the mainstay of bronchodilator therapy**. The primary agent is albuterol.
  - Albuterol is dosed as 2.5 mg by continuous flow (updraft) nebulization every 20 minutes until improvement or toxicity.
  - It can also be administered in a metered-dose inhaler (MDI) as 6–12 puffs at similar dosing intervals.
  - MDI plus spacer allows lower dose of β-adrenergic agonist to be used and is as effective as nebulized β-adrenergic agonist when performed under direct supervision.
- **Systemic corticosteroids** speed resolution of asthma exacerbations and should be administered to all patients with moderate or severe exacerbations, though the ideal dose is poorly defined.
  - **Methylprednisolone** 40–60 mg IV every 6 hours is the drug of choice for IV therapy.
  - **Oral corticosteroids** are as effective if given in equivalent doses (e.g., prednisone 60 mg PO every 6–8 hours).
  - Tapering should not begin until there is objective evidence of clinical improvement, generally 36–48 hours.
  - Patients initially on IV therapy should be switched to PO.
  - 7–14-day tapering dosage of prednisone is usually prescribed in combination with an inhaled corticosteroid (ICS) to be instituted at the beginning of the tapering schedule.

Second Line

- **Inhaled anticholinergic medications** like ipratropium can sometimes be used in treatment.
  - Ipratropium is dosed as 0.5 mg by continuous flow (updraft) nebulization every 2 hours in combination with β-agonist until improvement
  - Special circumstances in which parasympatholytic therapy may be of benefit:
    - COPD with asthmatic component
    - Patients with asthma triggered by ingestions of β-blocker
    - Patients on monoamine oxidase inhibitor (MAOI) therapy at risk for sympathomimetic toxicity secondary to impaired drug metabolism
- **Methylxanthines** including theophylline or aminophylline can be used, however with caution.
  - IV theophylline or aminophylline in combination with β-agonist results in no further bronchodilation than β-agonist alone.
  - Toxicity is increased with no benefit.
  - Routine use of methylxanthines in the management of acute asthma attacks is not recommended.
- **Magnesium sulfate** can be considered in severe exacerbations (FEV_1 or PEF <40% predicted) that fail to respond to initial treatment with β-agonists and may reduce hospital admission and improve lung function.[2]

- Magnesium sulfate is dosed as 2 g IV infused over 20 minutes and can be considered in severe exacerbations.
- This medication can also be considered in patients with toxicity-limiting β–adrenergic agonist therapy or respiratory failure.

- **Epinephrine** may rarely be needed for the treatment of asthma and can be administered as aqueous epinephrine 0.3 mL of 1:1000 solution subcutaneously every 20 minutes for up to 3 doses.
  - ECG monitoring is necessary
  - Should be avoided in patients with known or suspected coronary artery disease
- **Heliox** is a blend of helium and oxygen with a lower density than air. Heliox (70:30 or 80:20 helium:oxygen mixture) can be considered in patients with severe exacerbation (FEV_1 or PEF <40% predicted) who fail initial treatment with inhaled bronchodilators.
  - Heliox also appears most promising for patients with respiratory acidosis and short duration of symptoms.
  - It may also be helpful in avoiding mechanical ventilation.
- **Antibiotics** have been shown to be of no benefit when administered routinely for acute asthma exacerbations and are only recommended if indicated for treatment of comorbid conditions (e.g., pneumonia or bacterial sinusitis).

Other Nonpharmacologic Therapies

- Mechanical ventilation is considered in any patient with asthma admitted to the ICU as there is a relatively high morbidity and mortality among asthma patients undergoing invasive mechanical ventilation.[3]
- Noninvasive positive-pressure ventilation (NIPPV)
  - Improves alveolar ventilation and decreases work of breathing.
  - Has been shown to reduce the need for intubation in a selected group of patients with severe asthma.[4]
  - NIPPV should only be performed in an ICU setting by physicians with experience in noninvasive ventilation.
  - Heliox may be used in conjunction with NIPPV to further assist avoiding invasive ventilation.
- **Invasive positive-pressure ventilation**
  - Hyperinflation may result secondary to incomplete expiration of the machine-delivered tidal volumes resulting in intrinsic positive end-expiratory pressure (PEEP), also referred to as auto-PEEP.[5]
  - PEEP may impede venous return leading to decreased cardiac output and hypotension.
  - Strategies to minimize intrinsic PEEP, hemodynamic instability, and barotrauma include:
    - Reduced respiratory rate and tidal volume, which may result in permissive hypercapnia
    - Avoidance of ventilator-applied PEEP
    - Increased inspiratory airflow rates to maximize the duration of expiration.

Chronic, Daily Asthma Management

- The main goals of daily management are
  - Control of symptoms while maintaining normal activity and pulmonary function
  - Prevention of exacerbations
  - Minimization of medication toxicity
- The successful management requires four main components[6]:
  - Assessing and monitoring severity
  - Patient education
  - Control of triggers
  - Medication plan for both daily therapy and exacerbations

TABLE 9-2 CLASSIFYING ASTHMA SEVERITY

Components of Severity	Intermittent	Persistent: Mild	Persistent: Moderate	Persistent: Severe
Occurrence of symptoms	≤2 d/wk	>2 d/wk	Daily	Multiple times daily
Nighttime awakenings	≤2 times/mo	3–4 times/mo	>1 time/wk	Often 7 times/wk
PRN medication use for symptom control	≤2 d/wk	>2 d/wk	Daily	Multiple times daily
Limits on activity	None	Minor	Some	Significant
Lung function	Normal FEV_1 between exacerbations Or FEV_1 >80% FEV_1/FVC Normal	FEV_1 ≥80% FEV_1/FVC Normal	FEV_1 >60 but <80% FEV_1/FVC Decreased by ≤5%	FEV_1 <60% FEV_1/FVC Decreased by >5%
Exacerbations that require corticosteroids	0–1/yr		≥2/yr	

FEV_1, forced expiratory volume in 1 second; FVC, forced vital capacity; PRN, as needed.

Adapted from National Asthma Education and Prevention Program. Expert panel report 3 (EPR-3): guidelines for the diagnosis and management of Asthma-Summary Report 2007. *J Allergy Clin Immunol.* 2007;120:S94–S138.

- Asthma severity should be classified as intermittent or mild persistent, moderate persistent, or severe persistent at the first visit, please see Table 9-2.[6] If already on treatment, the dose of ICS that provides control can be used to assign severity.
- It is important to assess asthma control at each visit. Standardized questionnaires are available, including:
  - Asthma Control Test (ACT)[7]
  - Asthma Control Questionnaire (ACQ)[8]
  - Asthma Therapy Assessment Questionnaire (ATAQ)[9]
- An asthma action plan is a necessary component of the care of the patient with asthma.
  - The action plan is a written daily management plan that teaches patients how to avoid factors that aggravate their disease, how to manage daily medications, and how to recognize and deal with acute exacerbations.[6]
  - Patients are taught to avoid exposure to chronic irritants or allergens, specifically those that trigger their disease, including: dust mites, cockroaches, pet dander, viral URI, sinusitis, postnasal drainage, GERD, tobacco and wood smoke, cold air, exercise, aspirin, and NSAIDs.

- PEF provides objective measurement of airflow obstruction.
  - PEF should be measured early morning before any bronchodilator therapy.
  - Personal best PEF is identified as highest PEF when disease is under control.
  - PEF is then checked with any symptoms or when triggers are identified.
    - Green zone: 80–100% of best PEF
    - Yellow zone: 50–80% of best PEF
    - Red zone: <50% of best PEF
  - Evidence suggests that an asthma action plan based on symptoms alone is as effective as PEF-based plan.[10]

Medications

First Line

A Stepwise asthma treatment protocol for patients aged 12 and older is summarized in Table 9-3.[6]

- SABA[6]
  - SABAs, such as albuterol are a mainstay of asthma therapy, while they do not provide long-term control, they are necessary to provide quick relief of symptoms.
  - Can be used to judge the adequacy of control.

TABLE 9-3 ASTHMA MANAGEMENT FOR PATIENTS 12 YEARS OF AGE AND OLDER

Severity	Step	Preferred Treatment	Other	Notes
Intermittent	1	SABA PRN		Education, trigger control, and management of other conditions necessary at each step (steps 1–6)
Persistent: mild to severe	2	Low-dose ICS	Consider allergy referral for allergen immunotherapy for allergic asthma (steps 2–6)	
	3	Low-dose ICS + LABA or med-dose ICS		
	4	Med-dose ICS + LABA		
	5	High-dose ICS + LABA and consider omalizumab for allergic patients		
	6	High-dose ICS + LABA + oral corticosteroid and consider omalizumab for allergic patients		

SABA, short-acting bronchodilator; ICS, inhaled corticosteroid; LABA, long-acting bronchodilator.

Adapted from National Asthma Education and Prevention Program. Expert panel report 3 (EPR-3): guidelines for the diagnosis and management of Asthma-Summary Report 2007. *J Allergy Clin Immunol.* 2007;120:S94–S138.

- ICSs are another mainstay of asthma treatment and are safe and effective medications.
  - If delivered by MDI, a spacing device should be used and the patients should rinse their mouth with water thereafter to minimize the possibility of oral candidiasis and hoarseness.
  - Dosing is determined by severity of asthma and potency of the steroid preparation and comprehensive dosing guidelines can be found in the detailed Expert Panel Report-3.[6]
  - Patients with frequent β-agonist use or other signs of poor control will need the ICS dose increased by 50–100% until symptoms resolve. If symptoms are severe, there is nighttime awakening, or PEF <65% predicted, a short course of oral corticosteroids (prednisone 40–60 mg/d for 5–7 days) may be necessary to regain disease control.
  - ICS dose should be decreased by 25% every 2–3 months to lowest possible dose needed to maintain control of asthma. Of note, systemic absorption can occur in patients using prolonged high doses of ICS.
- **Long-acting β-adrenergic agonists (LABAs)**
  - LABAs such as salmeterol or formoterol added to low- or medium-dose ICS have been shown to improve lung function and symptoms in patients with asthma.
  - LABAs have been shown to decrease the necessary ICS dose in patients with moderate persistent asthma.
  - Combination therapy with ICS and LABAs (fluticasone/salmeterol, budesonide/formoterol, mometasone/formoterol) is available and may improve patient adherence.
  - Combination therapy should be considered in all patients with moderate and severe persistent asthma.
  - LABAs should not be given without ICSs, as there has been an association with increased mortality in this scenario.
- **Leukotriene antagonists**
  - Montelukast (10 mg PO daily) and zafirlukast (20 mg PO bid) provide effective control of mild persistent asthma in a subset of patients though these medications are not as effective as corticosteroids in improving asthma outcomes.
  - Leukotriene antagonists should be considered in patients with:
    - Aspirin-induced asthma
    - Exercise-induced asthma
    - Asthmatics with allergic rhinitis
    - Individuals who cannot master the use of an inhaler

Second Line

- **Methylxanthines**
  - The primary medication in this category is theophylline, which is a mild bronchodilator.
  - Sustained-release theophylline may be a useful adjuvant therapy in persistent asthma, especially for controlling nocturnal symptoms:
    - Serum concentrations must be monitored on a regular basis because of narrow therapeutic window and significant toxicities
    - Starting dose is generally ~10 mg/kg/d
    - Serum concentrations of 5–15 μg/mL are recommended
  - There are multiple potential drug interactions with theophylline that must be taken into account, especially with antibiotics.
- **Omalizumab** is a humanized monoclonal antibody to the Fc portion of the IgE antibody that prevents binding of IgE to its receptor on mast cells and basophils.
  - Omalizumab has been shown to decrease exacerbations in patients with severe asthma.[11]
  - It should be considered as adjunctive therapy in patients with:
    - Moderate to severe asthma inadequately controlled on high-dose ICS and LABA therapy **AND**
    - Objective evidence of sensitization to aeroallergens **AND**
    - IgE levels between 30 and 700 IU/mL

- **Mepolizumab** is a humanized monoclonal antibody that binds to and inhibits interleukin-5 and was recently approved by the U.S. Food and Drug Administration as an add-on medication for severe asthma. In patients with severe eosinophilic asthma on chronic oral corticosteroid, this therapy was shown to decrease corticosteroid dose, reduce asthma exacerbations, and improve control of asthma symptoms.[12]
- **Additional medications**: Methotrexate, cyclosporine, tacrolimus, and troleandomycin have all been studied and are not recommended, given their potential toxicity.

Other Nonpharmacologic Therapies

- Bronchial thermoplasty (BT) is an emerging treatment modality for patients with moderate to severe asthma.
- BT is performed by advancing a catheter through the bronchoscope to deliver a fixed duration and intensity of controlled thermal energy to the airway wall.
- Performed during three bronchoscopies ~3 weeks apart.
- There is increased risk of worsening asthma symptoms immediately post-BT.
- Over 1-year follow-up, patients undergoing BT compared to a sham procedure had[13]:
  - Improved quality of life
  - Fewer severe exacerbations
  - Fewer ER visits
  - Fewer days missed from work
- At 5-year follow-up patients undergoing BT continued to have[14]:
  - Fewer severe exacerbations
  - Fewer ER visits
- BT should be performed at centers with experience in complex bronchoscopy and management of difficult to treat asthma.

REFERENCES

1. Tsai TW, Gallagher EJ, Lombardi G, et al. Guidelines for the selective ordering of admission chest radiography in adult obstructive airway disease. *Ann Emerg Med.* 1993;22:1854–8.
2. Kew KM, Kirtchuk L, Michell CI. Intravenous magnesium sulfate for treating adults with acute asthma in the emergency department. *Cochrane Database Syst Rev.* 2014;5:CD10909.
3. Mansel JK, Stogner SW, Petrini MF, et al. Mechanical ventilation in patients with acute severe asthma. *Am J Med.* 1990;89:42–8.
4. Fernandez MM, Villagra A, Blanch L, et al. Non-invasive mechanical ventilation in status asthmaticus. *Intensive Care Med.* 2001;27:486–92.
5. Leatherman JW, Ravenscroft SA. Low measured auto-positive end-expiratory pressure during mechanical ventilation in patients with severe asthma: hidden auto-positive end-expiratory pressure. *Crit Care Med.* 1996;24:541–6.
6. National Asthma Education and Prevention Program. Expert panel report 3 (EPR-3): Guidelines for the diagnosis and management of Asthma-Summary Report 2007. *J Allergy Clin Immunol.* 2007;120:S94–S138.
7. Nathan RA, Sorkness CA, Kosinski M, et al. Development of the asthma control test: a survey for assessing asthma control. *J Allergy Clin Immunol.* 2004;113:59–65.
8. Juniper EF, O'Byrne PM, Guyatt GH, et al. Development and validation of a questionnaire to measure asthma control. *Eur Respir J.* 1999;14:902–7.
9. Vollmer WM, Markson E, O'Connor, et al. Association of asthma control with health care utilization and quality of life. *Am J Respir Crit Care Med.* 1999;160:1647–52.
10. Bhogal S, Zemek R, Ducharme FM. Written action plans for asthma in children. *Cochrane Database Syst Rev.* 2006;3:CD005306.
11. Humbert M, Beasley R, Ayres J, et al. Benefits of omalizumab as add-on therapy in patients with severe persistent asthma who are inadequately controlled despite best available therapy (GINA 2002 step 4 treatment): INNOVATE. *Allergy.* 2005;60:309–16.

12. Bel EH, Wenzel SE, Thompson PJ, et al. Oral glucocorticoid-sparing effect of mepolizumab in eosinophilc asthma. *N Engl J Med.* 2014;371:1189–97.
13. Castro M, Rubin A, Laviolette M, et al. Effectiveness and safety of bronchial thermoplasty in the treatment of severe asthma: a multicenter, randomized, double-blind, sham-controlled clinical trial. *Am J Respir Crit Care Med.* 2009;181:116–24.
14. Wechsler ME, Laviolette M, Rubin AS, et al. Bronchial thermoplasty: long-term safety and effectiveness in patients with severe persistent asthma. *J Allergy Clin Immunol.* 2013;132: 1295–302.

Chronic Obstructive Pulmonary Disease

10

John Dickinson and Roger D. Yusen

GENERAL PRINCIPLES

Definition

- Chronic obstructive pulmonary disease (COPD) is a common, preventable, treatable, and usually progressive condition characterized by persistent airflow limitation (i.e., not fully reversible) and an enhanced chronic inflammatory response to noxious particles or gases.
- Patients with COPD have emphysema and/or airways disease (e.g., chronic bronchitis).
  - Emphysema, defined pathologically, consists of nonuniform distal airway enlargement associated with destruction of the acini, loss of lung elasticity, and absence of significant parenchymal fibrosis.
  - Chronic bronchitis is defined clinically as cough productive of (e.g., at least 2 tablespoons of) sputum on most days of 3 consecutive months in 2 consecutive years, in the absence of other lung diseases.
  - COPD has characteristics that overlap with asthma, and both conditions may occur in the same patient (asthma copd overlap syndrome, ACOS).
  - Although asthma, bronchiectasis, obliterative bronchiolitis, and sarcoidosis often have associated expiratory airflow obstruction, they do not fall within the classification of COPD.

Classification

- The Global Obstructive Lung Disease 2015 (GOLD) classification of COPD bases its assessment on the patient's level of symptoms, exacerbation history, spirometric abnormality, and identification of comorbidities.[1]
- Postbronchodilator spirometric pulmonary function tests determine the grade of airflow limitation (Table 10-1).[1] Height, weight, gender, and sometimes race determine predicted normal values for the forced expiratory volume in 1 second (FEV_1) and forced vital capacity (FVC).

Epidemiology

- In the United States, ~5% of the population has COPD.[2]
- COPD has climbed ahead of stroke to become the third leading cause of death in the United States, following heart disease and cancer.[2]

Pathophysiology

- Inhaled particles that cause lung inflammation may induce parenchymal tissue destruction (e.g., emphysema) and cause airway disease (e.g., airway fibrosis) through the disruption of normal repair and defense mechanisms.
- Increased mucus production from goblet cell hyperplasia.
- Genetic disorders may create a predisposition to developing COPD.
- Role of airway infections in COPD:
  - Defective innate immune responses promote persistent airway bacterial colonization and recurrent airway infections.
  - Acute airway infections often lead to acute exacerbations and subsequently worsened lung function.

TABLE 10-1 2016 GOLD SEVERITY GRADE OF AIRFLOW LIMITATION FOR PATIENTS THAT HAVE COPD[a]

Stage	Characteristics
GOLD 1: mild	• FEV_1/FVC <70% • FEV_1 ≥80% predicted
GOLD 2: moderate	• FEV_1/FVC <70% • 50% ≤FEV_1 <80% predicted
GOLD 3: severe	• FEV_1/FVC <70% • 30% ≤FEV_1 <50% predicted
GOLD 4: very severe	• FEV_1/FVC <70% • FEV_1 <30% predicted

[a]Based on postbronchodilator FEV_1.

GOLD, Global Initiative for Obstructive Lung Disease; COPD, chronic obstructive lung disease; FEV_1, forced expiratory volume in 1 second; FVC, forced vital capacity.

From the Global Strategy for Diagnosis, Management, and Prevention of COPD, 2016, Available from http://www.goldcopd.org

  - Viral infections (e.g., influenza, rhinovirus, and adenovirus) and bacterial infection (e.g., *Haemophilus influenzae*, *Streptococcus pneumoniae*, *Moraxella catarrhalis*, and *Mycoplasma pneumoniae*) cause most exacerbations.

Risk Factors

- The risk of developing COPD correlates with the total lifetime burden of exposure of inhaled toxins.
  - The most important risk factor for the development of COPD is cigarette smoking, which is associated with the majority of cases. However, only a minority of smokers develop clinically significant COPD, suggesting that genetic predisposition and other environmental factors may be required for its development.
  - Cigar and pipe smokers are also at increased risk of developing COPD.
  - Occupational exposures and indoor air pollution may lead to COPD.
- Genetic disorders may lead to the development of COPD. α1-Antitrypsin deficiency (A1ATD) contributes to <1% of COPD cases.
  - α1-Antitrypsin inhibits neutrophil-derived elastase, an enzyme responsible for the destruction of lung parenchyma in emphysema.
  - Patients with A1ATD carry a genetic polymorphism that leads to decreased α1-antitrypsin serum levels.
  - A1ATD should be considered in a patient with emphysema who has:
    - COPD and a minimal smoking history.
    - Early onset COPD (<45 years).[1]
    - Family history of COPD.
    - Predominance of lower lobe emphysema seen on imaging studies.[1]

Associated Conditions

A number of extrapulmonary comorbidities have been identified in those with COPD such as cardiovascular disease, lung cancer, osteoporosis, skeletal muscle dysfunction, depression, and metabolic syndrome.

DIAGNOSIS

- Symptoms of dyspnea or chronic cough should lead to an evaluation.
- History of heavy smoking should prompt further evaluation in the appropriate clinical setting.
- Spirometry is required to make the diagnosis of COPD.

Clinical Presentation

Symptoms of COPD typically consist of increased dyspnea with exertion, decreased exercise tolerance, and increased sputum production.

History

- Chronic cough and sputum production may precede the development of COPD by many years.
- COPD may develop without chronic cough or sputum production.
- Dyspnea from COPD typically develops after the FEV_1 has significantly decreased (e.g., <60% of the predicted normal value) over many years.
- Clinicians should perform a thorough medical history assessment, and question patients regarding symptoms, risk factors, clinical course, comorbidities, medications, and family history.

Physical Examination

Physical examination findings suggestive of COPD do not become apparent until after COPD has significantly progressed, and include:

- Accessory muscle use, pursed lip breathing, and Hoover sign.
- Hyperinflation of the lungs associated with hyperresonant chest percussion.
- Decreased breath and heart sounds.
- Expiratory wheezes variably occur.
- Clubbing of the fingers not expected.
- Symptoms of cor pulmonale occur less commonly:
  - Elevated JVP.
  - Lower extremity edema.
  - Right ventricular precordial heave, increased S2 and P2 strength, right-sided S3, and tricuspid regurgitation.

Diagnostic Criteria

- Spirometry is used to diagnose COPD, and the FEV_1 determines the severity of the expiratory airflow obstruction based on the GOLD stages, see Table 10-1 for classification schema.[1]
- Peak expiratory flow measurement has high sensitivity but low specificity.
- Symptoms and examination findings assist with diagnosis.
- Imaging studies provide evidence of the presence or absence of emphysema.

Differential Diagnosis

- Asthma
- Bronchiectasis
- Reactive airways dysfunction syndrome
- Bronchiolitis obliterans
- Lymphangioleiomyomatosis (LAM)
- Sarcoidosis
- Langerhans cell histiocytosis
- Panbronchiolitis
- Fixed or variable airway obstruction in the upper airways

- Vocal cord dysfunction
- Congestive heart failure (will not cause expiratory airflow obstruction)
- TB

Diagnostic Testing

Laboratory Testing

- We suggest obtaining an arterial blood gas (ABG) if the patient has a low SpO_2 (e.g., <92%), FEV_1 very low (e.g., <35%), or signs of respiratory or right heart failure occur.
- CBC, to look for polycythemia.
- Complete metabolic panel, to look for elevated bicarbonate level.
- α1-Antitrypsin screening.[1]

Imaging

CXR posterioranterior and lateral to assess for emphysema or other conditions that could produce similar signs or symptoms.

Diagnostic Procedures

- Pulmonary function tests:
  - Spirometry: pre- and postbronchodilator (FEV_1/FVC <0.70 and scooping of the expiratory limb of the flow–volume curve).
  - Lung volumes (e.g., air trapping [elevated residual volume (RV)] and thoracic hyperinflation [e.g., elevated total lung capacity (TLC)]).
  - Diffusing capacity (e.g., reduced diffusing capacity of the lung for carbon monoxide [DLCO]).
- Pulse oximetry assessment at rest, with exercise, and possibly during sleep.
- Cardiac testing, when appropriate, to assist with a dyspnea evaluation.

TREATMENT

Acute Exacerbations

- COPD exacerbations are diagnosed clinically based on a worsening in respiratory symptoms beyond the expected day-to-day variation.
- COPD exacerbations typically increase (compared to baseline) one or more of the following:
  - Dyspnea
  - Cough and sputum production
  - Sputum purulence
- The first step taken when encountering a patient with an acute exacerbation should be a quick assessment to determine the need for hospitalization or intensive care unit (ICU) admission for impending respiratory failure (Table 10-2).

TABLE 10-2 INDICATIONS FOR ICU ADMISSION
Severe dyspnea that does not adequately respond to initial therapy
Mental status deterioration (e.g., confusion, coma, lethargy)
Persistently worse or worsening hypercapnia or respiratory acidosis
Persistently worse or worsening hypoxemia
Lack of adequate response to supplemental oxygen and/or noninvasive positive pressure ventilation

- Indications for inpatient admission include
  - Marked dyspnea
  - New physical findings such as cyanosis or peripheral edema
  - New or worsened hypoxemia/hypercapnia
  - Lack of adequate response to initial medical management
  - Consider hospital admission for those with advanced age or significant comorbidities
- Initial assessment
  - CXR
  - ECG
  - ABG, CBC, chemistry panel, brain natriuretic peptide (BNP), and cardiac enzymes.
    - ABG provides important information about alveolar gas exchange and acid–base status not obtained by pulse oximetry.
    - ABGs can differentiate between acute and chronic respiratory acidosis, and may indicate a need for assisted ventilation and ICU admission.
- Additional testing
  - Consider chest CT to evaluate for pulmonary embolism.
  - Spirometry is not recommended during an exacerbation.

Medications

- General considerations regarding **bronchodilator therapy**
  - First-line therapy for symptomatic management of a COPD exacerbation.
  - Multiple randomized controlled trials have demonstrated the similar efficacy of short-acting β2-agonists (SABA) and short-acting anticholinergic (SAAC) agents for rapidly improving symptoms during an acute COPD exacerbation.
  - Combination therapy using a SABA/SAAC has added benefits beyond either agent alone (reduction in hospital length of stay duration and increase in FEV_1).
  - Combination therapy with SABA/SAAC may also have a more rapid onset of action, longer duration of action, and fewer side effects (owing to smaller doses of each individual agent) than use of higher doses of a single agent.
  - Long-acting agents are typically not recommended for the management of acute exacerbations of COPD because of the risk of side effects in combination with high-dose short-acting bronchodilator therapy and a lack of demonstrated efficacy and safety in this setting. Long-acting agents should typically be initiated prior to hospital discharge.
- **Inhaled SABA**
  - Albuterol may be administered q30–60min as tolerated. Subsequent treatment frequency can be decreased, eventually to q4–6h, as the acute exacerbation begins to resolve.
  - β2-agonists may cause tremor, nervousness, tachycardia, tachyarrhythmias, and hypokalemia.
- **Inhaled SAACs**
  - Ipratropium may be dosed at 4–8 puffs or nebulized q4–6h for a COPD exacerbation.
  - Ipratropium is generally well tolerated and tends to produce fewer of the other side effects characteristic of β2-agonist agents.
  - Anticholinergic agents may cause dry mouth, dry eyes, bladder outlet obstruction/ urinary retention, and acute angle glaucoma exacerbation.
- **Corticosteroids**
  - Systemic administration of corticosteroids is recommended during acute exacerbations of COPD requiring hospitalization.
  - Corticosteroids minimize recovery time, decrease hospital length of stay, reduce the incidence of relapse, and improve lung function toward baseline.
  - A randomized trial of patients hospitalized for COPD exacerbations found that oral systemic corticosteroids were noninferior to IV corticosteroids.[3]

  - The most common adverse effect of systemic corticosteroid administration is hyperglycemia, but other acute adverse effects include but are not limited to systemic hypertension, insomnia, and mood changes.
  - A typical steroid regimen includes prednisone 30–40 mg PO per day followed by a taper over 10–14 days.
  - Outpatient management
    - Short courses of oral steroids in patients with moderate to severe COPD can improve the outcomes of patients with exacerbations discharged from the emergency department (ED).
    - Inhaled steroids currently do not have a role in the treatment of acute COPD exacerbations.
- **Antibiotics**
  - Current methods do not reliably differentiate bacteria-caused exacerbations from those produced by viruses.
  - Commonly implicated bacterial pathogens: *S. pneumoniae,* nontypeable *H. influenzae* and *Haemophilus parainfluenzae, Chlamydia pneumoniae,* and *M. catarrhalis.*
  - Sputum cultures in the absence of pneumonia or bronchiectasis are likely of little benefit.
  - Antibiotics (usually for 5–10 days) are recommended during a COPD exacerbation for those with[1]:
    - Increased sputum purulence and sputum volume and increased dyspnea **OR**
    - Have increased sputum purulence with only one other cardinal symptom **OR**
    - Requiring mechanical ventilation.
  - Because of rampant antibiotic resistance, particularly in *S. pneumoniae*, broader-spectrum antibiotic coverage is commonly recommended for acute exacerbations, using one of the following:
    - Amoxicillin/clavulanate
    - Respiratory fluoroquinolone (e.g., levofloxacin or moxifloxacin)
    - Macrolide antibiotic (e.g., azithromycin, erythromycin, or clarithromycin)
- **Methylxanthines**
  - The role of parenteral or oral methylxanthines (e.g., theophylline) during an acute exacerbation is unclear.
  - Considered third-line agents due to their narrow therapeutic window and potential for severe side effects

Other Nonpharmacologic Therapies

- **Oxygen**
  - Oxygen should be administered to achieve a PaO_2 of >55–60 mm Hg (≥89–90% oxyhemoglobin saturation on pulse oximetry).
  - Worsening hypercapnia may occur with oxygen administration in patients with baseline hypercapnia, and ABG should be checked ~30–60 minutes after starting oxygen therapy.
  - An increased or new requirement for supplemental oxygen may indicate the presence of a complicating condition such as pulmonary embolism, pneumonia, pneumothorax, or heart failure.
- **Noninvasive ventilation**
  - Noninvasive positive-pressure ventilation (NIPPV) is useful for improving oxygenation, decreasing hypercapnia, and relieving work of breathing in patients with acute COPD exacerbation and acute respiratory failure.
  - NIPPV decreases intubation and mortality rates.[4]
  - Methods of NIPPV
    - Continuous positive airway pressure ventilation (CPAP) improves oxygenation and work of breathing, but generally not an underlying acute respiratory acidosis.

TABLE 10-3 CRITERIA FOR NONINVASIVE POSITIVE PRESSURE VENTILATION

Inclusion criteria

Severe dyspnea, with signs of respiratory muscle fatigue or increased work of breathing (e.g., use of accessory muscles, paradoxical abdominal motion), or

pH 7.30–7.35 and $PaCO_2$ >45 mm Hg

Exclusion criteria

Altered mental status

Respiratory arrest

Cardiovascular instability

High aspiration risk

Recent facial or gastroesophageal surgery

Nasopharyngeal abnormalities

Extreme obesity

- Bilevel positive airway pressure ventilation (BiPAP) is the preferred method for treatment of respiratory failure associated with acute respiratory acidosis. The larger the gradient between high and low pressure settings, the greater the ventilatory support (improvement in PCO_2) provided by NIPPV.
  - Most patients tolerate NIPPV, which has been show to decrease mortality, the need for endotracheal intubation, and length of hospitalization.
  - To be effective, patients must be awake and cooperative with NIPPV. See inclusion and exclusion criteria for NIPPV in Table 10-3.
- **Follow-up**: For patients hospitalized for a COPD exacerbation, discharge plans should include reinforcement of smoking cessation, review of home medication regimen, assessment of metered dose inhaled (MDI) technique and training when needed, vaccination updates, education, oxygen assessment, and outpatient pulmonary rehabilitation, and healthcare provider follow-up.

CHRONIC COPD TREATMENT

Long-term management of COPD should aim to reduce symptoms and decrease risk for the frequency and severity of acute exacerbations, progression of disease, morbidity, side effects of therapy, and mortality. Of the medical therapies, randomized controlled trials have demonstrated that smoking cessation and the correction of hypoxemia with supplemental oxygen improve survival.

Medications

- General considerations regarding **bronchodilator therapy**
  - Bronchodilator therapy may control symptoms, increase exercise tolerance, improve lung function, and decrease the frequency and severity of exacerbations.
  - Studies have not shown that medications modify the long-term decline in lung function associated with COPD.
  - Clinicians should prescribe scheduled and on-demand bronchodilators.
  - Short-acting bronchodilators (SABA and/or SAAC) are preferred for those with mild symptoms and mild airflow obstruction and low risk of exacerbation.
  - Long-acting agents are recommended for those with more severe disease.
  - MDIs are preferred over nebulizers for outpatient management. However, for those with severe dyspnea, weakness, or poor coordination, nebulizers may be preferred.

- Different respiratory societies promote anticholinergic agents or β2-agonists as first-line treatment for those requiring scheduled bronchodilators.
- **Anticholinergic agents**
  - Ipratropium is effective as initial bronchodilator therapy.
  - It has a longer duration of action and less toxicity than available β2-agonists such as albuterol.
  - The usual dosage of 2 puffs q4–6h can be doubled or tripled to achieve maximal bronchodilation.
- **β2-agonists**
  - Albuterol is the mainstay β2-agonist.
  - Titrate up the standard albuterol dose of 2 puffs q4–6h for symptomatic relief.
- **Combination therapy**
  - Combination therapy with a β2-agonist and an anticholinergic provides a greater benefit in terms of symptoms and bronchodilation (FEV_1) than does either agent alone.
  - It is also convenient having both drugs in a single MDI.
  - Combination short-acting therapy (e.g., Combivent 2–4 puffs q6h) is recommended for patients with moderate to severe disease.
  - Patients often benefit from the use of combination short-acting therapy with a simultaneous long-acting β2-agonist (LABA).
- **Long-acting inhaled medical therapy**
  - LABAs and long-acting anticholinergics (LAACs) can reduce exacerbations and improve dyspnea on patients with moderate to severe disease.
  - The LABAs
    - Improve respiratory symptoms
    - Increase morning peak expiratory flows
    - Decrease the use of rescue bronchodilator therapy
  - Oral formulations of β2-agonists should be avoided, as they provide similar efficacy to inhaled agents with a higher risk of toxic side effects.
  - A recent randomized controlled trial in patients with moderate to severe COPD found that tiotropium (an LAAC agent) had greater efficacy than salmeterol for preventing COPD exacerbations.[5]
- **Inhaled corticosteroids**
  - Guidelines recommend long-term treatment with inhaled corticosteroids in patients with FEV_1 <50% or frequent (especially severe) exacerbations.
  - An LABA may be combined with an inhaled corticosteroid for convenience.
  - Inhaled maintenance corticosteroid therapy increases the FEV_1 and decreases the frequency and severity of exacerbations in patients with moderate to severe disease, though they do not slow the progression of disease.
  - Inhaled steroids should be administered after inhaled bronchodilator treatment, and patients should rinse the mouth and spit after each use to avoid thrush and hoarseness.
- **Systemic corticosteroids**
  - Patients with very severe COPD with frequent life-threatening infections may benefit from chronic low-dose steroids. The decision to institute chronic prednisone therapy should be individualized to the particular patient and readdressed at each subsequent clinic visit.
  - Prednisone at 5–10 mg/d is a typical long-term regimen.
  - Potential adverse effects include osteoporosis, hyperglycemia, systemic hypertension, muscle wasting, and bruising.
- **Methylxanthines**
  - Theophylline is a long-acting phosphodiesterase (PDE) inhibitor from the methylxanthine class and has demonstrated efficacy in the long-term management of COPD.[6] However, the risks of toxicity may outweigh the benefits.

- In our experience, theophylline may also improve morning respiratory symptoms when dosed at night.
- A common starting dose of long-acting theophylline for an average-sized patient is 200 mg PO q12h, with the usual therapeutic dose being between 400 and 900 mg/d.
- Serum levels should be checked 1–2 weeks after each dose adjustment, aiming for a level of 10 ± 2 μg/mL checked 4 hours after dosing, and monitored at least twice yearly.
- Continued inhalation of tobacco smoke lowers theophylline levels.
- Withdrawal of theophylline may lead to exacerbations of right heart failure.
- Clinicians should be aware of multiple potential drug interactions.

- **Vaccines**
  - Influenza vaccination decreases morbidity and mortality and should be administered annually to all patients that have COPD.
  - According to the Advisory Committee on Immunization Practices, all patients with COPD should receive the pneumococcal vaccine.[7] It is important to note that different formulations exist. A single revaccination can be given if the patient received the vaccine >5 years earlier and was aged <65 years at the time of primary vaccination.
- **PDE4 selective inhibitors**
  - The selective inhibition of PDE4 by more recently available medications (e.g., cilomilast and roflumilast) decreases bronchial constriction and inflammation and improves FEV_1 without the significant side effects associated with the nonselective PDE inhibitor theophylline.
  - Common side effects from PDE4 inhibitors include headache, nausea, and weight loss.
  - A recent randomized trial demonstrated that roflumilast, a PDE4 inhibitor, reduced exacerbations and improved lung function in patients with moderate to severe COPD.[8]
- **Chronic antibiotic treatment**
  - The macrolide class of antibiotics (azithromycin, erythromycin, and clarithromycin) has increasingly been studied in lung disease for both its antimicrobial and immune regulatory function.
  - A randomized trial demonstrated that addition of a macrolide antibiotic to inhaled medical therapy reduced the number of COPD exacerbations.[9]
  - Side effects of chronic macrolide therapy include QTc prolongation, hearing loss, and a theoretical risk of developing resistance infections.
- **Mucolytics, antioxidant agents, and vasodilators** have not been shown to be of benefit in COPD.
- **Nedocromil and leukotriene modifiers**, used frequently for the treatment of asthma, have not been adequately tested for the treatment of COPD and are therefore not recommended at this time.
- **Antitussives are not specifically recommended** in COPD because of the protective role of coughing in clearing secretions.[1]

Other Nonpharmacologic Therapies

- **Oxygen therapy**
  - Long-term supplemental oxygen therapy (>15 h/d) decreases mortality and improves physical and mental function in hypoxemic patients who have COPD.[10]
  - Oxygen therapy reduces the sensation of dyspnea and increases oxygen-carrying capacity to the heart, skeletal muscles, and the brain.
  - Experimental evidence suggests that hyperoxemia induces cellular oxidative stress via imbalance in oxidants and antioxidants, and it may hasten airway dysfunction and parenchymal destruction.
  - Thus, supplemental oxygen therapy should only be used in a goal-targeted fashion.

TABLE 10-4 INDICATIONS FOR LONG-TERM SUPPLEMENTAL OXYGEN ADMINISTRATION

Continuous administration
Resting PaO_2 ≤55 mm Hg or arterial oxygen saturation (SaO_2) ≤88%
Resting PaO_2 of 56–59 mm Hg or SaO_2 ≤89%, if patient has polycythemia (Hct ≥55%) or evidence of cor pulmonale

Noncontinuous administration (criteria for oxygen supplementation at rest not met)
PaO_2 ≤55 mm Hg or SaO_2 ≤88% during exertion
PaO_2 ≤55 mm Hg or SaO_2 ≤88% during sleep

- Assessment for oxygen therapy
  - A baseline room-air ABG should be performed routinely in patients with an FEV_1 <40% or clinical signs suggesting respiratory failure and/or right heart failure.
  - A monitored exercise oxygen assessment may identify increased needs of supplemental oxygen with activity.
  - Patients with evidence of sleep-disordered breathing, and possibly those with severe to very severe COPD not using supplemental oxygen at rest, should undergo evaluation of oxygenation during sleep.
  - Patients receiving long-term oxygen therapy should undergo routine reevaluation at least once yearly, and more frequently in the setting of changing clinical conditions (e.g., during an exacerbation and about a month after an exacerbation).
- Treatment
  - Supplemental oxygen is prescribed based on PaO_2 or SpO_2 at rest, during sleep, and with exertion (Table 10-4).
  - Desaturation is more common during sleep in patients with COPD, and patients requiring supplemental oxygen during exertion often need it during sleep.
  - While the exact amount required nocturnally might be measured with home overnight pulse oximetry, it is reasonable to set the oxygen to be delivered during sleep as 1 L/min greater than that required during rest when awake.
  - Though the use of oxygen for patients who have isolated nocturnal desaturation remains controversial, it is typically prescribed for this indication.
- Oxygen delivery systems
  - Continuous flow, dual-prong nasal cannula serves most patients regardless of activity level. Patients rarely require higher concentrations of oxygen, and in these cases, the use of a reservoir system with an oxymizer or high-flow nasal cannula may be most cost-effective.
  - In all cases, whenever an oxygen prescription is written, it should state the delivery system required (liquid, compressed gas, or concentrator), the delivery device required (e.g., nasal cannula), the required oxygen flow rates (liters per minute), and settings for rest, sleep, and exercise.

- **Pulmonary rehabilitation**
  - Exercise training is the foundation of pulmonary rehabilitation, and an exercise program may return a patient to a more functional and satisfactory life.
  - Pulmonary rehabilitation (as defined by the American Thoracic Society) is a multidisciplinary program of care for patients with chronic respiratory impairment that is individually tailored and designed to optimize physical and social performance and autonomy.
  - Patients with COPD who should be referred to a comprehensive rehabilitation program include those who have severe dyspnea despite optimal medical management, have reduced exercise tolerance, and experience a restriction in activities.

- Pulmonary rehabilitation[11]
  - Improves exercise tolerance
  - Improves dyspnea
  - Improves quality of life
- Pulmonary rehabilitation components include medical therapy, supplemental oxygen, exercise, education, psychosocial/behavioral intervention, and outcome assessment.
- A cautious approach toward exercise is required for patients with conditions such as coronary artery disease or pulmonary hypertension.

Surgical Management

- Surgical options for the treatment of COPD include **bullectomy, lung volume reduction surgery (LVRS), and lung transplantation.**
- **Bullectomy** in carefully selected patients with giant bullous disease may improve lung function and decrease symptoms.[12]
  - Generally, patients with bullae that occupy at least 50% of the hemithorax with other areas of relatively preserved lung are the best candidates for bullectomy.
  - A chest CT scan helps to determine the location and the extent of emphysema.
- **LVRS** performed by experienced surgeons in appropriately selected patients can improve functioning and quality of life, and increase survival.[13]
  - Patients with predominantly upper lobe disease achieve the best results.
  - Target areas for resection consist of focal areas of emphysematous lung that are accessible to surgical resection.
  - Poor candidates for LVRS include patients with an FEV_1 ≤20%, and either a very low DLCO or homogeneously distributed disease (without target areas).
  - **Endoscopic lung volume reductions via devices, biologic agents, or other approaches** continue to undergo evaluation, but surgical approach (i.e., LVRS) has shown the greatest efficacy.
- **Lung transplantation** may improve quality of life in patients and may confer a survival benefit in patients with very severe COPD.[14]
  - The International Society of Heart and Lung Transplantation (ISHLT) provides guidance regarding indications for lung transplantation.[15]
  - Patients with COPD and BODE (BMI, airway Obstruction by FEV_1, Dyspnea by the Medical Research Council Dyspnea scale, and Exercise capacity by 6 minute walk distance) score of 7–10, low FEV_1 (e.g., <25%), hypercapnia, pulmonary arterial hypertension, and severe clinical course may be appropriate for a transplant evaluation.
  - Lung transplantation is typically not an option for elderly patients (age >70–75 years) or those with significant comorbidities.

Lifestyle/Risk Modification

- **Smoking Cessation**
  - Smoking cessation should be discussed with all smokers during every office visit and during hospitalizations (see Chapter 11, for details).
  - This simple and cost-effective intervention is the most effective way to reduce the risk of developing COPD and the rate of decline in lung function.
  - Standard interventions include counseling, providing smoking cessation literature, and pharmacotherapy:
    - **Nicotine replacement therapies**, available in multiple forms (e.g., gum, transdermal patch, inhaler, nasal spray, sublingual tablet, and lozenge) increase abstinence and reduce relapses.
    - **Bupropion and nortriptyline** are antidepressants that, in combination with smoking cessation counseling, increase long-term abstinence rates.

- **Varenicline**, a nicotinic acetylcholine receptor partial agonist increases abstinence. It is typically started 1 week prior to an agreed upon smoking stop date, then uptitrated to goal dose of 1 mg bid for duration of up to 12 weeks. Varenicline therapy has an increased incidence of mood disorders, agitation, and suicide idealization in comparison to placebo.

PROGNOSIS

- COPD causes significant morbidity and mortality.
- Worsened expiratory airflow obstruction has an increased risk of exacerbations and death.
- Previously treated exacerbations predict recurrent exacerbations.
- The BODE score[16] and other validated scoring systems classify COPD severity and predict mortality and other adverse outcomes.

REFERENCES

1. Global Initiative for Chronic Obstructive Lung Disease (GOLD). Global strategy for the diagnosis, management and prevention of COPD, updated 2015. Available at http://www.goldcopd.org/uploads/users/files/GOLD_Report_2015_Apr2.pdf. Accessed 24/11/15.
2. Qaseem A, Wilt TJ, Weinberger SE, et al. Diagnosis and management of stable chronic obstructive pulmonary disease: a clinical practice guideline update from the American College of Physicians, American College of Chest Physicians, American Thoracic Society, and European Respiratory Society. *Ann Intern Med.* 2011;155:179–91.
3. de Jong YP, Uil SM, Grotjohan HP, et al. Oral or IV prednisolone in the treatment of COPD exacerbations: a randomized, controlled, double-blind study. *Chest.* 2007;132:1741–7.
4. Plant PK, Owen JL, Elliott MW. Early use of non-invasive ventilation for acute exacerbations of chronic obstructive pulmonary disease on general respiratory wards: a multicentre randomised controlled trial. *Lancet.* 2000;355:1931–5.
5. Vogelmeier C, Hederer B, Glaab T, et al. POET-COPD Investigators. Tiotropium versus salmeterol for the prevention of exacerbations of COPD. *N Engl J Med.* 2011;364:1093–103.
6. Murciano D, Auclair MH, Pariente R, et al. A randomized, controlled trial of theophylline in patients with severe chronic obstructive pulmonary disease. *N Engl J Med.* 1989;320:1521–5.
7. Kim DK, Bridges CB, Harriman KH on behalf of the Advisory Committee on Immunization Practices. Advisory committee on immunization practices recommended immunization schedule for adults aged 19 years or older—United States, 2015. *Ann Intern Med.* 2015;162:214–23.
8. Rabe KF, Bateman ED, O'Donnell D, et al. Roflumilast–an oral anti-inflammatory treatment for chronic obstructive pulmonary disease: a randomised controlled trial. *Lancet.* 2005;366:563–71.
9. Seemungal TA, Wilkinson TM, Hurst JR, et al. Long-term erythromycin therapy is associated with decreased chronic obstructive pulmonary disease exacerbations. *Am J Respir Crit Care Med.* 2008;178:1139–47.
10. Long term domiciliary oxygen therapy in chronic hypoxic cor pulmonale complicating chronic bronchitis and emphysema. Report of the Medical Research Council Working Party. *Lancet.* 1981;1:681–6.
11. Casaburi R, ZuWallack R. Pulmonary rehabilitation for management of chronic obstructive pulmonary disease. *N Engl J Med.* 2009;360:1329–35.
12. Palla A, Desideri M, Rossi G, et al. Elective surgery for giant bullous emphysema: a 5-year clinical and functional follow-up. *Chest.* 2005;128:2043–50.
13. Naunheim KS, Wood DE, Mohsenifar Z, et al. Long-term follow-up of patients receiving lung-volume-reduction surgery versus medical therapy for severe emphysema by the National Emphysema Treatment Trial Research Group. *Ann Thorac Surg.* 2006;82:431–43.
14. Lahzami S, Bridevaux PO, Soccal PM, et al. Survival impact of lung transplantation for COPD. *Eur Respir J.* 2010;36:74–80.
15. Weill D, Benden C, Corris PA, et al. A consensus document for the selection of lung transplant candidates: 2014–an update from the Pulmonary Transplantation Council of the International Society for Heart and Lung Transplantation. *J Heart Lung Transplant.* 2015;34:1–15.
16. Celli BR, Cote CG, Marin JM, et al. The body-mass index, airflow obstruction, dyspnea, and exercise capacity index in chronic obstructive pulmonary disease. *N Engl J Med.* 2004;350:1005–12.

Smoking Cessation

11

Sundeep Viswanathan and Amy McQueen

GENERAL PRINCIPLES

Epidemiology

- Cigarette smoking causes over 400,000 deaths annually in the United States. In 2012, 18.1% of adults smoked cigarettes.[1]
- Rates of smoking vary based on ethnicity, region, socioeconomic status, and education. Smoking rates are also higher among people with disabilities, substance use problems, mental health disorders, and HIV/AIDS and people on Medicaid.
- Second- and third-hand smoke represent an underappreciated and definite risk to the household members of smokers and the general public.

Pathophysiology

- Nicotine stimulates acetylcholine receptors in the brain and activates the sympathetic nervous system, leading to elevated circulating levels of norepinephrine, epinephrine, vasopressin, growth hormone, cortisol, and endorphins. Nicotine also stimulates specific dopaminergic reward centers in the brain leading, to its psychological addiction. These result in increases in heart rate, blood pressure, cardiac stroke volume, and coronary blood flow.
- Other effects of nicotine use include arousal early in the day, relaxation during stressful situations, and an increased metabolic rate with reduced hunger leading to body weight reduction.
- Most smoking cessation attempts fail. Nicotine is addictive, and people become physiologically (and psychologically) dependent on its effects. People who quit experience withdrawal symptoms with the peak varying from 24 hours to 4 weeks after quitting. Withdrawal symptoms include anxiety, impatience, restlessness, irritability, hostility, difficulty in concentrating, nicotine cravings, headaches, insomnia, depression, dysphoria, and hunger. Patients with a previous history of major depression, bipolar disorder, or alcohol and drug abuse may be especially susceptible to withdrawal and relapse.
- Psychological addiction can continue for months to years following quitting. Daily activities related to smoking such as eating, drinking, sex, being around other smokers, and driving can act as triggers for nicotine cravings.

Associated Conditions

- There are multiple known carcinogens in cigarette smoke, resulting in a high risk of lung, oral, esophageal, laryngeal, and urothelial cancers.
- The risk of lung cancer increases in relation to the amount an individual smokes and the age at which he or she started smoking.
- Cigarette smoking alters immunity in the lung as well as the structure and function of the airways. Smokers have a lower forced expiratory volume over 1 second (FEV_1) and an accelerated rate of FEV_1 decline when compared with nonsmokers. Cigarette smoking has resulted in a high prevalence of chronic obstructive pulmonary disease (COPD). It is also an important trigger for asthma attacks.
- There is evidence that smoking contributes to vascular endothelial damage, coronary vasospasm, and increased platelet aggregation. Cigarette smoking is a known risk factor

for coronary artery disease, hypertension, and stroke. Smoking also alters the senses of taste and smell.

- Smoking cessation mitigates some of these risks but does not drop the risk down to a lifelong nonsmoker.

DIAGNOSIS

- Studies have shown that physicians continue to do a poor job in identifying current smokers and urging them to quit despite the data behind the benefits of smoking cessation. Barriers include a lack of perceived training and awareness of resources on the part of physicians, low expectations that patients will actually quit, and low reimbursements for time spent discussing smoking cessation.
- Clinicians can use the Modified Fagerström Test for Nicotine Dependence to grade patients' dependence.[2] Patients should be considered **highly dependent** on nicotine if they smoke >20 cigarettes per day, smoke their first cigarette of the day within 30 minutes of awakening, or if during a previous quit attempt they developed strong cravings or withdrawal symptoms. Because nicotine is an addictive substance, patients can be expected to cycle through multiple periods of relapse and remission. Physicians should support each quit attempt as they would for patients in alcohol or drug rehabilitation.

Diagnostic Criteria

- The following steps, initially developed by the National Cancer Institute as the "Four A's" program, can be used in most outpatient settings to identify smokers and aid quitting. The Four A's have been expanded to the Five A's by the Clinical Practice Guidelines for Treating Tobacco Use and Dependence.[3]
- **Ask: Systematically identify all tobacco users at every visit.** Ask at every visit about smoking: *Do you smoke? Have you considered quitting? Are you ready to quit? What can I do to help you quit?* Consider expanding documentation of vital signs to include tobacco use.
- **Advise: Strongly urge all tobacco users to quit** at every visit. The goal is to present compelling evidence about the importance of quitting and to educate the patient about methods for quitting and the help available. Clear, strong, and personalized advice based on both the patient's health and his or her social situation works best. For example, tie tobacco use to current illness or if the patient lives with children, the adverse effects of smoking on children.
- **Assess: Determine willingness to make quit attempt** by asking the patient to make a quit attempt at this time. If he or she is willing to try quitting, provide assistance and further information. Schedule a return visit to prepare a plan for smoking cessation. If the patient not ready to quit, continue to educate him or her about the risk of smoking and offer to schedule a follow-up visit to continue the discussion. However, even among smokers who report no plans to quit, pharmacotherapy use has been associated with increased quit attempts, fewer cigarettes smoked, and greater abstinence rates.[4]
- **Assist: Aid the patient in quitting** with the development of a quit plan. Give consideration to drawing up a contract for the patient to sign in a similar fashion to a narcotics contract or asthma management plan. Discuss the patient's motivation for quitting and the benefits and drawbacks of quitting. Identify roadblocks to quitting, and discuss strategies for overcoming these. Encourage the patient to discuss the plan with family and friends and enlist their support. Suggest the patient remove all tobacco-related products from the house as the quit date approaches.
  - The smoker also may want to avoid alcohol because it is a cue for many patients to smoke.
  - Initiating an exercise plan should be encouraged, with the goal being twofold: (a) occupying the patient's free time, leaving less time to smoke, and (b) helping avoid

the weight gain associated with nicotine withdrawal. The average weight gain with smoking cessation is 2–3 kg, and it may be delayed by use of pharmacologic agents.
  - Provide pharmacologic therapy after assessment of the individual's dependence and risk factors. Patients also benefit from counseling and/or scheduled follow-up. Most states have free telephone quit lines that patients can call for information and help with quitting. Encourage total abstinence as the ultimate goal, but acknowledge that even cutting down the number of cigarettes by 50% has some benefits and may improve later quit success. Similarly, nicotine replacement, even for long periods, is considered safer than smoking.
  - With patients who have had previous failed quit attempts, the discussion should center on the reasons for the failure and developing strategies to cope with these problems. Common reasons for failure include withdrawal, cravings, stress, illness, and situational factors.
- **Arrange: Arrange follow-up visits** to confirm and maintain abstinence. The physician, a counselor, or even office staff can perform the follow-up. Focus on positive health benefits of cessation and congratulate the patient on quitting. Assess and treat withdrawal symptoms as needed. Educate patients about the numerous resources available to them to help them stay quit. If patients relapse, offer encouragement, discuss reasons for failure, and offer continued support.

TREATMENT

- Achieving smoking cessation centers around a combination of counseling and behavior modification, strong social support, a knowledgeable and motivated patient, and pharmacologic therapies.
- Although the medication labels and inserts caution against using multiple nicotine products concurrently, research has shown that first-line agents can be used in combination safely and often with greater efficacy.[5]
- Results of the best single or combination of agents have varied across meta-analyses and trials.
- Common combinations include
  - Bupropion + patch OR
  - Patch + gum, lozenge, or nasal spray the following, which suggest a benefit of treating nicotine dependence through multiple mechanisms (i.e., steady delivery of patch + ad-lib use of faster-acting nicotine replacement therapies for acute cravings)

Medications

Several first-line therapies are available either by prescription or over-the-counter. Selecting the right first-line method should be made on an individual basis. The impact of comorbidities, contraindications, drug interactions, patient preference, ease and understanding of use, patient's previous history of failed attempts, cost, and severity of addiction should all be taken into consideration.

- **Nicotine replacement therapy** (NRT)
  - NRT works via direct absorption into the circulation through the buccal mucosa, nasal mucosa, or skin. NRT should be considered for any smoker attempting cessation, but it is **contraindicated in anyone with unstable angina or within 2 weeks of a coronary event.** There is however no increased cardiovascular risk in patients with known cardiovascular disease.
  - It has not been approved for use during pregnancy, but because circulatory levels are lower than those achieved by actual cigarette smoking, NRT should in theory cause less uterine vasoconstriction, and therefore be safer, than smoking.

- NRT may be used in a step-down method, but doing so may prolong the total duration of therapy. There is a low potential for dependence because blood nicotine levels achieved with any method of NRT are lower than levels achieved through cigarette smoking. NRT also does not produce tar and carbon monoxide, which are other substances linked to the ill effects of smoking.
- Underuse (not overuse) of NRT is a substantial problem which hinders quit success, and some research shows that smokers are more concerned about nicotine addiction than the harms from smoking, so healthcare professionals should inform patients of the relative harms.
- The recommended course of treatment varies by NRT product, but research has shown that some people (especially heavy smokers) may benefit from longer periods and combinations of NRT until they are confident they will not relapse.
- In general, it is advised that patients start NRT on their quit date and not smoke while on NRT. However, some studies have shown positive effects of starting the patch a week before the quit date. Patients using NRT should be encouraged not to give up if they relapse and have a cigarette. In these cases, the patient may benefit from a higher dose of NRT or a combination of products to be able to stay off cigarettes.
- **Nicotine patch**
  - There are two types of nicotine patches available: a 24-hour release form and a 16-hour release form. They are applied to the skin and changed every day over a total period of about 8–10 weeks. The maximum strength of the 24-hour patch is 21 mg, whereas the maximum strength of the 16-hour patch is 15 mg. Peak action is within 2–9 hours of application. The 21-mg patches are frequently used for 4–6 weeks followed by a short taper (14 mg/d for 2–4 weeks, then 7 mg/d for 2–4 weeks) to wean the patient off of the patches completely.
  - Advantages of the patch include convenience and a minimal need for instruction.
  - Disadvantages include mild itching or erythema at the application site and possible allergy to the adhesive. Alternative delivery methods should be considered in patients with eczema or skin conditions. Some patients also develop sleep disturbances, anxiety, appetite disturbances, generalized rash, headache, nausea, vertigo, or dyspepsia.
  - The 24-hour patch is believed to be more effective against early morning urges but has also been associated with a greater incidence of sleep disturbances. Some of the side effects can be mitigated by removing the patch at bedtime or lowering the dose of the patch in those who experience nicotine overdose symptoms.
  - Six-month quit rates with the patch range from 22% to 42%, whereas permanent cessation rates range from 5% to 28%.
- **Nicotine gum and lozenges**
  - Nicotine gum was the first NRT approved for use in the United States and is readily available over-the-counter. The gum is chewed briefly until a tingling sensation is noted, then is "parked" in the mouth. The location of parked gum should be rotated regularly. Each piece of gum is used for about 30 minutes and the effects of the absorbed nicotine peak within 20–40 minutes. Maximum dosing recommendations are 30 pieces of the 2-mg gum, or 20 pieces of the 4-mg gum, per day. It is suggested that patients start with a fixed dose per day (e.g., 1 piece every 1–2 hours) then progressively wean themselves over a total period of about 12 weeks.
  - The most obvious advantage of this method is that gum chewing is socially acceptable in most settings and the gum can be chewed whenever a patient has a craving.
  - The disadvantages include a higher level of instruction for proper use and difficulty of use for people with temporomandibular joint problems or dentures, or those who are edentulous. Other disadvantages include air swallowing, hiccups, indigestion, nausea, stomachache, burning sensation in the throat, and a sore jaw. The gum has also been noted to have a bad taste.

        - Because absorption of the nicotine is based on pH in the oral cavity, ingestion of coffee and carbonated beverages before use may lead to poor absorption. Food intake can also disrupt the absorption. Oftentimes people do not use the correct dosage or amount of the gum during the day to stave off cravings, so education by healthcare personnel is essential. Alternatively, combining a patch and gum or lozenge may be more beneficial than use of either type of NRT alone.
        - Nicotine lozenges have a similar nicotine delivery system as the gum; dosing is similar. The lozenge should require less instruction than the gum, but have similar efficacy. Patients should not chew or swallow the lozenge, but allow it to dissolve completely in the mouth, which takes about 20–30 minutes. As with the gum, patients should move the lozenge around their mouth and "park" it occasionally.
    - **Nicotine inhaler**
        - A nicotine inhaler consists of nicotine plugs inside hollow cigarette-like rods (a long cartridge). The nicotine levels peak in 10–15 minutes after inhalation. Although it is called an inhaler, 95% of the nicotine is absorbed in the mouth and esophagus, not in the lung. The usual dosing is 6–16 nicotine cartridges per day. One cartridge (10-mg nicotine) is used up after about 20 minutes of active puffing. The recommended duration of treatment is 12 weeks followed by a 6–12-week weaning period.
        - This form of NRT is especially good for cravings because of the quicker onset of action. It also satisfies the hand-to-mouth ritual of cigarette smoking.
        - The major disadvantages of this method include awkwardness of using an inhaler in certain social settings, cough, and throat irritation. Patients need a prescription in order to get nicotine inhalers.
    - **Nicotine nasal spray**
        - The nasal spray most closely resembles the effects of actual cigarette smoking because of the high peak blood levels obtained and the rapid onset of action in 5–7 minutes. The levels of nicotine in the blood obtained with this method, although higher than all other forms of NRT, are still lower than levels achieved with cigarette smoking. Maximum dosing is 1 spray per nostril every 1–2 hours, not to exceed 30–40 times per day, for 3 months followed by a tapering period up to 3 months.
        - The advantage of the nasal spray is that users are able to satisfy cravings rapidly.
        - The disadvantages include local irritation of the nose, eyes, and throat, as well as headache, burning sensation, sneezing, and watery eyes. Some patients are also embarrassed to use the spray in public. A cold or nasal congestion can also negatively affect absorption. Nicotine nasal spray should be avoided in patients with asthma. Patients need a prescription in order to get nicotine nasal spray.
    - **Nonnicotine pharmacotherapies**: Bupropion and varenicline are considered first-line therapies and both require a prescription and close physician monitoring. Both are associated with more adverse side effects than NRT which subsequently affects adherence and quit rates.
    - **Bupropion**
        - The effectiveness of bupropion in smoking cessation is believed to be related to the dopaminergic and noradrenergic effects of the drug. The noradrenergic modifications may limit nicotine withdrawal symptoms, while the dopaminergic modulation may affect areas of the brain that are involved with the reinforcing properties of addictive drugs such as nicotine. Medication should commence 1 week before quitting, at a dose of 150 mg daily for 3 days, and then be increased to 150 mg bid for 7–24 weeks. Although approved at higher doses for use as an antidepressant, 300 mg/dis the maximum dose indicated for smoking cessation. Patients already on bupropion for depression should not be given bupropion for smoking cessation.
        - Bupropion is in pregnancy category B. It is contraindicated in patients with a seizure history, as it lowers seizure threshold, and it should not be used by patients

with anorexia nervosa or bulimia nervosa, patients undergoing alcohol withdrawal, or patients who have used an MAOI in the previous 2 weeks.
    - Side effects include insomnia, dry mouth, nervousness, difficulty concentrating, rash, and constipation.
    - A blinded, randomized, placebo-controlled trial demonstrated an 18% success rate with bupropion alone and a 22% success rate with a combination of bupropion and a nicotine patch.[6] The difference between the groups was not statistically significant, however.
  - **Varenicline**
    - Varenicline is a partial agonist of the nicotinic acetylcholine receptor and helps with reducing nicotine withdrawal symptoms and blocking nicotine from binding to the receptor, therefore taking away the pleasurable effects of smoking. A meta-analysis demonstrated that varenicline was associated with greater abstinence (6 months or greater) compared to bupropion or NRT alone, but not when either was used in combination with other cessation aids.[7]
    - The starting dose of varenicline is 0.5 mg daily 1 week before the quit date. The dosage is increased to 0.5 mg bid on days 4–7, and finally increased to 1 mg bid until the end of treatment (3–6 months).
    - Side effects include nausea, strange dreams, neuropsychiatric disorders including depression and mania, and a small, increased risk of cardiovascular adverse events in patients who have cardiovascular disease. Psychiatric risks include changes in behavior, depressed mood, hostility, and suicidal thoughts or actions.
    - Care shoud be implemented in following patients at a high neuropsychiatric or cardiovascular risk with surveillance and careful screening. Caution is advised in patients with renal insufficiency.
    - NRT can be used in combination with varenicline in patients who have failed monotherapy.
  - Other therapies include
    - **Nortriptyline**, a tricyclic antidepressant, and other antidepressants are being investigated for efficacy in smoking cessation and have shown modest results. Side effects include dry mouth and sedation. Currently, bupropion remains the only antidepressant that has a smoking cessation indication.
    - **Anxiolytics** such as **benzodiazepines and buspirone** have been used in patients demonstrating increased anxiety during smoking cessation. Although there is no proven benefit for the use of these drugs in smoking cessation, they may be helpful in selected individuals.
    - Some physicians have tried to diminish withdrawal symptoms through the use of **clonidine**. There is little evidence to support the use of clonidine in smoking cessation.
    - There is no convincing evidence that **naloxone or naltrexone** is effective in smoking cessation.

Other Nonpharmacologic Therapies

- **Behavioral counseling**
  - Nonpharmacologic therapies are a helpful adjunct to medical therapy, and there is ample evidence that counseling improves a patient's chance of quitting. Most studies of smoking cessation have a counseling component or, at the very minimum, regular appointments with counselors to reinforce and remind patients of their goal to quit.
  - Counseling and support are now available through a variety of media and locations based on patient preference.
  - Any amount of counseling is known to be effective, even if it is simply a physician advising a smoker to quit. Studies have demonstrated that brief interventions by physicians, often no longer than 3–10 minutes, can increase cessation rates.

  - There seems to be a **dose–response relationship between counseling intensity and effectiveness.** High-intensity counseling lasting >30 minutes or at more than two visits is even more effective than brief interventions.
  - The components of successful smoking cessation counseling therapy are variable and center mostly on cognitive behavior therapy. Some of the ideas discussed include self-management or patient awareness of personal cues and patterns that encourage smoking and how to avoid them. Relapse prevention can also be important, for example, some patients may need to avoid going to bars or drinking alcoholic beverages if such activities trigger a relapse to smoking. Avoiding other smokers is often helpful.
  - Smoking cessation groups are often organized by hospitals or workplaces with the assistance of the American Lung Association and can be very helpful. They allow smokers to share their difficulties in a group setting. Most states have telephone quit lines that patients can call at any time to get assistance with quitting.
  - Several websites and computer-based programs can be used in the privacy of one's own home and have been found to be helpful in maintaining abstinence. Resources online include www.becomeanex.org, www.ffsonline.org, and www.smokefree.gov. Accessed 12/10/15.
  - Hospitalized smokers provide a unique opportunity for aggressive inpatient counseling by medical personnel. Most US medical campuses are now smoke-free. Patients can be closely monitored for nicotine withdrawal side effects. NRT can be instrumental in the hospital and should be offered to patients by admitting physicians.
- **Alternative therapies**
  - Other aids that are used commercially but are unproven include hypnosis, auricular therapy, acupuncture or acupressure, biofeedback, relaxation or meditation, herbal remedies, teas, or supplements.
  - Other nicotine products are available commercially and are not regulated by the FDA, but may be increasingly used by smokers trying to quit or replace cigarettes (i.e., electronic cigarettes).
  - Nicotine fading involves systematized cutting back and some studies have shown that patients who are able to successfully cutback have a higher likelihood of quitting.

MONITORING/FOLLOW-UP

- Nicotine affects the metabolism of several medications including warfarin (increased metabolism), heparin (increased clearance), and theophylline (decreased levels) and physicians should carefully review the medication list of patients who are quitting or have recently quit.
- For previous smokers who quit in the distant past, no further intervention is needed. They should, however, be congratulated on their achievement.
- For smokers who quit within the past year, reinforcement is given along with reeducation on the benefits of having quit. Discuss any problems that might have been encountered and their possible solutions. Again, congratulations are in order.

PROGNOSIS

- Many of the health risks of smoking are drastically reduced upon cessation of tobacco smoking.
- The risk of smoking relapse remains high and physicians should be understanding about relapses. Physicians and patients need to evaluate the causes for relapse and underscore the importance of trying to quit again.

REFERENCES

1. Agaku IT, King BA, Dube SR. Current cigarette smoking among adults—United States, 2005–2012. *MMWR Morb Mort Wkly Rep.* 2014;63:29–34.
2. Heatherton TF, Kozlowski LT, Frecker RC, et al. The Fagerström test for nicotine dependence: a revision of the Fagerström Tolerance Questionnaire. *Br J Addict.* 1991;86:1119–27.
3. Fiore MC, Bailey WC, Cohen SJ, et al. Treating tobacco use and dependence. Quick reference guide for clinicians. Rockville, MD: US Department of Health and Human Services; 2000. www.surgeon-general.gov/tobacco/tobaqrg.htm
4. Hughes JR, Rennard SI, Fingar JR, et al. Efficacy of varenicline to prompt quit attempts in smokers not currently trying to quit: a randomized placebo-controlled trial. *Nicotine Tob Res.* 2011;13(10):955–64.
5. Zapawa LM, Hughes JR, Benowitz NL, et al. Cautions and warnings on the US OTC label for nicotine replacement: what's a doctor to do? *Addictive Behaviors.* 2011;36:327–32.
6. Fiore MC, Baker TD, Bailey WC, et al. A clinical practice guideline for treating tobacco use and dependence: 2008 update. A U.S. Public Health Service Report. *Am J Prev Med.* 2008;35(2):158–76.
7. Cahill K, Stevens S, Perera R, et al. Pharmacological interventions for smoking cessation: an overview and network meta-analysis. *Cochrane Database Syst Rev.* 2013;5:CD009329.

Community-Acquired Pneumonia

12

Jake M. Chanin and Carlos A. Q. Santos

GENERAL PRINCIPLES

- Community-acquired pneumonia (CAP) is a significant cause of morbidity and mortality in the United States.
- CAP ranks highly among all causes of death. The exact mortality rate varies widely depending on the treatment setting (outpatient vs. inpatient vs. intensive care unit [ICU]), the presence or absence of associated comorbidities, and the age of the patient.
- It causes over 1 million hospitalizations annually.
- Administration of appropriate antimicrobials and management for severe pneumonia have a significant benefit on patient survival.
  - Nearly half of all cases do not have an identified etiologic agent.
  - Early empiric treatment is essential, and bacterial resistance must be considered.
- The most widely recognized guidelines for the treatment of CAP include those of the American Thoracic Society, the Infectious Diseases Society of America, and the Canadian Infectious Disease Society and Canadian Thoracic Society.

Definition

- CAP is a primary infection of lung parenchyma. Bacterial or viral invasion causes inflammation and alveolar infiltration that result in focal consolidation.
- CAP is distinctive from health care–associated pneumonia (HCAP) and hospital-acquired pneumonia (HAP) in that the infection is acquired in the community.

Classification

- Typical bacterial: *Streptococcus pneumoniae, Staphylococcus aureus, Haemophilus influenzae,* Group A streptococci, *Moraxella catarrhalis,* mixed anaerobes (aspiration), and aerobic gram-negative organisms.
- Atypical bacterial: *Legionella pneumophila, Mycoplasma pneumoniae, Chlamydophila pneumoniae.*
- Viral: Influenza A and B, respiratory syncytial virus (RSV), adenovirus, rhinoviruses, rubeola, varicella.

Epidemiology

Pneumonia and influenza combine to be the eighth leading cause of death in the United States. In 2008, there were over 56,000 deaths due to pneumonia and influenza.[1] The rate of deaths due to pneumonia is increasing. Pneumonia is more common in the winter months and elderly. Men and African-Americans are slightly more affected than women and Caucasians.

Etiology

- The most common etiology for CAP is *S. pneumoniae.*
- Frequently, pneumonia is preceded by an upper airway infection or viral illness.

Pathophysiology

- Lobar pneumonia is characterized by consolidation of a large portion of lung. Consolidation of airspaces is caused by host inflammatory infiltration in response to bacterial infection of lung tissue.

- Bronchopneumonia similarly involves acute inflammation, but the consolidated areas are patchy and often multilobar or bilateral. This pattern is more common to atypical viral pneumonias or mycoplasmal pneumonias.

Risk Factors

- Predisposing comorbid conditions: chronic obstructive pulmonary disease (COPD), heart failure, chronic renal disease, and chronic bronchitis.
- Host factors: advanced age, tobacco use, prior history of pneumonia, recent viral respiratory infection.
- Immunosuppressed states: HIV infection, chemotherapy, solid organ and stem cell transplant recipients.
- Mechanical: dysphagia, lung cancer, mechanical obstruction of bronchus, hiatal hernia, radiation esophagitis.
- Aspiration risk factors: alcoholism and drug intoxication, altered mental status, seizure disorder, stroke, procedural sedation, and anesthesia.
- Mucus clearance: cystic fibrosis, Kartagener syndrome, immotile cilia syndrome, Young syndrome.

Prevention

Prevention should include major risk factor modifications such as smoking cessation and vaccination against influenza and pneumococcus.

DIAGNOSIS

The gold standard for diagnosis of pneumonia is a posteroanterior and lateral CXR demonstrating new pulmonary infiltration. Clinical signs and symptoms should correlate with active infection and pulmonic consolidation.

Clinical Presentation

- Patients will typically complain of fever, chills, productive cough, shortness of breath, and chest pain.
- Physical examination findings include fever, tachypnea, tachycardia, abnormal breath sounds including rhonchi or crackles, increased tactile fremitus, dullness to percussion, and reduced chest movement.

Differential Diagnosis

- The differential diagnosis for pneumonia includes pathology that causes radiographic consolidations that can mimic pneumonia. This includes acute heart failure exacerbation and other causes of pulmonary edema, malignancy, pulmonary embolism (PE), septic embolism, and foreign body.
- Multiple different bacteria, viruses, and fungi can cause acute pneumonia.

Diagnostic Testing

The primary objective is to identify the causative agent. Other laboratory testing should be undertaken to assess the severity of illness. Typical studies include basic laboratory chemistries, blood cell counts, and cultures.

Laboratories

- Initial inpatient and outpatient studies should include blood cultures, complete blood count (CBC) with differential, basic metabolic profile (BMP), and liver function tests (LFT).
- Blood cultures are positive in 5–18% of hospitalized patients.[2,3] Ideally blood cultures should be obtained before antibiotics are given, but this should not delay administration of early empiric treatment.

- HIV testing should be considered among patients age 15 years and older.
- Urine studies such as urine pneumococcal and *Legionella* antigen assays can assist in microbe identification.
- For patients with suspected influenza, nasopharyngeal viral culture and immunofluorescence, or polymerase chain reaction (PCR) should be obtained. For *M. pneumonia,* PCR or serology can aid in diagnosis.
- Gram stain and sputum culture have been commonly used in the evaluation of CAP. Due to limitations in Gram stain and culture of sputum, we no longer recommend it in the initial care of uncomplicated CAP. Sputum analysis should be considered in patients who fail initial treatment with antibiotics, require ICU-level care, have cavitary lesions on CXR, or have a history of alcoholism or immunosuppression.

Imaging

- Plain CXR is the imaging study of choice. Pneumonic infiltrates can "fluff up" after volume resuscitation in volume-depleted patients.
- CT and MRI are not required for the diagnosis of pneumonia.
- CT scan should be performed when clinical symptoms do not suggest infection as the cause of radiographic infiltrate (e.g., malignancy). CT can also be used to evaluate empyema, cavitary disease, interstitial lung disease, and in patients who fail to respond to antibiotics.
- MRI can provide additional information about mass lesions and lymphadenopathy.

Diagnostic Procedures

- Invasive diagnostic procedures such as bronchoscopy and bronchoalveolar lavage are rarely required or recommended but can be of use in nonresponders, critically ill patients, or immunocompromised hosts.
- Diagnostic thoracentesis should be performed for pleural effusions that layer >10 mm on a lateral decubitus radiograph. Sampling of fluid helps rule out empyema, which would require tube thoracostomy. Pleural fluid testing should include cell count and differential, protein, lactate dehydrogenase, pH, glucose, Gram stain, and culture.
- Tracheal aspiration should be performed on patients requiring intubation.

TREATMENT

- Care should be triaged to inpatient versus outpatient treatment. Patients should also be evaluated for severity of illness, for example, patient requiring ICU admission versus admission to a medical floor.
- CURB-65 criteria (0–1 points: outpatient; 2 points: medical floor admission; ≥3 points: ICU-level care)[4]
  - Confusion
  - Uremia (blood urea nitrogen [BUN] >20 mg/dL)
  - Respiratory rate (>30 breaths/min)
  - Blood pressure (systolic <90 mm Hg or diastolic <60 mm Hg)
  - Age ≥65 years
- Criteria for determining severity of CAP (ICU admit is recommended for patients with ≥1 major criteria or ≥3 minor criteria)[5]
  - Major criteria
    - Invasive mechanical ventilation
    - Septic shock with the need for vasopressors
  - Minor criteria
    - Respiratory rate ≥30 breaths/min
    - PaO_2/FiO_2 ratio ≤250
    - Multilobar infiltrates
    - Confusion/disorientation
    - Uremia (BUN >20 mg/dL)

    - Leukopenia (white blood cell [WBC] count <4000 cells/mm^3)
    - Thrombocytopenia (platelet count <100,000 cells/mm^3)
    - Hypothermia (core temperature <36°C)
    - Hypotension requiring aggressive fluid resuscitation

Medications

- **Outpatient, previously healthy**[5]
  - Macrolide (any of the following)
    - Azithromycin 500 mg PO × 1, then 250 mg PO daily × 4 days
    - Clarithromycin 500 mg PO bid or clarithromycin XL 1000 mg PO daily
    - Erythromycin 250–500 mg PO q6h
  - Doxycycline 100 mg PO bid
- **Outpatient with comorbidities**[5] (e.g., heart/lung/liver/renal disease, diabetes, alcoholism, malignancy, asplenia, immunosuppressed, prior use of antibiotics)
  - Respiratory quinolone (any of the following)
    - Levofloxacin 750 mg PO daily
    - Moxifloxacin 400 mg PO daily
  - β-Lactam (any of the following) **PLUS** macrolide **OR** doxycycline
    - Amoxicillin 1 g PO tid
    - Amoxicillin-clavulanate 875 mg/125 mg PO bid
    - Cefpodoxime 200 mg PO bid
    - Cefuroxime 500 mg PO bid
- **Inpatient therapy non-ICU**[5]
  - Respiratory quinolone (any of the following)
    - Levofloxacin 750 mg IV daily
    - Moxifloxacin 400 mg IV daily
  - β-Lactam (any of the following) **PLUS** macrolide (e.g., azithromycin 500 mg IV daily) **OR** doxycycline 100–200 mg IV bid
    - Cefotaxime 1 g IV q8h
    - Ceftriaxone 1 g IV q24h
    - Ampicillin/sulbactam 3 g IV q6h
    - Ertapenem 1 g IV q24h
- **Inpatient therapy ICU**[5]
  - IV β-lactam **PLUS**
  - IV respiratory quinolone **OR** IV azithromycin

Other Nonpharmacologic Therapies

Pulmonary hygiene with cough assist devices or chest physiotherapy can aid in the medical management of pneumonia.

Duration of Therapy

- Minimum duration should be 5 days.
- Antibiotics should not be tapered until the patient has been afebrile for 48–72 hours, symptoms are improving, and the WBC count is decreasing.
- Patients may be switched to oral antibiotics once improvement is noted clinically and they are stable enough to take oral medicines.

Surgical Management

- If present, an empyema should be drained with thoracostomy tube placement.
- Drainage of lung abscess is controversial. Chest physiotherapy should be used to promote natural expectoration. Complications of percutaneous or surgical drainage can include bronchopleural fistula and pneumothorax.

MONITORING/FOLLOW-UP

- Infiltrate on CXR will persist longer than clinical symptoms of pneumonia.
- Routine follow-up CXR is not recommended. However, there is evidence to suggest that follow-upradiography in select groups (e.g., >50 years old, tobacco users) may reveal other diagnosesincluding malignancy.[6,7]

OUTCOME/PROGNOSIS

- Treatment failure
  - Occurs in 10–15% of cases, and mortality is increased nearly 5-fold in some studies.[8]
  - It is important to distinguish clinical deterioration from failure in symptomatic improvement.
- Clinical deterioration
  - Within 72 hours: typically resistant organisms, alternate diagnosis (consider PE, acute respiratory distress syndrome [ARDS], pulmonary vasculitis syndromes, polymicrobial infection due to aspiration), severe illness, and natural progression of disease to respiratory and/or multiorgan failure.
  - After 72 hours: nosocomial infections, severe comorbid conditions, PE, myocardial infarction (MI), renal failure.
- Failure in symptomatic improvement
  - Within 72 hours: typically normal response.
  - After 72 hours: resistant organisms or inappropriate antibiotic selection, local complications (parapneumonic effusion or empyema), alternate diagnosis (pulmonary edema, malignancy, vasculitis, PE), drug fevers.
- Overall mortality from pneumonia ranges based on severity of disease and host factors. In one meta-analysis ranged from 5.1% in hospitalized and ambulatory patients to 36.5% in patients requiring ICU care.[9]

REFERENCES

1. Miniño AM, Murphy SL, Xu J, et al. Deaths: final data for 2008. *Natl Vital Stat Rep.* 2011; 59(10):1–126.
2. Campbell SG, Marrie TJ, Anstey R, et al. The contribution of blood cultures to the clinical management of adult patients admitted to the hospital with community-acquired pneumonia: a prospective observational study. *Chest.* 2003;123:1142–50.
3. Waterer GW, Wunderink RG. The influence of the severity of community-acquired pneumonia on the usefulness of blood cultures. *Respir Med.* 2001;95:78–82.
4. Lim WS, van der Eerden MM, Laing R, et al. Defining community acquired pneumonia severity on presentation to hospital: an international derivation and validation study. *Thorax.* 2003;58:377–82.
5. Mandell LA, Wunderink RG, Anzueto A, et al. Infectious Diseases Society of America/American Thoracic Society consensus guidelines on the management of community-acquired pneumonia in adults. *Clin Infect Dis.* 2007;44(Suppl 2):S27–72.
6. Tang KL, Eurich DT, Minhas-Sandhu JK, et al. Incidence, correlates, and chest radiographic yield of new lung cancer diagnosis in 3398 patients with pneumonia. *Arch Intern Med.* 2011;171:1193–8.
7. Little BP, Gilman MD, Humphrey KL, et al. Outcome of recommendations for radiographic follow-up of pneumonia on outpatient chest radiography. *AJR Am J Roentgenol.* 2014;202:54–9.
8. Menendez R, Torres A. Treatment failure in community-acquired pneumonia. *Chest.* 2007; 132(4):1348–55.
9. Fine MJ, Smith MA, Carson CA. Prognosis and outcomes of patients with community acquired pneumonia: a meta-analysis. *JAMA.* 1996;275:134–41.

Hospital-Acquired Pneumonia

13

Cristina Vazquez Guillamet
and Marin H. Kollef

GENERAL PRINCIPLES

Definition

- **Hospital-acquired** pneumonia (HAP) is pneumonia occurring >48 hours after admission to the hospital.[1]
- **Ventilator-acquired pneumonia** (VAP) is pneumonia occurring >48 hours after intubation of the trachea and initiation of mechanical ventilation.[1]
- **Health care–associated pneumonia** (HCAP) is pneumonia in patients presenting from the community with the following risk factors:
  - **Risk factors** originally derived from risk factors for health care–associated bacteremia with a **resistant pathogen**[1–3]:
    - Hospitalization for ≥2 days in an acute care facility within 90 days of infection
    - Presentation from a nursing home or long-term care facility
    - Attending a hospital or hemodialysis clinic
    - Receiving IV antibiotic therapy, chemotherapy, or wound care within 30 days of infection
    - Family member with multidrug-resistant pathogen
  - Pneumonia-specific risk factors associated with drug-resistant pathogens[4]:
    - Recent hospitalization (within 90 days) for ≥2 days or recent antibiotic use
    - Immunosuppression
    - Nonambulatory status
    - Tube feeding
    - Use of gastric acid suppressive agents

Epidemiology

- HAP/VAP is the most clinically significant hospital-acquired infection and the leading cause of death from all nosocomial infections. The incidence of HAP is estimated to be between 5 and 10 cases per 1000 admissions and is substantially higher in mechanically ventilated patients, ~10–20% of patient mechanically ventilated for >48 hours.[1,5]
- The rise in hospital-associated infections due to antibiotic-resistant bacteria has resulted from the increasingly recognized administration of inadequate antimicrobial regimens.
- Inadequate initial antibiotic treatment of HCAP/HAP/VAP increases the risk of hospital mortality and may also predispose to the emergence of antibiotic-resistant bacteria.[6]
- Patients with HAP and HCAP have mortality rates of 15–20%, which is significantly worse than patients with community-acquired pneumonia (CAP).[7]
- VAP appears to be an independent determinant of mortality in critically ill patients requiring mechanical ventilation, and mortality rates range from 25–50% in different series.[8] However, patients who develop VAP have a higher severity of illness and have longer ICU and hospital stays. In an analysis of 4479 patients from a multicenter database, using a model taking into account severity of illness and other confounding factors, the 30-day attributable mortality for VAP was 4.4%.[9] A meta-analysis found the overall attributable mortality of VAP to be 13%.[10]

- More importantly, emerging clinical data suggest that the application of new management strategies for the prevention and treatment of VAP could result in improved patient outcomes.

Etiology

- Infectious organisms that commonly result in HCAP/HAP/VAP are generally different from those that are most commonly associated with CAP.
- HAP can be divided into early- or late-onset infections and more or less likely to be associated with drug-resistant organisms.
- **Early-onset HAP** occurs between days 2 and 4 of hospitalization.
  - These infections are **usually due to common community-acquired pathogens** such as *Streptococcus pneumoniae*, methicillin-sensitive *Staphylococcus aureus*, and *Haemophilus influenzae*.
  - Specific risk factors have been associated with certain pathogens. Aspiration has been associated with mouth anaerobes, gram-negative enteric bacilli, and *S. aureus*.
- **Late-onset HAP** occurs after 4 days of hospitalization. It is associated with **more virulent organisms** such as methicillin-resistant *S. aureus*, *Pseudomonas aeruginosa*, and *Acinetobacter* species.
- In certain areas of the world, antimicrobial resistance is common and increasing. In one large, international study of HAP and VAP, multidrug resistance rates for *Acinetobacter* species and *P. aeruginosa* were 82.0% and 42.8%, respectively. Extensively drug-resistance rates were 51.1% and 4.9%.[11]
- Patients with HCAP may be at risk for infection with the same organisms that are responsible for late-onset HAP.

Pathophysiology

- The pathogenesis of HAP and VAP is linked to two separate but related processes:
  - **Colonization of the aerodigestive tract** with pathogenic organisms
  - **Aspiration** of contaminated secretions
- The most common **sources of pathogens** are[1]
  - Microaspiration of oropharyngeal secretions
  - Aspiration of esophageal/gastric contents
  - Inhalation of infected aerosols
  - Hematogenous spread from distant infection
  - Exogenous penetration from the pleural space
  - Direct inoculation (e.g., resulting from intubation)
- Bacterial colonization of the oropharynx is universal and *S. pneumoniae,* various anaerobes, and, occasionally, *H. influenzae* are found in the oropharynx of normal subjects.
- However, colonization with gram-negative bacilli, notably virulent organisms such as *P. aeruginosa* and *Acinetobacter* species, is rare in healthy individuals.
- It is known that oropharyngeal and tracheal colonization with *P. aeruginosa* and enteric gram-negative bacilli increases with length of hospital stay and with severity of illness.
- **Aspiration** of oropharyngeal secretions is not uncommon, even in healthy individuals. In one study, ~45% of healthy subjects were shown to aspirate during sleep.[12] However, the rate of aspiration is higher in patients with impaired levels of consciousness and inability to adequately protect their airway.
- **Factors promoting aspiration** include
  - Abnormal swallowing for any reason
  - Reduced levels of consciousness
  - Blunted gag reflex
  - Delayed gastric emptying
  - Decreased gastrointestinal (GI) motility
  - Supine position

TABLE 13-1 RISK FACTORS FOR NOSOCOMIAL PNEUMONIA

Aspiration	Colonization of the Aerodigestive Tract
Witnessed aspiration	Chronic obstructive pulmonary disease
Supine positioning	Use of histamine type-2 antagonists
Coma	Tracheostomy
Enteral nutrition	Prior antibiotic exposure
Reintubation	Age >60 yrs
Tracheostomy	Acute respiratory distress syndrome
Acute respiratory distress syndrome	
Head trauma	
Intracranial pressure monitoring	

- Reflux and aspiration of nonsterile gastric contents (especially when antacids are used) is also a possible mechanism of pathogen entry into the lungs, although its role is generally less significant than that of oropharyngeal microbial colonization.[13,14]
- The stomach has been implicated, particularly in late-onset VAP, as a potential reservoir for the aspiration of contaminated secretions.[15]

Risk Factors

- A number of risk factors for the development of HCAP/HAP/VAP have been described.
- These risk factors generally promote either aspiration or colonization of the aerodigestive tract with pathogenic bacteria (see Table 13-1).[16]

Prevention

A number of pharmacologic and nonpharmacologic interventions have been studied as modalities to minimize HAP and VAP. The strategies with best clinical evidence include those in Table 13-2.[1,17–21]

TABLE 13-2 STRATEGIES FOR PREVENTING HOSPITAL-VENTILATOR-ASSOCIATED PNEUMONIA

Strategies
Effective hand washing by hospital personnel
Protective gowns and gloves
Avoiding large gastric volumes
Avoiding invasive ventilation when possible
Oral (nonnasal) intubation
Stress ulcer prophylaxis using non–pH-lowering agents in intubated patients
Interrupting sedation daily
Assessing readiness for extubation daily
Maintaining integrity of ventilator circuit
Maintaining proper endotracheal tube cuff pressure
Oral decontamination with chlorhexidine
Head elevation (30–45 degrees)
Avoiding unnecessary antibiotics
Adequate initial empiric antibiotic therapy

DIAGNOSIS

Clinical Presentation

- HAP or VAP is suspected when a patient develops[1]:
  - New or progressive pulmonary infiltrate
  - Fever
  - Leukocytosis
  - Purulent tracheobronchial secretions
- However, a number of noninfectious causes of fever and pulmonary infiltrates can also occur in these patients, making clinical criteria nonspecific for the diagnosis of HAP/VAP, and a number of studies have demonstrated the limitations of using clinical parameters alone for establishing the diagnosis of VAP.[22–24] Compared to autopsy findings **the accuracy of clinical criteria alone is only moderate at best** but the conclusion that clinical diagnosis of VAP is markedly inferior to other methods has not been universal.[25,26]
- Clinical criteria for the diagnosis of VAP have also been used in an effort to manage antibiotic therapy more effectively. One group of investigators used the **Clinical Pulmonary Infection Score** to limit the duration of antibiotic therapy for patients at low risk for VAP.[25] The Clinical Pulmonary Infection Score is a simple scoring system evaluating temperature, blood leukocyte count, tracheal secretions, oxygenation, and pulmonary infiltrates. Such a strategy may allow improved use of empiric antibiotics for patients with suspected VAP; however, a subsequent study failed to confirm the diagnostic accuracy of this approach.[27]
- Noninfectious causes of fever and pulmonary infiltrates that can mimic HAP/VAP include chemical aspiration without infection, atelectasis, pulmonary embolism, acute respiratory distress syndrome (ARDS), pulmonary hemorrhage, lung contusion, infiltrative tumor, radiation pneumonitis, and drug or hypersensitivity reactions.

Diagnostic Testing

- The limitations and inaccuracies in clinical decision-making have been the motivation for using other techniques to diagnose VAP.
- These techniques include a variety of methods for sampling material from the airways and alveoli, including bronchoscopic and nonbronchoscopic techniques. Cultures should be obtained in a timely manner, but empiric therapy should not be withheld in severely ill patients.
- **Bronchoscopic sampling of the lower airways**, using either a protected specimen brush or bronchoalveolar lavage, is currently accepted as the most accurate method of diagnosing VAP, short of direct tissue examination.[28–31]
  - Quantitative or semiquantitative cultures are usually performed on the bronchoscopic specimens, with the diagnosis of VAP being made when some appropriate threshold is exceeded.
  - From a practical standpoint, quantitative cultures between 100 and 1000 colony-forming units (cfu)/mL for **protected brush specimens** and between 1000 and 10,000 cfu/mL for **bronchoalveolar lavage specimens** should probably be considered positive.
  - It is important to note that few studies have shown that lower airway specimens obtained with bronchoscopic sampling meaningfully influence patient outcomes.
- **Tracheal aspirates** can be obtained with ease from endotracheal tubes (ETT), making them an attractive alternative diagnostic technique for patients with suspected VAP.
  - Tracheal aspirates are **nonspecific for establishing the diagnosis of VAP** because tracheobronchial bacterial colonization is common in critically ill patients as a consequence of biofilm formation on the surface of ETT.[32]
  - As a result, tracheal aspirates have been of limited utility because of the increased accuracy of specimens obtained by bronchoscopy.
  - Nevertheless, tracheal aspirate specimens have reasonable overall sensitivity for the identification of pathogens associated with VAP.

TREATMENT

Medications

- There are two overriding principles that make up the strategy of antibiotic treatment of HAP.
    - The first is to **provide an adequate initial antimicrobial regimen** that is likely to be active against the pathogen(s) causing infection.
    - The second is to **limit the unnecessary use of antibiotics**.
- **Deescalation** is a strategy that attempts to unify these two principles into a single strategy that optimizes patient outcomes while minimizing the emergence of antibiotic resistance.[1]
- The first goal of antibiotic deescalation requires the **administration of an adequate empiric regimen** to patients with suspected HAP.
    - Decisions regarding antibiotic selection often occur in the absence of identified pathogens. It is, therefore, imperative that clinicians be aware of both the microorganisms likely to be associated with infection and adequate antimicrobial options in their patient population.
    - The most common pathogens associated with the administration of **inadequate** antimicrobial treatment in patients with HAP include potentially antibiotic-resistant **gram-negative bacteria** (*P. aeruginosa, Acinetobacter* species, *Klebsiella pneumoniae,* and *Enterobacter* species) and ***S. aureus,*** especially strains with methicillin resistance.[1]
    - It is also important to recognize that the predominant pathogens associated with hospital-associated infections may **vary between hospitals** as well as **between specialized units within individual hospitals.** Therefore, clinicians should be aware of the prevailing bacterial pathogens in their hospitals and their associated antimicrobial susceptibilities.
    - This awareness should help in the selection of empiric antibiotic regimens that are less likely to provide inadequate treatment for hospital-associated infections.
    - Recommended therapies are summarized in Table 13-3.[1]
- The second goal of antibiotic deescalation is to avoid the **unnecessary administration of antibiotics.**
    - Physicians practicing in the hospital setting are frequently faced with the dilemma of caring for acutely ill patients with suspected nosocomial infection owing to the presence of nonspecific clinical findings (fever, leukocytosis, hemodynamic instability).
    - Failure to provide treatment with an adequate initial antimicrobial regimen may result in greater morbidity, whereas unnecessary antibiotic treatment can lead to colonization or infection with antibiotic-resistant pathogens. Original criteria to identify patients at risk for HCAP caused by resistant pathogens proved to be too inclusive thus leading to antibiotic overuse and worse outcomes. Recently developed pneumonia-specific risk factors may allow for a more accurate stratification.[33,34]
- The third goal of antibiotic deescalation is **tailoring therapy based on the patient's culture results.**
    - Tailoring therapy will help to avoid unnecessary broad-spectrum antibiotic usage and is a strategy to help decrease the incidence of antibiotic-resistant organisms.
    - In those patients with negative culture results or that lack drug-resistant organisms, it is generally felt to be desirable and safe to deescalate therapy.[35,36]
- **Duration of therapy**
    - Despite the thoroughness of many guidelines, durations of therapy remain an imprecise science.
    - Treatment for 7–10 days has been advocated for treatment of *S. aureus* or *H. influenzae* infection.
    - Longer courses of antibiotics have been proposed for gram-negative necrotizing pneumonias or with isolation of *Pseudomonas* spp.

TABLE 13-3 THERAPY FOR HAP

Early-onset HAP (or no specific risk factors for MDR organisms[a])
Organisms:
Enteric gram-negatives, including *Enterobacter* spp., *Escherichia coli*, *Klebsiella* spp., *Proteus* spp., *Serratia marcescens*; also *Streptococcus pneumoniae*, *Haemophilus influenzae*, and methicillin-sensitive *Staphylococcus aureus*
Therapy:
Nonantipseudomonal third-generation cephalosporin (e.g., ceftriaxone) or β-lactam/β-lactamase inhibitor combination (e.g., ampicillin/sulbactam) or fluoroquinolone (e.g., levofloxacin or moxifloxacin)
For penicillin-allergic patients, fluoroquinolone or clindamycin plus aztreonam[b]
Late-onset HAP (or with risk factors for MDR[a])
Organisms:
Any of the above organisms plus *Pseudomonas aeruginosa*, *Acinetobacter baumannii*, methicillin-resistant *S. aureus*
Therapy:
Antipseudomonal β-lactam (e.g., cefepime, ceftazidime, meropenem, piperacillin/tazobactam) plus antipseudomonal fluoroquinolone (e.g., levofloxacin, or moxifloxacin) or aminoglycoside ± vancomycin or linezolid
For *Acinetobacter baumannii* and other extensively resistant organisms (e.g., *P. aeruginosa* and *Klebsiella* spp.) consider inhaled or IV colistin ± minocycline in addition to a carbapenem

[a]See text for MDR organism risk factors.

[b]Many patients with penicillin allergy can safely be given a cephalosporin or carbapenem. Consider allergy consultation in such patients.

HAP, hospital-acquired pneumonia; MDR multidrug resistant.

- The results of a large randomized trial comparing 8 days of adequate antibiotic therapy for VAP to 15 days of treatment showed similar efficacy. However, the longer course of antibiotic therapy was associated with statistically greater emergence of multidrug-resistant bacteria.[37]
- In a study of patients with serious infections in the intensive care unit, the antibiotic course for those with VAP was safely shortened to 7.3 days using a procalcitonin-based discontinuation protocol.[38] However, procalcitonin assays are not currently in widespread clinical use.

REFERENCES

1. American Thoracic Society, Infectious Diseases Society of America. Guidelines for the management of adults with hospital-acquired, ventilator-associated, and healthcare-associated pneumonia. *Am J Resp Crit Care Med.* 2005;171:388–416.
2. Friedman ND, Kaye KS, Stout JE, et al. Health care–associated bloodstream infections in adults: a reason to change the accepted definition of community-acquired infections. *Ann Intern Med.* 2002; 137:791–7.
3. Kollef MH, Morrow LE, Baughman RP, et al. Health care—associated pneumonia (HCAP): a critical appraisal to improve identification, management, and outcomes—proceedings of the HCAP Summit. *Clin Infect Dis.* 2008;46:S296–334.

4. Shindo Y, Ito R, Kobayashi D, et al. Risk factors for drug-resistant pathogens in community-acquired and healthcare-associated pneumonia. *Am J Respir Crit Care Med.* 2013;188:985–95.
5. Peleg AY, Hooper DC. Hospital-acquired infections due to gram-negative bacteria. *N Engl J Med.* 2010;362:1804–13.
6. Kollef MH, Sherman G, Ward S, et al. Inadequate antimicrobial treatment of infections. A risk factor for hospital mortality among critically ill patients. *Chest.* 1999;115:462–74.
7. Kollef MH, Shorr A, Tabak YP, et al. Epidemiology and outcomes of health care-associated pneumonia: results from a large US database of culture-positive pneumonia. *Chest.* 2005;128:3854–62.
8. Chastre J, Fagon JY. Ventilator-associated pneumonia. *Am J Respir Crit Care Med.* 2002;165:867–903.
9. Bekaert M, Timsit JH, Vansteelandt S, et al. Attributable mortality of ventilator-associated pneumonia: a reappraisal using casual analysis. *Am J Respir Crit Care Med.* 2011;184:1133–9.
10. Melsen WG, Rovers MM, Groenwold RH, et al. Attributable mortality of ventilator-associated pneumonia: a meta-analysis of individual patient data from randomised prevention studies. *Lancet Infect Dis.* 2013;13:665–71.
11. Chung DR, Song JH, Kim SH, et al. High prevalence of multi-drug resistant non-fermenters in hospital-acquired pneumonia in Asia. *Am J Respir Crit Care Med.* 2011;184:1409–17.
12. Huxley EJ, Viroslav J, Gray WR, et al. Pharyngeal aspiration in normal adults and patients with depressed consciousness. *Am J Med.* 1978;64:564–8.
13. du Moulin GC, Paterson DG, Hedley-Whyte J, et al. Aspiration of gastric bacteria in antacid-treated patients: a frequent cause of postoperative colonization of the airway. *Lancet.* 1982;1: 242–5.
14. Prod'hom G, Leuenberger P, Koerfer J, et al. Nosocomial pneumonia in mechanically ventilated patients receiving antacid, ranitidine, or sucralfate as prophylaxis for stress ulcer. A randomized controlled trial. *Ann Intern Med.* 1994;120:653–62.
15. Atherton ST, White DJ. Stomach as a source of bacteria colonizing respiratory tract artificial ventilation. *Lancet.* 1978;2:968–9.
16. Cook DJ, Kollef MH. Risk factors for ICU-acquired pneumonia. *JAMA.* 1998;279:1605–6.
17. Kollef MH. Epidemiology and risk factors for nosocomial pneumonia. Emphasis on prevention. *Clin Chest Med.* 1999;20:653–70.
18. Bouadma L, Mourvillier B, Deiler V, et al. A multifaceted program to prevent ventilator-associated pneumonia: impact on compliance with preventive measures. *Crit Care Med.* 2010;38:789–96.
19. Berenholtz SM, Pham JC, Thompson DA, et al. Collaborative cohort study of an intervention to reduce ventilator-associated pneumonia in the intensive care unit. *Infect Control Hosp Epidemiol.* 2011;32:305–14.
20. Kollef MH. Prevention of ventilator-associated pneumonia or ventilator-associated complications: a worthy, yet challenging, goal. *Crit Care Med.* 2012;40:271–7.
21. Klompas M, Branson R, Eichenwald EC, et al. Strategies to prevent ventilator-associated pneumonia in acute care hospitals: 2014 update. *Infect Control Hosp Epidemiol.* 2014;35:915–36.
22. Andrews CP, Coalson JJ, Smith JD, et al. Diagnosis of nosocomial bacterial pneumonia in acute, diffuse lung injury. *Chest.* 1981;80:254–8.
23. Fagon JY, Chastre J, Hance AJ, et al. Evaluation of clinical judgment in the identification and treatment of nosocomial pneumonia in ventilated patients. *Chest.* 1993;103:547–53.
24. Kirtland SH, Corley DE, Winterbauer RH, et al. The diagnosis of ventilator pneumonia: a comparison of histologic, microbiologic, and clinical criteria. *Chest.* 1997;112:445–57.
25. Fàbregas N, Ewig S, Torres A, et al. Clinical diagnosis of ventilator associated pneumonia revisited: comparative validation using immediate post-mortem lung biopsies. *Thorax.* 1999;54:867–73.
26. Tejerina E, Esteban A, Fernández-Segoviano P, et al. Accuracy of clinical definitions of ventilator-associated pneumonia: comparison with autopsy findings. *J Crit Care.* 2010;25:62–8.
27. Fartoukh M, Maitre B, Honore S, et al. Diagnosing pneumonia during mechanical ventilation: the clinical pulmonary infection score revisited. *Am J Respir Crit Care Med.* 2003;168:173–9.
28. Fagon JY, Chastre J, Hance AJ, et al. Detection of nosocomial lung infection in ventilated patients: use of a protected specimen brush and quantitative culture techniques in 147 patients. *Am Rev Respir Dis.* 1988;138:110–6.
29. Niederman MS, Torres A, Summer W. Invasive diagnostic testing is not needed routinely to manage suspected ventilator-associated pneumonia. *Am J Respir Crit Care Med.* 1994;150:565–9.
30. Heyland DK, Cook DJ, Marshall J, et al. The clinical utility of invasive diagnostic techniques in the setting of ventilator-associated pneumonia. *Chest.* 1999;115:1076–84.
31. Fagon JY, Chastre J, Wolff M, et al. Invasive and noninvasive strategies for management of suspected ventilator-associated pneumonia. A randomized trial. *Ann Intern Med.* 2000;132:621–30.

32. Adair CG, Gorman SP, Feron BM, et al. Implications of endotracheal tube biofilm for ventilator-associated pneumonia. *Intensive Care Med.* 1999;25:1072–6.
33. Shorr AF, Zilberberg MD, Micek ST, et al. Prediction of infection due to antibiotic-resistant bacteria by select risk factors for health care-associated pneumonia. *Arch Intern Med.* 2008;168:2205–10.
34. Kollef MH. Health care-associated pneumonia: perception versus reality. *Clin Infect Dis.* 2009; 49:1875–7.
35. Niederman MS, Soulountsi V. De-escalation therapy: is it valuable for the management of ventilator-associated pneumonia? *Clin Chest Med.* 2011;32:517–34.
36. Nair GB, Niederman MS. Ventilator-associated pneumonia: present understanding and ongoing debates. *Intensive Care Med.* 2015;41:34–48.
37. Chastre J, Wolff M, Fagon JY, et al. Comparison of 8 vs 15 days of antibiotic therapy for ventilator-associated pneumonia in adults: a randomized trial. *JAMA.* 2003;290:2588–98.
38. Bouadma L, Luyt CE, Tubach F, et al. Use of procalcitonin to reduce patient's exposure to antibiotics in intensive care units (PRORATA trial): a multicenter randomized controlled trial. *Lancet.* 2010;375:463–74.

Tuberculosis

14

Jonathan Baghdadi and
Carlos C. Daughaday

GENERAL PRINCIPLES

Classification

- Active infection can occur with initial exposure to *Mycobacterium tuberculosis* (MTB) or following reactivation of latent disease.
- Latent infection occurs when the body has suppressed the primary infection but failed to eradicate the mycobacteria, which find an intracellular reservoir within macrophages.

Epidemiology

- Approximately one-third of the world's population is estimated to carry MTB.[1] Most infections are latent. According to the World Health Organization (WHO), highest incidence regions (sub-Saharan Africa, India, Southeast Asia, and Micronesia) have rates from 100/100,000 to over 500/100,000. Worldwide in 2014 there were 9.6 million new cases of TB and 1.5 million TB deaths. HIV patients accounted for 13% of new cases and 27% of deaths.[2]
- In the United States, 9421 cases (2.96 per 100,000 incidence rate) were reported to the Centers for Disease Control and Prevention (CDC) in 2014.[1] Two-thirds of these cases occurred in non–US-born individuals.
- Incidence temporarily surged in the early 1990s with the spread of HIV/AIDS and increased immigration from endemic areas but has since been decreasing.[3]
- Globally, it is estimated that 5% of TB cases in 2014 (about 480,000 cases) were caused by multidrug-resistant (MDR) organisms.[4]
- In 2013, 1.3% of US cases were MDR-TB.[5]

Pathophysiology

- Infection is transmitted by deposition of small airborne particles (<5 microns in diameter) containing MTB in an alveolus. Approximately 5% of exposed patients develop primary infection, which is usually self-limited.
  - Local inflammation forms caseating granulomas with lymphadenopathy.
  - In immunocompromised hosts, hematogenous spread can cause diffuse extrapulmonary disease.
- In a small group of patients, rupture of a subpleural caseous focus causes pleuritis.
  - Tuberculous proteins trigger a delayed hypersensitivity reaction.
  - Pleural fluid cultures are commonly negative.
  - An untreated, isolated tuberculous effusion typically resolves spontaneously but patients are at higher risk for developing reactivation TB within the next 2 years.
- **Following primary infection, 5–10% of immunocompetent individuals experience reactivation of disease.** Immunocompromised state, drug use, and medical comorbidities increase risk of reactivation.[6]

Risk Factors

- **The most important risk factor is exposure** to MTB. Exposure risks include close contacts of those with active infection, foreign-born persons from endemic areas, residents of high-risk congregate settings (such as correctional facilities and homeless shelters), healthcare workers caring for high-risk patients, and illicit drug abusers.[6]
- Patients with HIV infection, other immunocompromised states (including tumor necrosis factor-α inhibitor use, glucocorticoid use, and posttransplant status), chronic medical illnesses (e.g., diabetes mellitus, silicosis, and chronic kidney disease requiring dialysis), alcoholism, malnutrition, and findings on CXR to suggest previously cleared disease (e.g., granulomas, apical fibronodular changes) are at increased risk for developing active disease once exposed.[7,8]
- A 2007 metaanalysis suggested that exposure to tobacco smoke is also a modest risk factor.[9]

Prevention

- Inpatients with suspected pulmonary TB should be placed in negative-pressure isolation until ruled out for disease.
- Patients with exclusively extrapulmonary disease are not contagious. These patients do not need to be placed on airborne precautions unless immunocompromised, in which case they should likewise be ruled out for concurrent active pulmonary TB.

DIAGNOSIS

Clinical Presentation

- Primary infection typically takes the form of a self-limited respiratory illness.
  - The most common symptoms are chest pain and subacute, low-grade fever.
  - Pleuritic pain may represent a tuberculous effusion.
- Reactivation can have a variable and unimpressive presentation.
  - The most common history involves productive cough, fatigue, and weight loss for at least 2–3 months.
  - Fever, night sweats, dyspnea, chest pain, and hemoptysis are classic but are each present in less than one-third of patients.
- Chest findings are variable and depend on the nature of disease.
  - Alveolar infiltrates may manifest as rales.
  - Tubular breath sounds may be audible over areas of complete consolidation.
  - Dullness to percussion may indicate pleural thickening or effusion.
  - Breath sounds may be soft or hollow (amphoric) locally over cavities.
- Examination of the extremities may reveal digital clubbing.

Differential Diagnosis

- TB should be suspected in any individual presenting with cough for >2 weeks and (a) classic symptoms, (b) risk factors for exposure, or (c) immunocompromise.
- High-risk patients with abnormalities on imaging should provide sputum for evaluation even when asymptomatic.
- Consider TB in patients who fail treatment for community-acquired pneumonia (CAP).
- Other relatively common differential diagnostic items for pulmonary TB include fungal infections (see Chapter 15), nontuberculous mycobacterial infections (e.g., *M. avium* complex, *M. kansasii*), lung abscess/septic emboli, sarcoidosis, and cancer.

Diagnostic Testing

Tuberculin Skin Test

- **The tuberculin skin test** (TST) is used to diagnose latent TB infection (LTBI).
- Patients at risk of exposure and those at risk for developing TB if exposed should be tested. **Individuals without these risk factors should not be routinely tested** because a positive TST is less likely to represent true LTBI. The decision to test implies a de facto decision to treat if the test is positive.
- TST involves intradermal injection of a standardized dose of 5 tuberculin units purified protein derivative. The injected material forms a 5–10-mm wheal immediately.
- The reaction to the TB proteins should be measured 48–72 hours later.
- **The area of induration, not erythema, determines a positive or negative test.**
- Interpretation of the skin test is stratified by level of risk (Table 14-1).[10,11] Positive tests are defined as:

TABLE 14-1 TUBERCULIN SKIN TEST INTERPRETATION

Induration (mm)	Risk Factors for TB Infection
≥5	HIV infection Recent close contacts of active TB infection CXR consistent with prior TB Patients status post organ transplantation Other immunocompromised patients (including those on TNF-α antagonists or those on ≥15 mg/d prednisone or equivalent)
≥10	Children <5 yrs old Infants, children, and adolescents exposed to adult at high risk Persons born in endemic areas arrived in the United States ≤5 yrs ago Injection drug users Patients with chronic medical illness known to increase the risk of reactivation (i.e., silicosis, chronic kidney disease requiring dialysis, diabetes mellitus, leukemia, lymphoma, head and neck cancer, lung cancer, ≥10% below IBW, gastrectomy, or jejunoileal bypass) Residents and employees of high-risk congregate settings (i.e., hospitals, long-term care facilities, residential facilities for those with HIV/AIDS, homeless shelters, and correctional facilities) Mycobacteriology laboratory personnel
≥15	All others tested, presumably those with no known risk factors (who perhaps should not have been tested; the CDC does not recommend testing for latent TB in those without known risk factors)

TB, tuberculosis; TNF, tumor necrosis factor; IBW, ideal body weight; CDC, Centers for Disease Control and Prevention.

Adapted from Centers for Disease Control and Prevention; National Center for HIV/AIDS, Viral Hepatitis, STD, and TB Prevention; Division of Tuberculosis Elimination. Latent tuberculosis infection: a guide for primary health care providers. Atlanta: Centers for Disease Control and Prevention, 2013. Available at http://www.cdc.gov/tb/publications/ltbi/default.htm.

  - An area of induration with diameter ≥5 mm in those at highest risk of developing active infection—persons with HIV, immunocompromise, close contact with active TB, or radiographic findings consistent with prior TB.
  - A reaction ≥10 mm in those at risk of exposure—persons born in endemic areas, injection drug users, healthcare workers, and residents of congregate settings—and those with chronic medical conditions that place them at intermediate risk of progression to active disease, such as diabetes mellitus, renal failure, or silicosis.
  - A reaction ≥15 mm for persons without risk factors. In general, the CDC does not recommend screening such individuals, however, administrative constraints sometimes required such testing.
- **A positive TST should be followed by CXR.** Symptoms or radiographic findings suggestive of active TB should prompt attempts to isolate the organism as described above. If cultures and Gram stain of sputum samples are negative, LTBI is present.
- A false-positive TST can occur when the test is repeated within 1 month of a previous TST in the absence of a new exposure. This so-called **booster reaction** is due to immunologic stimulation by the first test in those with remote exposure. It should not be interpreted as a new conversion. Two-step testing is recommended only in persons who will be tested periodically, typically healthcare workers at the time of hiring. If either the first or second test (1–3 weeks later) is positive the individual is considered previously infected (i.e., prior to the current employment) and treated appropriately for latent TB.[11]
- Patients with history of **bacille Calmette–Guérin (BCG)** vaccination may have a false-positive TST. However, due to the variability of the host response to BCG and the inconsistency of its protection against MTB, these patients should be treated as if the test were positive.[11]
- False-positive TST may occur with nontuberculous mycobacteria.
- **An increase in size of tuberculin reaction >10 mm in the setting of new or ongoing exposure represents conversion.**
- Falsely negative TSTs may occur in adults with cutaneous anergy in immunocompromised patients or overwhelming TB infection. As many as a quarter of patients with active TB may have a negative TST.

Laboratories

- In cases of pulmonary parenchymal TB, sputum analysis by **acid-fast bacillus stain** (AFB) **and mycobacterial cultures** is paramount. Cultures are necessary to determine drug susceptibility, to differentiate MTB from nontuberculous mycobacteria, and because smears alone miss up to 50% of positive samples.[8]
  - With newer laboratory techniques using rapid radiometric culture assays, culture results may finalize within 1–2 weeks.
  - If sputum cannot be obtained or analysis is nondiagnostic, bronchoscopy with bronchoalveolar lavage (BAL), transbronchial lung biopsies, and brushings may facilitate diagnosis either of TB or an alternative process.
  - Caseating granulomas on histopathology are strongly suggestive of TB while cultures are pending.
- The **interferon-γ release assay** (IGRA) is an alternative test for LTBI that measures the in vitro release of interferon-γ by leukocytes in response to various MTB proteins.
  - Two products are currently U.S. Food and Drug Administration (FDA) approved, QuantiFERON-TB Gold In-Tube (QFT-GIT, Qiagen) and T-SPOT (Oxford Diagnostic Laboratories).[12,13]
  - As with the TST, only those who would benefit from the treatment of latent infection should be tested. And also as with the TST, IGRA cannot distinguish latent from active MTB infection.

- Based on a single blood sample, results are typically available within 24 hours. Shorter turn-around time may make IGRA preferable in patients for whom follow-up is uncertain.
- TST can only be positive or negative, while **IGRA results may be indeterminate**. At present, cut points are not based on pretest risk as they are with the TST.
- The sensitivity of the QFT-GIT is about 80% and the T-SPOT 88% compared with 70% for the TST. The estimated specificity is 97–99%.[13,14] Sensitivity is likely less in HIV-infected persons.
- A major advantage of the IGRA is that prior history of **BCG vaccination will not produce a false-positive result**. The genome for BCG does not contain coding for the stimulating proteins.[13]
- Infection with *M. marinum* or *M. kansasii* can result in a positive IGRA but most other nontuberculous mycobacteria do not.[13,15]
- As IGRA is an in vitro test there is no possibility of a booster phenomenon.

- **Nucleic acid amplification** (NAA) may facilitate rapid diagnosis of active TB but does not replace AFB smear and culture.[16]
  - Specificity is poor when applied to AFB smear-negative specimens but high with smear-positives.
  - NAA can indicate a high likelihood of MTB in conjunction with positive smears but can neither diagnose nor exclude TB in the absence of smear data.
  - NAA may detect genetic material from either living or dead organisms, thus cannot be used to track the efficacy of treatment.
  - Several next-generation NAA tests are in development.[8]

Imaging

- **A positive TST should be followed by CXR.**
- CT scanning is more sensitive than CXR for the detection and characterization of the radiographic findings of TB and improves diagnostic accuracy.[17]
- In **primary infection**, hilar adenopathy is said to be the most consistent finding but airspace consolidation may also be seen. Pleural effusion is an occasional manifestation of primary TB. Miliary TB occurs in 2–6% of cases. [17]
- **Reactivation** TB presents radiographically most commonly as focal or patchy heterogeneous consolidation in the apical and posterior segments of the upper lobes and the superior segments of the lower lobes. Ill-defined nodules and linear opacities are also fairly common. Cavitation is seen in a significant minority of patients. Lymphadenopathy is not very common (5–10%) and pleural effusion can be seen in 15–20% of cases. A few patients present with mass-like lesions, a tuberculoma.[17]
- The ability to distinguish primary infection from reactivation by radiographic appearance has been seriously questioned.[18]
- Atypical radiographic presentations are more common in patients with impaired immunity including lower lung disease, adenopathy, and effusions.[18]
- In HIV-infected patients with CD4 ≤200/μL more mediastinal and hilar lymphadenopathy and less cavitation may be seen. Extrapulmonary involvement is also more common.[17]
- In latent or cleared disease, healed parenchymal lesions appear radiographically as calcified nodules (Ghon lesions) and may remain associated with ipsilateral hilar adenopathy (Ranke complex).

TREATMENT

- A joint effort on the part of clinicians and public health workers is required to treat active infection and prevent spread of disease.
- **Cases of TB should be reported to local public health authorities** to ensure adequate therapy of the individual, to evaluate close contacts, and to track potential outbreaks.

TABLE 14-2 REGIMENS FOR THE TREATMENT OF LATENT TUBERCULOSIS INFECTION

Regimen	Duration (mo)	Daily Oral Dose (max dose)	Twice Weekly Dose (max dose)[a]	Weekly Dose (max dose)[a]	Comments
INH	9	10–15 mg/kg (300 mg)	20–30 mg/kg (900 mg)		Preferred regimen in most adults Recommended regimen for children Recommended regimen for pregnant women
INH	6	10–15 mg/kg (300 mg)	20–30 mg/kg (900 mg)		Acceptable for HIV-negative adults **Not** recommended for HIV-positive persons, children, or those with fibrotic changes on CXR Recommended regimen for pregnant women
RIF[b]	4	10–20 mg/kg (600 mg)			For persons intolerant to INH and contacts of patients with TB resistant to INH but sensitive to RIF
INH, RPT[c]	3			INH: 15 mg/kg (900 mg) RFP: dosing weight dependent, 900 mg for >50 kg	**Not** recommended for children <2 yrs, HIV-infected persons on antiretroviral therapy, or pregnant women[22]
RIF, PZA	2	RIF: 10 mg/kg (600 mg) PZA: 15–20 mg/kg (2 g)	RIF: 10 mg/kg (600 mg) PZA: 50 mg/kg (4 g)		**Not** generally recommended due to the risk of severe liver injury[23]

[a]Intended only for directly observed therapy.

[b]Multiple drug interactions with HIV medications; consult a reputable prescribing resource.

[c]Drug interactions between RPT and HIV medications have not been sufficiently studied; multiple other drug interactions; RPT stains secretions.

INH, isoniazid; RPT, rifapentine; RIF, rifampin.

Adapted from Centers for Disease Control and Prevention (CDC); American Thoracic Society. Targeted tuberculin testing and treatment of latent tuberculosis infection. *MMWR Recomm Rep.* 2000;49:1–51.

- Several general principles guide treatment:
  - Duration of therapy is prolonged because MTB is a slow-growing organism.
  - Multiple agents reduce the development of drug resistance.
  - Culture and susceptibility data are followed to ensure drug activity.
  - To improve adherence, the shortest sufficient course of therapy is necessary.
  - **Directly observed therapy** (DOT) **is the preferred method of treatment for most patients** and offers the highest chance of successful completion of therapy. While DOT decreases dropout from treatment, it may not improve microbiologic failure, development of resistance, or relapse rate.[19,20]

Medications

Latent Infection

Before initiating therapy for LTBI, **careful evaluation to rule out active TB is necessary.** Table 14-2 details multiple accepted treatment regimens.[21,22,23]

First-Line Treatment for Active TB

- First-line antituberculous drugs are listed in Table 14-3.[24] These agents are proven to be effective and are relatively well tolerated.
- Combination therapy reduces the risk of drug resistance and limits shedding of the organism in the community by rapidly decreasing the burden of MTB in the host.
- The success rate for treatment is between 90% and 95%.[19]
- With LTBI, the burden of organisms is small enough to allow monotherapy with isoniazid (INH).

TABLE 14-3 FIRST-LINE ANTITUBERCULOSIS AGENTS

Drug	Daily (max dose)	Twice Weekly (max dose)	Thrice Weekly (max dose)	Adverse Reactions	Monitor
EMB	15–25 mg/kg (1 g)	50 mg/kg	25–30 mg/kg	Optic neuritis, rash	Visual acuity, color vision
INH	5 mg/kg (300 mg)	15 mg/kg (900 mg)	15 mg/kg (900 mg)	Rash, hepatitis, neuropathy, drug interactions	LFTs
PZA	15–30 mg/kg (2 g)	50–70 mg/kg (4 g)	50–70 mg/kg (3 g)	Rash, hepatitis, hyperuricemia	Uric acid, LFTs
RFB	5 mg/kg (300 mg)	5 mg/kg (300 mg)	Unknown	Rash, hepatitis, thrombocytopenia, uveitis	CBC, LFTs
RIF	10 mg/kg (600 mg)	10 mg/kg (600 mg)	10 mg/kg (600 mg)	Rash, hepatitis, drug interactions	CBC, LFTs

INH, isoniazid; RIF, rifampin; RFB, rifabutin; PZA, pyrazinamide; EMB, ethambutol; LFTs, liver function tests.

Adapted from American Thoracic Society; Centers for Disease Control and Prevention; Infectious Diseases Society of America. Treatment of tuberculosis. *MMWR Recomm Rep.* 2003;52:1–77.

TABLE 14-4 TREATMENT REGIMENS FOR ACTIVE TUBERCULOSIS

	Minimum Duration (wks)	Induction	Interval and Duration	Maintenance	Interval and Duration
1	26	INH, RIF, PZA, EMB	qday × 8 wks, or 5 d/wk[a] × 8 wks	INH, RIF	qday × 18 wks[b], or 5 d/wk[a] × 18 wks[b], or Twice weekly for 18 wks[b,c], or Once weekly for 18 wks[d,e]
2	26	INH, RIF, PZA, EMB	qday × 2 wks then twice weekly × 6 wks, or 5 d/wk[a] × 2 wks then twice weekly × 6 wks	INH, RIF	Twice weekly × 18 wks[b,c]Once weekly × 18 wks[d,e]
3	26	INH, RIF, PZA, EMB	Thrice weekly × 8 wks	INH, RIF	Thrice weekly × 18 wks[b]
4	39	INH, RIF, EMB	qday × 8 wks, or 5 d/wk[a] × 8 wks	INH, RIF	qday × 31 wks, or 5 d/wk[a] × 31 wks, or Twice weekly × 31 wks

[a]Intended for directly observed therapy only.

[b]Extend maintenance phase of treatment to 31 weeks in patients with cavitation on the initial CXR and positive cultures at the end of the 8-week induction phase.

[c]Not recommended for HIV-positive patients with CD4 <100/μL.

[d]Substitute rifapentine for rifampin due to its longer half-life.

[e]To be used only in HIV-negative patients with negative smears at the end of the 8-week induction phase and who do not have cavitation on the initial CXR; if such patients have a positive sputum culture at the end of the 8-week induction phase then the maintenance phase should continue for 31 weeks.

TB, tuberculosis; INH, isoniazid; RIF, rifampin; PZA, pyrazinamide; EMB, ethambutol.

Adapted from American Thoracic Society; Centers for Disease Control and Prevention; Infectious Diseases Society of America. Treatment of tuberculosis. *MMWR Recomm Rep.* 2003;52:1–77.

- INH targets extracellular organisms growing rapidly along cavity walls and in a liquid necrotic medium.
- Rifampin's (RIF) rapid onset of action allows it to kill slower-growing extracellular organisms found in caseous material during intermittent spurts of growth.
- Pyrazinamide (PZA) works best in an acid pH, allowing it to target slowly growing organisms within macrophages.
- No drug targets dormant organisms until they begin to grow.
- **Treatment regimens consist of a 2-month initial phase followed by a 4–7-month continuation phase.**
- Response to therapy is monitored with monthly sputum samples until cultures have cleared.
- The duration and timing of therapy depends on the patient's HIV status and CD4 count, organism susceptibility, and response to therapy on serial sputum samples.
- Table 14-4 shows different regimens that may be used depending on patient characteristics.[24]
  - The initial phase consists of INH, RIF, PZA, and ethambutol (EMB) for 2 months.
    - In HIV-negative patients, EMB can be discontinued if culture results show MTB that is susceptible to the other three agents.
    - Patients taking INH should receive vitamin B6 supplementation (25–50 mg daily) to prevent development of neuropathy.
  - The continuation phase consists of dual therapy with INH and RIF.
    - Except in cases of severe immunocompromise, intermittent dosing is appropriate.
    - Higher doses of INH, PZA, and EMB are required if these medications are not taken daily (see Table 14-3).[24]
    - The dose of RIF remains unchanged regardless of timing.
  - In HIV-positive patients, rifabutin is an alternative to rifampin that is less likely to interact with antiretroviral agents.

Second-Line Treatment for Active TB

Second-line agents, listed in Table 14-5, are less effective, more toxic, or less characterized.[24–29] The use of these agents is largely dependent on susceptibility.

SPECIAL CONSIDERATIONS

HIV Coinfection

- TB is an AIDS-defining diagnosis and, therefore, a clear indication to start antiretroviral therapy (ART) regardless of CD4 count.
- Although some patients may experience worsening of their TB symptoms as part of the immune reconstitution inflammatory syndrome (IRIS), prompt initiation of antiretrovirals is associated with improved treatment outcomes.[30] This is particularly true in those with CD4 <50/μL; initiation of ART after 2 weeks of anti-TB therapy improves survival.[31]
- HIV patients are as likely to respond to anti-TB therapy as the general population.
- Total duration of treatment is the same but more frequent medication dosing is typical. Once-weekly dosing schedules should not be used.
- Choice of anti-TB regimen may be complicated by drug interactions with antiretroviral therapies. Infectious disease consultation is generally warranted in such patients.
  - RIF decreases blood levels of protease inhibitors and nevirapine.
  - Rifabutin is a more expensive alternative for patients on these antiretrovirals.[24]
  - RIF is preferable for concurrent use with efavirenz and has no interactions with nucleoside reverse-transcriptase inhibitors.

TABLE 14-5 SECOND-LINE ANTITUBERCULOSIS AGENTS

Drug	Oral Dose (max dose)	Adverse Reactions	Monitor	Comments
Amikacin	IV/IM: 15 mg/kg/d (1 g)	Ototoxicity, renal dysfunction, dizziness	Hearing tests, renal function	Dose reduction after response, for those ≥60 reduce dose to 10 mg/kg/d, dose adjustment also required for those with significant renal dysfunction
Bedaquiline[25]	400 mg/d × 2 wks then 200 mg 3 × weekly	GI upset, hepatotoxicity, QT prolongation	QT interval, LFTs, drug interactions	FDA approved 2012, may be associated with increased mortality[26]
Capreomycin	IV/IM: 15 mg/kg (1 g)	Ototoxicity, renal dysfunction	Hearing tests, renal function	Dose reduction after response, for those ≥60 reduce dose to 10 mg/kg/d, dose adjustment also required for those with significant renal dysfunction
Ciprofloxacin	1500 mg/d	GI upset, hypersensitivity, QT prolongation	Drug interactions	Not FDA approved for TB therapy
Clofazimine[27–29]	50–100 mg/d	GI upset; skin, hair, corneal, secretion discoloration	Drug interactions	Not FDA approved for TB therapy, unclear efficacy
Cycloserine	10–15 mg/kg/d (1 g)	Rash, depression, psychosis, seizures, headaches	Mental status	Pyridoxine may reduce CNS effects

Ethionamide	15–20 mg/kg (1 g)	Hepatotoxicity, GI upset, metallic taste	LFTs	May cause hypothyroidism, pyridoxine may reduce CNS effects
Kanamycin	IV/IM: 15 mg/kg (1 g)	Ototoxicity, renal dysfunction	Hearing tests, renal function	Dose reduction after response, for those ≥60 reduce dose to 10 mg/kg/d, dose adjustment also required for those with significant renal dysfunction
Levofloxacin	500–1000 mg/d	GI upset, hypersensitivity, QT prolongation	Drug interactions	Not FDA approved for TB therapy
Moxifloxacin	400 mg/d	GI upset, hypersensitivity, QT prolongation	Drug interactions	Not FDA approved for TB therapy
Para-aminosalicylic acid	8–12 g of granules per day	Hepatotoxicity, GI upset, hypersensitivity	LFTs, thyroid function tests	May cause hypothyroidism
Streptomycin	IM: 15 mg/kg/d(1 g)	Ototoxicity, vestibular dysfunction, renal dysfunction	Hearing tests, renal function	Dose reduction after response, for those ≥60 reduce dose to 10 mg/kg/d, dose adjustment also required for those with significant renal dysfunction

GI, gastrointestinal; LFTs, liver function tests; FDA, U.S. Food and Drug Administration; TB, tuberculosis; CNS, central nervous system.

Adapted from American Thoracic Society; Centers for Disease Control and Prevention; Infectious Diseases Society of America. Treatment of tuberculosis. *MMWR Recomm Rep.* 2003;52:1–77.

Drug Resistance

- All cultures growing MTB should be evaluated for drug susceptibility.
  - With INH resistance, RIF, PZA, and EMB should be given for 6 months.[24] A fluoroquinolone may also be added to this regimen.
  - With RIF resistance, patients may be given INH, PZA, and streptomycin for 9 months or INH, PZA, and EMB for 12–18 months. Streptomycin may be added to the latter during the first 2–3 months or a fluoroquinolone may be added for the entire duration.[24]
- Isolates resistant to two agents are defined as MDR. Expert consultation is advised.
  - The necessary therapy is complex and must be individualized.
  - Insufficient data are available on the effectiveness of various second-line regimens.
  - When possible, at least three drugs with efficacy should be given.
  - This regimen should be continued until sputum cultures are negative, followed by at least 12 months of two-drug therapy.
- Surgical resection, when feasible, can offer significantly improved cure rates; however, drug therapy is still necessary to sterilize remaining disease.

Pregnancy

- Antituberculous therapy is indicated during pregnancy for the well-being of both the pregnant patient and the fetus.
- Treatment involves an initial phase with INH, RIF, and EMB followed by continuation with INH and RIF (Table 14-4, regimen 4).[24]
  - Streptomycin and many of the second-line agents are contraindicated.
  - PZA should be avoided due to lack of evidence for its safety.
  - Treatment is safe during breastfeeding.

PATIENT EDUCATION

Patients with TB will likely benefit from a review of the basic principles of disease.

- Because TB is contagious, close contacts need to be evaluated.
- Because the organism is slow growing, a prolonged course of treatment is required. Due to emerging resistance, adherence to treatment is critical.
- While taking INH, patients should be advised to avoid alcohol. Acetaminophen and other potentially hepatotoxic agents should be used sparingly.
- Patients taking EMB should be advised to contact their physician if they develop visual disturbances.

MONITORING/FOLLOW-UP

- During therapy, patients should be monitored for medication adherence, for improvement or persistence of symptoms, and for signs of hepatitis. Routine monitoring of hepatic transaminases is not necessary unless the patient has baseline hepatic dysfunction as risk factors for hepatotoxicity.[24]
  - Up to 20% of persons taking INH develop a mild, asymptomatic transaminitis.
  - These laboratory abnormalities tend to resolve even when INH is continued.
  - If liver enzymes are elevated >3–5 times the upper limit of normal, INH should be stopped.
- CXR should be obtained at initiation and completion of therapy to serve as baseline for future reference.

- Sputum samples should be taken for AFB stain and MTB culture on a monthly basis until two consecutive samples are culture negative, documenting adequate response to therapy. A final sputum culture should be obtained at the completion of therapy to document cure.[24]
- **DOT**, often arranged in conjunction with the local public health department, is the treatment method of choice for most patients. DOT is particularly important when adherence is a concern and may involve incentives for the patient to take his or her medicines.

REFERENCES

1. Centers for Disease Control and Prevention. TB incidence in the United States, 1953–2014. Available at http://www.cdc.gov/tb/statistics/tbcases.htm. Accessed 14/12/15.
2. World Health Organization. Global tuberculosis report 2015. 20th ed. Geneva: World Health Organization, 2015. Available at http://www.who.int/tb/publications/global_report/en/. Accessed 14/12/15.
3. Taylor Z, Nolan CM, Blumberg HM, et al. Controlling tuberculosis in the United States. Recommendations from the American Thoracic Society, CDC, the Infectious Diseases Society of America. *MMWR Recomm Rep.* 2005;54:1–81.
4. World Health Organization. Multidrug-resistant tuberculosis (MDR-TB) 2015 update. Available at http://www.who.int/tb/challenges/mdr/en/. Accessed 14/12/15.
5. Scott C, Kirking HL, Jeffries C, et al. Tuberculosis trends—United States, 2014. *MMWR Morb Mortal Wkly Rep.* 2015;64:265–9.
6. Deiss RG, Rodwell TC, Garfein RS. Tuberculosis and illicit drug use: review and update. *Clin Infect Dis.* 2009;48:72–82.
7. Dooley KE, Chaisson RE. Tuberculosis and diabetes mellitus: convergence of two epidemics. *Lancet Infect Dis.* 2009;9:737–46.
8. Dheda K, Barry CE 3rd, Maartens G. Tuberculosis. *Lancet.* 2015;pii: S0140-6736(15)00151-8. doi: 10.1016/S0140-6736(15)00151-8.
9. Bates MN, Khalakdina A, Pai M, et al. Risk of tuberculosis from exposure to tobacco smoke: a systematic review and meta-analysis. *Arch Intern Med.* 2007;167:335–42.
10. Centers for Disease Control and Prevention. Screening for tuberculosis and tuberculosis infection in high-risk populations: recommendations of the Advisory Council for the Elimination of Tuberculosis. *MMWR Recomm Rep.* 1995;44:19–34.
11. Centers for Disease Control and Prevention; National Center for HIV/AIDS; Viral Hepatitis, STD, and TB Prevention; Division of Tuberculosis Elimination. Latent tuberculosis infection: a guide for primary health care providers. Atlanta: Centers for Disease Control and Prevention, 2013. Available at http://www.cdc.gov/tb/publications/ltbi/default.htm. 12/14/2015.
12. Mazurek GH, Jereb J, Vernon A, et al. Updated guidelines for using interferon gamma release assays to detect Mycobacterium tuberculosis infection—United States, 2010. *MMWR Recomm Rep.* 2010;59:1–25.
13. Belknap R, Daley CL. Interferon-gamma release assays. *Clin Lab Med.* 2014;34:337–49.
14. Diel R, Loddenkemper R, Nienhaus A. Evidence-based comparison of commercial interferon-gamma release assays for detecting active TB: a metaanalysis. *Chest.* 2010;137:952–68.
15. Arend SM, van Meijgaarden KE, de Boer K, et al. Tuberculin skin testing and in vitro T cell responses to ESAT-6 and culture filtrate protein 10 after infection with Mycobacterium marinum or M. kansasii. *J Infect Dis.* 2002;186:1797–807.
16. Centers for Disease Control and Prevention (CDC). Updated guidelines for the use of nucleic acid amplification tests in the diagnosis of tuberculosis. *MMWR Morb Mortal Wkly Rep.* 2009;58:7–10.
17. Jeong YJ, Lee KS. Pulmonary tuberculosis: up-to-date imaging and management. *AJR Am J Roentgenol.* 2008;191:834–44.
18. Rozenshtein A, Hao F, Starc MT, et al. Radiographic appearance of pulmonary tuberculosis: dogma disproved. *AJR Am J Roentgenol.* 2015;204:974–8.
19. Zumla A, Raviglione M, Hafner R, et al. Tuberculosis. *N Engl J Med.* 2013;368:745–55.
20. Pasipanodya JG, Gumbo T. A meta-analysis of self-administered vs directly observed therapy effect on microbiologic failure, relapse, and acquired drug resistance in tuberculosis patients. *Clin Infect Dis.* 2013;57:21–31.

21. Centers for Disease Control and Prevention (CDC); American Thoracic Society. Targeted tuberculin testing and treatment of latent tuberculosis infection. *MMWR Recomm Rep.* 2000;49:1–51.
22. Centers for Disease Control and Prevention (CDC). Recommendations for use of an isoniazid-rifapentine regimen with direct observation to treat latent Mycobacterium tuberculosis infection. *MMWR Morb Mortal Wkly Rep.* 2011;60:1650–3.
23. Centers for Disease Control and Prevention (CDC); American Thoracic Society. Update: adverse event data and revised American Thoracic Society/CDC recommendations against the use of rifampin and pyrazinamide for treatment of latent tuberculosis infection—United States, 2003. *MMWR Morb Mortal Wkly Rep.* 2003;52:735–9.
24. American Thoracic Society; Centers for Disease Control and Prevention; Infectious Diseases Society of America. Treatment of tuberculosis. *MMWR Recomm Rep.* 2003;52:1–77.
25. Centers for Disease Control and Prevention. Provisional CDC guidelines for the use and safety monitoring of bedaquiline fumarate (Sirturo) for the treatment of multidrug-resistant tuberculosis. *MMWR Recomm Rep.* 2013;62:1–12.
26. Diacon AH, Pym A, Grobusch MP, et al. Multidrug-resistant tuberculosis and culture conversion with bedaquiline. *N Engl J Med.* 2014;371:723–32.
27. Mitnick CD, Shin SS, Seung KJ, et al. Comprehensive treatment of extensively drug-resistant tuberculosis. *N Engl J Med.* 2008;359:563–74.
28. Van Deun A, Maug AK, Salim MA, et al. Short, highly effective, and inexpensive standardized treatment of multidrug-resistant tuberculosis. *Am J Respir Crit Care Med.* 2010;182:684–92.
29. Dooley KE, Obuku EA, Durakovic N, et al. World Health Organization group 5 drugs for the treatment of drug-resistant tuberculosis: unclear efficacy or untapped potential? *J Infect Dis.* 2013;207:1352–8.
30. Panel on Opportunistic Infection in HIV-Infected Adults and Adolescents. Guidelines for the prevention and treatment of opportunistic infections in HIV-infected adults and adolescents: recommendation from the Centers for Disease Control and Prevention, the National Institutes of Health, and the HIV Medicine Association of the Infectious Diseases Society of America. Available at https://aidsinfo.nih.gov/guidelines/html/4/adult-and-adolescent-oi-prevention-and-treatment-guidelines/0. Accessed 14/12/15.
31. Uthman OA, Okwundu C, Gbenga K, et al. Optimal timing of antiretroviral therapy initiation for HIV-infected adults with newly diagnosed pulmonary tuberculosis: a systematic review and meta-analysis. *Ann Intern Med.* 2015;163:32–9.

Fungal Pulmonary Infections

15

Catherine Chen

INTRODUCTION

- Infections of the lung with both opportunistic and endemic fungi are increasingly common and are a result of the increasing population of immunocompromised hosts, due to AIDS, chemotherapy, organ transplantation, and chronic steroid use. Patients with neutropenia or lymphocytic deficiencies are predisposed to mycotic infection and pulmonary involvement is the most common form of invasive fungal disease.
- This chapter examines the clinical presentation, diagnostic approach, and treatment of the most common fungal infections of the lung.
- There are three primary forms of fungi that infect the lungs:
  - Yeasts, which appear as budding forms, include species of *Candida*, *Cryptococcus* species, and *Pneumocystis jirovecii.*
  - Molds, which appear as hyphae, include *Aspergillus* and the zygomycota—*Mucorales*, *Fusarium*, and *Scedosporium.*
  - Dimorphic fungi appear as both budding forms in tissue and hyphae in cultures incubated at 25°C, and include *Histoplasma*, *Blastomyces*, and *Coccidioides.*
- This review of fungal pulmonary infections is not intended to be exhaustive; rather, the most common and emerging fungal infections will be reviewed.

ASPERGILLOSIS

- Aspergillus is a ubiquitous soil-dwelling organism with a worldwide distribution that is found in dust, compost, foods, spices, and rotted plants. Inhalation of the spores is common, but disease is rare.
- *Aspergillus fumigatus* is the most commonly implicated organism but any of the *Aspergillus* species, including *A. flavus*, can cause disease.
- Risk factors for developing infection include neutropenia, prolonged steroid use, AIDS, use of chemotherapy, hematopoietic or solid-organ transplantation, chronic granulomatous disease, and pre-existing lung disease.[1,2]
- The *Aspergillus* species cause a spectrum of clinical syndromes in the lung.[1,2]
  - Aspergilloma typifies the saprophytic processes of the lung.
  - Pulmonary aspergillosis may be categorized as saprophytic, invasive, or allergic.
  - Invasive pulmonary aspergillosis (IPA) develops as a bronchopneumonia or invasive sinusitis, and may be complicated by hemorrhage, invasion of adjacent structures, or dissemination to extrathoracic organs.
  - Chronic necrotizing aspergillosis (CNA) is a more indolent form of invasive infection.
  - Allergic conditions include allergic bronchopulmonary aspergillosis (ABPA).

Aspergilloma:
General Principles

- An aspergilloma is the **most common form of pulmonary aspergillosis.**[1]
- Also called a fungus ball, the aspergilloma is composed of fungal hyphae, mucus, inflammatory cells, fibrin, and tissue debris.

- It usually occurs in patients with **pre-existing cavitary lung disease**. Rare cases of de novo aspergilloma in patients without pre-existing cavitary lung disease have been reported.[1,3]
- Risk factors include TB, sarcoidosis, neoplasm, cystic fibrosis, or severe emphysema.

Diagnosis

- Most patients with aspergilloma have few clinical symptoms.
- When symptoms develop, **hemoptysis** is the most common and is usually mild but may occasionally be severe. Bleeding usually occurs from bronchial vessels lining the lung cavity.[1,3]
- Patients may also experience chest pain, dyspnea, malaise, and fever.

Diagnostic Testing

Laboratories

- Sputum cultures for *Aspergillus* are positive in only 50% of cases due to the limited communication between the cavity and the bronchial tree.[1]
- Serum IgG antibodies are very sensitive but may be negative in patients on corticosteroid therapy.[1,3]
- *Aspergillus* antigen has been found in the bronchoalveolar lavage (BAL) fluid of patients with aspergilloma, but the diagnostic utility is variable.

Imaging

- On CXR, aspergillomas classically appear as an upper lobe intracavitary mass surrounded by a radiolucent crescent, known as a crescent sign.
- However, these radiographic findings may also appear in other conditions, including neoplasm, abscess, cystic echinococcosis, and granulomatosis with polyangiitis.

Treatment

- Treatment of aspergilloma is usually considered only when patients become symptomatic and there is no consensus on treatment of choice.[1,3,4]
- Inhaled, intracavitary and endobronchial instillations of antifungal agents have been attempted, and have failed to demonstrate benefit in the clinical course, morbidity, or mortality.
- Oral itraconazole therapy has been shown to reduce the size of aspergillomas.
- Administration of amphotericin B percutaneously into the aspergilloma may be effective in patients with massive hemoptysis, with resolution of hemoptysis in several days.
- Bronchial artery embolization should be considered as a temporizing measure in patients with life-threatening hemoptysis.
- Surgical resection should be considered in patients who have recurrent hemoptysis, but resection is often limited by the underlying lung disease.

Invasive Pulmonary Aspergillosis: General Principles

- IPA is characterized by **direct vascular invasion** by the fungus, **often with dissemination to other organs**.
- It is a rapidly progressive, **frequently fatal** disease that occurs **primarily in immunocompromised hosts**.
- Aspergillus has a propensity for vascular invasion, resulting in vascular thrombosis, infarction, and tissue necrosis. It can also invade into adjacent structures, including the intercostal muscles, ribs, and pericardium.

- Risk factors for IPA include prolonged neutropenia or neutrophil dysfunction, hematopoietic stem cell and solid organ transplantation, prolonged and high-dose corticosteroid therapy, hematologic malignancy, advanced AIDS, and cytotoxic therapy.[1,2]

Diagnosis

- IPA should be suspected in immunocompromised hosts with high fevers that do not respond to treatment with broad-spectrum antibiotics.
- The most common clinical manifestations include pleuritic pain, hemoptysis, pulmonary hemorrhage, and cavitation.[1,2]
- Diagnosis of IPA is difficult due to its nonspecific clinical manifestations, and a high index of suspicion must be present in patients with risk factors. As a result, diagnostic criteria have been proposed, incorporating histologic, microbiologic, and antigenic findings. The criteria are summarized in Table 15-1.[1]

TABLE 15-1 DIAGNOSTIC CRITERIA FOR THE DIAGNOSIS OF IPA

Major Criteria	**Minor Criteria**
Halo sign	Symptoms of lower respiratory tract infection
Air-crescent sign	Pleural rub
Cavity within an area of consolidation	Any new infiltrate not fulfilling major criteria
	Pleural effusion
Diagnosis	**Criteria**
Proven IPA	Histopathologic examination of lung tissue showing hyphae or biopsy specimen with evidence of associated tissue damage **OR** Positive culture for *Aspergillus* from a sample obtained by sterile procedure from the lung and clinically or radiographically abnormal site consistent with infection
Probable IPA	Host risk factor[a] **AND** Positive *Aspergillus* culture from sputum or BAL, or positive galactomannan assay **AND** One major or two minor criteria
Possible IPA	Host risk factor[a] **AND** Positive *Aspergillus* culture from sputum or BAL or positive galactomannan assay **OR** One major or two minor criteria

[a]Prolonged neutropenia or neutrophil dysfunction, hematopoietic stem cell and solid organ transplantation, prolonged and high-dose corticosteroid therapy, hematologic malignancy, advanced AIDS, and cytotoxic therapy.

IPA, invasive pulmonary aspergillosis; BAL, bronchoalveolar lavage.

Adapted from Zmeili OS, Soubani AO. Pulmonary aspergillosis: a clinical update. *Q J Med.* 2007; 100:317–34.

Diagnostic Testing

- Isolation of *Aspergillus* from the sputum has a positive predictive value of 80–90% in immunosuppressed patients; however, negative sputum studies occur in 70% of patients with confirmed IPA.[1]
- Serum and BAL fluid testing for **galactomannan** antigen is available but the operating characteristics of such testing are variable, with specificity being better than sensitivity.[2,5–7] However, some medications, including β-lactam antibiotics, may be associated with a false-positive result, and antifungals with activity against *Aspergillus* may be associated with a false-negative result. Serum polymerase chain reaction (PCR) testing may also be available in the near future.[2,8]
- CXR findings are nonspecific, and may show patchy infiltrates or nodular opacities.[1]
- The imaging modality of choice is **high-resolution CT scanning**, which may reveal multiple nodules and an area of infiltrate surrounded by a rim of air, representing pulmonary necrosis, known as the halo sign.[1,3]
- Histopathologic diagnosis of lung tissue, obtained from thoracoscopic or open lung biopsy, remains the gold standard.
- Histologic examination demonstrates vascular invasion by septate, acute-angle–branching hyphae.
- Bronchoscopy with BAL is particularly helpful in patients with diffuse lung involvement, and has a sensitivity and specificity of 50% and 97%, respectively.[1]

Treatment

- Despite the introduction of new antifungal agents, the mortality of IPA remains high. Therapy should be initiated as soon as there is clinical suspicion of IPA.
- **The current treatment of choice is voriconazole** at 6 mg/kg IV bid on day 1, followed by 4 mg/kg IV daily for an additional 6 days. After 6 days of IV therapy, switching to voriconazole 200 mg PO bid can be considered.[1,2,4]
- **Amphotericin B** is also a first-line therapy, recommended dose 1–1.5 mg/kg/d; however, it is associated with nephrotoxicity and electrolyte disturbances. In patients who cannot tolerate amphotericin B due to renal dysfunction, the less toxic lipid formulations may be tried.[1,2,4]
- Optimal duration of therapy is unknown, but patients may be switched to oral itraconazole for at least 6–12 weeks only after immunosuppression has ended and there has been resolution of the lesions.
- **Posaconazole, caspofungin, micafungin, and anidulafungin** may also be used as salvage therapy in patients who do not respond to standard antifungal therapy.[2,4]
- Combination therapy has not been shown to be more effective than single-agent therapy.
- **Surgical resection** of infected tissue should be considered when there is massive hemoptysis or localized focus of infection, especially if further immunosuppression is planned.

Chronic Necrotizing Aspergillosis: General Principles

- CNA is a more indolent form of invasive infection characterized by local invasion of lung tissue. Unlike IPA, CNA is **slowly progressive and vascular invasion or extrathoracic dissemination is unusual**.
- CNA most commonly affects elderly patients with **underlying chronic lung disease**, particularly chronic obstructive pulmonary disease (COPD). Other risk factors include pulmonary TB, prior lung resection, prior radiation therapy, pneumoconiosis, and cystic fibrosis.[1,3]

- Patients with mild immunosuppression due to diabetes mellitus, chronic liver disease, corticosteroid therapy, alcohol abuse, and connective tissue disease, are also at increased risk.[1,3]

Diagnosis

- Patients with CNA typically present with constitutional symptoms, including fever, malaise, fatigue, and weight loss of 1–6 months' duration.
- Patients may also have chronic productive cough and hemoptysis of varying severity.
- Occasionally, patients are asymptomatic and the diagnosis is made incidentally.
- Patients must meet all of the following criteria in order for the diagnosis to be made[1]:
  - Chronic pulmonary or systemic symptoms, including at least one of: weight loss, productive cough, or hemoptysis.
  - No overt immunocompromising conditions.
  - Cavitary pulmonary lesion with evidence of paracavitary infiltrates, new cavitary formation, or expansion of cavity size over time.
  - Elevated levels of inflammatory markers.
  - Isolation of *Aspergillus* from pulmonary or pleural cavity, or positive serum *Aspergillus* precipitins test.
  - Exclusion of other pulmonary pathogens.

Diagnostic Testing

- **Serum IgG antibodies** to *A. fumigatus* are variably positive during the course of the disease.
- **CXR and chest CT** show consolidation, pleural thickening, and cavitary lesions in the upper lobes. Aspergilloma may be seen in half of patients. The radiographic findings may progress over weeks to months.
- As with IPA, diagnosis requires the **histologic demonstration of tissue invasion** by the fungus as well as the growth of *Aspergillus* on culture. However, transbronchial biopsy specimens and percutaneous aspirates have poor yield, and thoracoscopic or open lung biopsy is rarely performed, resulting in delayed diagnosis.[1]

Treatment

- **Voriconazole** 200 mg PO bid is the current primary therapy for CNA, but both itraconazole 400 mg daily and amphotericin B 0.5–1 mg/kg daily are considered first-line therapies as well. The duration of therapy is usually prolonged but optimal duration and criteria for discontinuing therapy are currently unclear.[1,4]
- Markers for response to therapy include weight gain, improved energy levels, improved pulmonary symptoms, decreasing inflammatory markers, decreasing total serum IgE levels, and reduction in cavity size.[3]
- **Surgical resection** can be considered in a very limited population, including young healthy patients with limited disease and good pulmonary reserve, patients not tolerating antifungal therapy, and patients with residual localized disease despite antifungal therapy.

Allergic Bronchopulmonary Aspergillosis

General Principles

- Unlike the previously discussed forms of pulmonary aspergillosis, ABPA is a **hypersensitivity reaction** rather than a true infection.
- The pathogenesis is not completely understood, but specific IgE-mediated type I hypersensitivity reactions, specific IgG-mediated type III hypersensitivity reactions, and abnormal T-lymphocyte cellular immune responses have all been implicated.[9]
- It most commonly occurs in patients with **asthma or cystic fibrosis**.[9]

Diagnosis

- Patients with ABPA usually present with episodic wheezing, occasional productive cough, fever, and chest pain.
- Patients may also complain of expectoration of thick brown plugs, which are *Aspergillus*-laden mucoid bronchial casts.
- Patients in whom ABPA is suspected should undergo a specific diagnostic evaluation, outlined below in Figure 15-1.[9]
- Patients with ABPA can be classified as those with **central bronchiectasis** (ABPA-CB) and those without (ABPA-**seropositive**).
- The minimal diagnostic criteria for ABPA-CB include asthma, skin reactivity to *Aspergillus* antigens, serum IgE >1000 IU/mL, elevated serum *A. fumigatus*-specific IgG and IgE, and central bronchiectasis.[9,10]
- The minimal diagnostic criteria for ABPA-seropositive include asthma, skin reactivity to *Aspergillus* antigens, serum IgE >1000 IU/mL, history of transient pulmonary infiltrates, and elevated serum *A. fumigatus*-specific IgG and IgE.[9,10]

Diagnostic Testing

- Early detection of ABPA prior to the development of irreversible bronchiectasis can help to minimize the severity of disease. A delay in diagnosis may result in irreversible pulmonary damage.

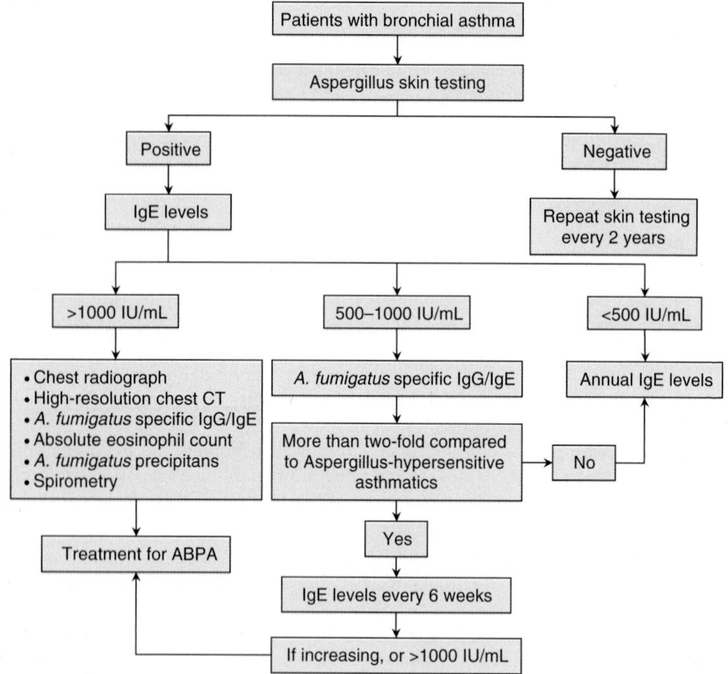

FIGURE 15-1. Diagnostic evaluation for allergic bronchopulmonary aspergillosis (ABPA). (Adapted from Agarwal R. Allergic bronchopulmonary aspergillosis. *Chest.* 2009;135:805–26.)

- **Serum IgE and IgG levels** are useful in diagnosing ABPA.
- The CXR may be clear or show **transient migratory infiltrates** in the upper lobes that occur during acute exacerbations. The ring sign and tram lines are radiographic findings that signify the thickened and inflamed bronchi.
- The **chest CT** scan may show mucoid impaction, bronchial thickening, or bronchiectasis, usually in a central upper lobe distribution.

Treatment

- **Glucocorticoids are the mainstay in treatment of ABPA.**[4,9]
- Although there is little data to guide the dosing or duration of therapy, lower doses of glucocorticoids have been associated with more frequent relapses.
- Current recommendations are to treat with prednisone 0.5 mg/kg/d PO daily for 2 weeks, followed by a slow taper over 3–6 months.
- Itraconazole, 200 mg bid, has been used as a steroid-sparing agent.[4]
- Total serum IgE can be used as a marker of disease activity, and should be checked 6–8 weeks after starting glucocorticoid therapy, then every 8 weeks for 1 year after that to determine a baseline serum IgE level.
- Although oral itraconazole has been shown to reduce IgE levels, it has not been demonstrated to improve lung function.

BLASTOMYCOSIS

General Principles

- Blastomycosis is a fungal infection caused by the dimorphic fungus *Blastomyces dermatitides*, which exists as a mold in nature and converts to a broad-based budding yeast at body temperature.
- It appears to be most commonly found in moist soil close to bodies of fresh water, and is traditionally thought to be endemic in the Ohio and Mississippi river valleys, but the epidemiology is not well delineated.[11–13]
- Like many of the other fungal pulmonary infections, infection most commonly occurs when the conidia are aerosolized and inhaled, although cases of transmission by the bite of an infected animal have also been documented.[11,13]
- Hosts with impaired cell-mediated immunity are at greater risk of developing disseminated disease.
- Unlike histoplasmosis, blastomycosis does not appear to be a self-limited disease, and must be treated once diagnosis is made as mortality rates approach 60% in untreated disease.

Diagnosis

Clinical Presentation

History

- Clinical presentations of blastomycosis infection are **highly variable**, and range from mild to fatal disseminated disease.[11–13]
- Most primary infections are asymptomatic or mild and resolve without treatment. Of those who are symptomatic, the illness most frequently manifests as a mild, self-limited pulmonary infection.[12]
- Patients who are ill enough to come to medical attention present with cough, fever, night sweats, weight loss, chest pain, dyspnea, myalgias, and hemoptysis. Patients with widely disseminated or miliary disease may present with acute respiratory distress syndrome (ARDS).
- Other common sites of dissemination include the bone, joints, genitourinary system, and central nervous system (CNS), but blastomycosis can involve virtually any organ.

Physical Examination

- Approximately half of patients with disseminated disease have either ulcerative or verrucous skin lesions, which are tender and frequently confused for panniculitis.[11–13]
- Verrucous lesions have a raised, irregular border over an abscess in the SC tissue, with crusting and drainage.
- Ulcerative lesions have sharp, heaped-up borders and the base contains exudate.

Diagnostic Testing

- Diagnosing blastomycosis remains difficult due to the nonspecific symptoms, and delays in diagnosis are common. Blastomycosis is often not considered until the patient has failed to respond to standard treatment for bacterial infections and becomes gravely ill.
- **Culture** of sputum, BAL fluid, tracheal secretions, or of the skin lesions is the definitive diagnostic test but it may take **up to 4–5 weeks for the organism to be isolated from culture.**
- **Microscopic examination** of sputum, aspirate, or tissue shows the classic broad-based budding yeast, and can lead to more rapid diagnosis.
- A **urine antigen** assay has a reported sensitivity of 93% and a specificity of 79% but histoplasmosis, paracoccidioidomycosis, and other fungal infections may result in false positives.[11,12]
- Serologic testing has traditionally not been useful but advances in technology made testing more sensitive and specific.
- CXR frequently demonstrates alveolar or mass-like infiltrate, often with cavitation, and can sometimes be mistaken for malignancy.

Treatment

- In patients with non-CNS, non–life-threatening disease, **itraconazole** 200 mg PO daily for 6–12 months is recommended; this may be increased to 200 mg PO bid for patients not responding to therapy.[4,11–13]
- In patients with severe, life-threatening disease, **amphotericin B** 0.7–1.0 mg/kg daily for 1–2 weeks remains the mainstay of therapy. Lipid formulations may be used at 3–5 mg/kg daily.[4] Once satisfactory clinical response has been documented, patients may be switched to itraconazole for a total of 1 year of therapy.
- CNS disease requires amphotericin B for 4–6 weeks prior to being switched to itraconazole.
- In immunosuppressed patients, lifelong suppressive therapy is recommended if the immunosuppression cannot be corrected.

CANDIDIASIS

General Principles

- *Candida* is a dimorphic fungus that is a common human saprophyte, found normally in the gastrointestinal (GI) tract and other mucocutaneous regions.
- Although *Candida albicans* is the major pathogenic species, other *Candida* organisms can also cause infection, such as *C. parapsilosis* and C. *glabrata.*[14,15]
- **Isolated pulmonary candidiasis is rare and pulmonary involvement is usually secondary to disseminated candidiasis.**[16] When primary pulmonary candidiasis occurs, it is usually the result of aspiration from the oropharynx.
- Risk factors for developing disseminated candidiasis include intensive care unit hospitalization, hematologic and solid organ malignancy, hematopoietic stem cell and solid organ transplantation, use of central venous catheters, antibiotic therapy, total parenteral nutrition, and prior fungal colonization.[14,15]

Diagnosis

- Symptoms of pulmonary candidiasis are nonspecific, and include cough productive of purulent sputum and hemoptysis.
- Signs of disseminated candidiasis include skin lesions, endophthalmitis, and high fevers not responsive to broad-spectrum antibiotic therapy.

Diagnostic Testing

- Because the oropharynx is colonized with *Candida*, isolation of *Candida* spp. from the sputum has modest operating characteristics and is nondiagnostic.[14,17,18]
- CXR may show a focal or diffuse patchy infiltrate with primary disease. A military nodular pattern is more common in disseminated disease.
- Definitive diagnosis of pulmonary candidiasis requires obtaining tissue via bronchoscopic or open lung biopsy and **histologic documentation of invasion of the bronchi or lungs**.
- Isolation of the organism from bronchial washings or BAL fluid is more representative but may also be contaminated/colonized.[19] In the correct clinical setting, repeated heavy growth of the organism from bronchial washings or BAL fluid may be used to diagnose candidiasis.

Treatment

- **Fluconazole** is the current treatment of choice in sensitive organisms at doses of 400 mg daily for 2–4 weeks. When using fluconazole for the treatment of candidiasis, speciation and susceptibility information is important as drug resistance is becoming common.[14,15,20]
- In patients who have failed fluconazole, IV amphotericin B in doses of 0.5–1.5 mg/kg daily may be used. Lipid preparations of amphotericin B may be used if amphotericin B is not tolerated.
- The echinocandins have also been shown to be effective, and have shown promise as a potential first-line agent for invasive candidiasis.

COCCIDIOIDOMYCOSIS

General Principles

- *Coccidioides immitis* is a dimorphic fungus that is endemic to the southwestern region of the United States.
- Infection occurs with the inhalation of arthroconidia, and has five primary manifestations: **acute pneumonia, chronic progressive pneumonia, pulmonary nodules and cavities, extrapulmonary nonmeningeal disease, and meningitis.**[21,22]
- AIDS, organ transplantation, use of tumor necrosis factor-α (TNF-α) antagonists, malignancy, and pregnancy are risk factors for acquiring coccidioidomycosis. Those of Filipino or African-American descent are at greater risk for developing disseminated disease.[21–23]

Diagnosis

- Approximately 60% of patients who become infected with *Coccidioides* are asymptomatic, and of those who are symptomatic, the vast majority develops acute **pneumonia.**[21,24]
- Symptoms develop 1–3 weeks after exposure, and are nonspecific, including fever, sore throat, cough, fatigue, and pleuritic chest pain; rarely, patients present with ARDS.
- It is sometimes associated with rashes, most classically erythema nodosum and erythema multiforme in a necklace pattern around the neck.[22]

- Approximately 1–4% of patients fail to recover from the acute pneumonia, and continue to have chronic progressive pneumonia, characterized by fever, weight loss, and productive cough.[21–23]
- Over the course of infection, the pneumonic process may consolidate to form a pulmonary **nodule or a cavity**. Patients may present with hemoptysis, cough, fever, night sweats, weight loss, and localized chest wall pain, but the majority of patients are asymptomatic.
- In ≤5% of immunocompetent hosts, coccidioidal infection evolves into **disseminated disease**.[22] The most common sites of dissemination include the skin, bones, joints, lymph nodes, and meninges. Dissemination is often not diagnosed until several months after the initial pulmonary symptoms. Patients with meningitis often present with headache, mental status changes, and neurologic deficits, most commonly cranial nerve palsies. Prognosis, even in immunocompetent hosts, is grave if not diagnosed and treated promptly.

Diagnostic Testing

Laboratories

- Diagnosis of coccidioidomycosis can be made in three ways: **identification of the spherules** in a cytology or biopsy specimen, **isolation of the organism from culture**, or a **serologic test** that is positive for *Coccidioides*.[22,23]
- Identifying spherules in sputum, BAL fluid, or other body fluid is indicative of disease, as *Coccidioides* is not a colonizing organism.[22]
- Active cultures of pathogenic *Coccidioides* pose an infection risk for laboratory personnel.
- An IgM antibody to coccidioidin may be measured with several different methods, and IgG complement fixing antibody can be quantified. The IgG is present at lower titers in early disease, and higher in disseminated disease. A titer ≥1:16 should prompt investigation for disseminated disease.[21,22] Negative serology does not rule out coccidiomycosis due to less than perfect sensitivity. Titers should also be quantified in the cerebrospinal fluid (CSF) if meningitis is suspected.

Imaging

- CXRs in acute pneumonia most frequently reveal dense, upper lobe infiltrates; hilar and mediastinal lymphadenopathies are not uncommon. In chronic pneumonia, CXRs may show persistent infiltrates, fibrosis, cavitation, hilar lymphadenopathy, and pleural changes.
- In cavitary disease, CXR classically shows a thin-walled lesion without an air–fluid level. In 90% of patients the cavities are solitary and in 70% they are usually 2–4 cm in size.[23]
- In disseminated disease, CXR most commonly shows diffuse reticulonodular infiltrates, although miliary infiltrates, nodules, and cavities may be seen.

Treatment

- In immunocompetent patients with mild symptoms, antifungal therapy is not indicated.[4]
- In immunocompetent patients with moderate pulmonary disease, an oral azole may be used, most commonly **fluconazole** 400 mg daily or **itraconazole** 400–600 mg daily.[4,21,22,24]
- In patients with disseminated disease or severe pulmonary disease, IV **amphotericin B** 0.5–1.5 mg/kg/d or its lipid formulations should be used until the patient has clinically stabilized, at which time they may be switched to maintenance therapy with an oral azole for at least 12–18 months.[4,21,22,24]
- Fluconazole is not efficacious in bone and joint disease.
- If the patient is immunosuppressed, they may require lifelong suppressive therapy with an oral azole.[4]
- In patients who are asymptomatic but have nodules or cavitary lesions, CXRs to monitor the size of the lesions are indicated; in the event that the patient becomes symptomatic, surgical resection may be indicated.

CRYPTOCOCCOSIS

General Principles

- Cryptococcosis is an opportunistic infection caused by *Cryptococcus neoformans* or *C. gatti*, an encapsulated, budding yeast.
- *C. neoformans* is found worldwide, and are especially abundant in soil that is contaminated with pigeon droppings.
- Cryptococcosis occurs when fungal cells are inhaled, and in the absence of a robust immune response, the fungus can disseminate to CNS, resulting in meningitis or meningoencephalitis.
- Risk factors for developing clinically significant disease include HIV infection, diabetes mellitus, chronic liver disease, hematologic malignancies, solid organ or hematopoietic stem cell transplantation, corticosteroid therapy, use of TNF-α antagonists, sarcoidosis, and connective tissue diseases.[25–28]

Diagnosis

- The majority of immunocompetent hosts infected by *Cryptococcus* are asymptomatic. Those with symptoms frequently complain of nonproductive cough, fever, malaise, chest pain, dyspnea, night sweats, and hemoptysis. Immunocompetent patients may have a self-limited disease that resolves over weeks to months, even without antifungal therapy.
- In the immunocompromised host, cryptococcal infection is often disseminated at the time of diagnosis, and patients most commonly present CNS findings, particularly meningoencephalitis, in addition to fever and cough. A very small minority of immunosuppressed patients presented with pulmonary symptoms, although severe cases may present with acute respiratory failure.[25–28]

Diagnostic Testing

- Definitive diagnosis of pulmonary cryptococcosis requires **culture** and identification of the organism from a sterile specimen but sensitivity may be poor.
- **Cryptococcal antigen** is found in the serum and CSF after the disease has become disseminated, and is of limited utility in immunocompetent patients with localized pulmonary disease. This test seems to be more sensitive in those with significant immunocompromise.[25,28]
- **Cultures of BAL fluid** increase the yield to almost 90%, and microscopic examination of the BAL smear with India ink may allow for rapid diagnosis. Testing of BAL fluid or sputum samples for cryptococcal antigen has yielded inconsistent results.[26,28]
- Radiographic findings of pulmonary cryptococcosis are variable, and dependent on the degree of immunosuppression in the patient.[25,26,28]
  - In immunocompetent patients, solitary or multiple pulmonary nodules and airspace consolidation are the most common finding on CXR.
  - In immunosuppressed patients, diffuse, interstitial, and lobar infiltrates are the most common findings.
  - Cavitation of pulmonary nodules and consolidations are more likely in patients with immunocompromise.

Treatment

Because the risk of dissemination and recurrence is related to host immunity, treatment is based upon the status of patient immune function as well as the severity of disease. Treatment recommendations are outlined in Table 15-2.[29]

TABLE 15-2 TREATMENT RECOMMENDATIONS FOR PULMONARY CRYPTOCOCCOSIS

Disease Severity	Immune Status	Recommended Treatment
Mild to moderate		Fluconazole 400 mg daily for 6–12 mo[a]
Severe or progressive[b]	HIV positive[c]	**Induction:** amphotericin B 0.7–1 mg/kg daily **PLUS** flucytosine (100 mg/kg daily in 4 divided doses) for 2 wks (4–6 wks if intolerant to flucytosine) **OR** Liposomal amphotericin B 3–4 mg/kg **PLUS** flucytosine (100 mg/kg daily in 4 divided doses) for 2 wks (4–6 wks if intolerant to flucytosine) **Consolidation:** fluconazole 400 mg daily for 8 wks **Maintenance:** fluconazole 200 mg daily for ≥1 yr **OR** itraconazole 400 mg daily for ≥1 yr
	Organ transplant recipient	**Induction:** liposomal amphotericin B 3–4 mg/kg daily **PLUS** flucytosine (100 mg/kg daily in 4 divided doses) for 2 wks **OR** Liposomal amphotericin B 6 mg/kg daily for 4–6 wks **OR** Amphotericin B 0.7 mg/kg daily for 4–6 wks **Consolidation:** fluconazole 400–800 mg daily for 8 wks **Maintenance:** fluconazole 200–400 mg daily for 6–12 mo
	Non–HIV infected and non transplant	**Induction:** amphotericin B 0.7–1 mg/kg daily **PLUS** flucytosine (100 mg/kg daily in 4 divided doses) for ≥4 wks (≥6 wks if intolerant to flucytosine) **OR** Liposomal amphotericin B 3–4 mg/kg with flucytosine if possible for ≥4 wks **Consolidation:** fluconazole 400–800 mg daily for 8 wks **Maintenance:** Fluconazole 200 mg daily for 6–12 mo

[a]For immunocompetent patients, itraconazole 200 mg bid, voriconazole 200 mg bid, and posaconazole 400 mg bid acceptable if patient intolerant to or inappropriate for fluconazole.
[b]In immunocompromised patients must rule out meningitis.
[c]Possible alternative induction therapies include amphotericin B plus fluconazole, fluconazole plus flucytosine, fluconazole, and itraconazole.
Adapted from Perfect JR, Dismukes WE, Dromer F, et al. Clinical practice guidelines for the management of cryptococcal disease: 2010 update by the infectious diseases society of America. *Clin Infect Dis.* 2010;50:291–322.

FUSARIOSIS

General Principles

- *Fusarium* species are colorless septate molds that are widely distributed in soil, plant parts and debris, and water biofilms.
- *F. solani*, *F. oxysporum*, and *F. moniliforme* are the most common pathogenic species.
- Localized disease occurs in immunocompetent individuals and **disseminated disease occurs almost exclusively in immunocompromised patients**. Pulmonary involvement usually occurs in the context of disseminated disease.[30]
- In immunocompetent patients, keratitis and onychomycosis are the most common infections. In 2005 and 2006, an outbreak of *Fusarium* keratitis was associated with Bausch & Lomb ReNu with MoistureLoc multipurpose contact lens solution, resulting in its voluntary recall and permanent removal from the market.[31]
- Risk factors include hematologic malignancies (particularly acute myeloid or lymphocytic leukemia), hematopoietic stem cell or solid organ transplantation, and profound neutropenia.[30,32]
- Despite aggressive therapy, mortality remains as high as 100% in patients with disseminated disease and persistent neutropenia.[30]

Diagnosis

- Onychomycosis and keratitis are the most common clinical presentations in immunocompetent hosts.
- Lung involvement is similar to that seen with aspergillosis including allergic disease (i.e., allergic bronchopulmonary fusariosis), allergic pneumonitis, cavity colonization, and pneumonia.[32]
- Disseminated infection presents with fever and myalgias, and about 70% of patients have characteristic bulls-eye cutaneous lesions that can mimic ecthyma gangrenosum.[30,32]
- Patients with pulmonary involvement may also have pleuritic chest pain, nonproductive cough, and shortness of breath.
- While isolation of the organism in culture is helpful in diagnosis, *Fusarium* species can also be a contaminant.
- **Blood cultures are positive in about 40% of cases with invasive disease.**[30]
- CXR findings are variable, may show nonspecific alveolar or interstitial infiltrates, cavities, and nodules.
- Diagnosis of fusariosis relies upon **histopathologic examination of the affected tissue**, which shows hyaline, acute-branching, septate hyphae, and sickle-shaped multiseptate macroconidia.

Treatment

- For localized disease, topical antifungals in conjunction with oral voriconazole may be sufficient.
- In disseminated disease, susceptibility testing is necessary to optimize therapy, as species-dependent resistance to amphotericin B and the azoles may occur. As a result, the most effective therapy for fusariosis has not been defined.
- **Liposomal amphotericin B, voriconazole, and posaconazole** have all been used with some success.[32]
- Combination therapies have been used but it is unclear if they are more efficacious than monotherapy.
- Local debridement may be necessary for skin lesions.
- If at all possible, immunosuppression should be mitigated.

HISTOPLASMOSIS

General Principles

- *Histoplasmosis capsulatum* is a dimorphic fungus that has a worldwide distribution and is endemic in the southeastern, mid-Atlantic, and central United States.
- It grows as a mold in the soil, and as budding yeast in tissues at 37°C.
- Humans become infected when the soil is disturbed and the microconidia are inhaled. Clusters of cases have occurred associated with known high-risk activities such as cleaning chicken coops, exposure to bird roosts (particularly starlings), caving, and using guano fertilizer.[33]
- Severity of the illness depends upon both the host immunity and degree of exposure.
- HIV infection with a CD4 count <150/μL, use of immunosuppressive agents (particularly TNF-α antagonists), hematologic malignancies, and solid organ transplantation are risk factors for disseminated histoplasmosis.[33,34]

Diagnosis

- **The vast majority of patients with acute histoplasmosis either have no symptoms or only very mild pulmonary symptoms for which they never seek medical care.** Those who do seek medical attention are frequently diagnosed with atypical pneumonia. It is occasionally associated with erythema nodosum.[34]
- Patients who develop severe pneumonia present with fevers, chills, chest pain, cough, dyspnea, and hypoxia, and the clinical course can rapidly progress to ARDS.
- A subset of elderly patients with emphysema is at increased risk of developing chronic cavitary pulmonary histoplasmosis.[33] Patients usually present with fever, fatigue, anorexia, weight loss, productive cough, hemoptysis, and other symptoms mimicking reactivation pulmonary TB.
- A few patients (almost always with significant immunocompromise) develop progressive disseminated disease.[34]

Diagnostic Testing

- The definitive diagnostic test for histoplasmosis remains **culture** of the organism with use of a specific DNA probe for verification, but **growth may take 4–6 weeks.**[33,34]
- Detection of *H. capsulatum* polysaccharide **antigen in urine** is the preferred rapid test, with a sensitivity of >90% in patients with disseminated disease.[34,35] Sensitivity is likely less in those with nondisseminated pulmonary disease is up to 75%.[34] While the specificity has been reported as 99%, false positives can occur in patients with other fungal infections.[33] Antigen testing can also be done on serum and when done in conjunction with urine testing may improve diagnostic yield.[36]
- **Complement fixation and immunodiffusion assays of antibodies** against histoplasmosis in the serum may be useful in patients who are not immunosuppressed and in those with chronic infection but may be negative in the first month after infection.[34]
- The **CXR** frequently shows patchy infiltrates with hilar or mediastinal lymphadenopathy in mild histoplasmosis. The CXR or **chest CT** scan usually shows diffuse reticulonodular infiltrates in severe pneumonia. In cavitary disease, CXR and CT scan reveal unilateral or bilateral upper lobe infiltrates and cavities, as well as extensive fibrosis in the lower lung fields.
- Pathologic specimens demonstrate 2–4-μm oval budding yeast on silver or periodic acid–Schiff staining.[33,34]

Treatment

- Treatment of immunocompetent patients with mild-to-moderate acute pulmonary histoplasmosis is often not necessary. For patients who have symptoms for

>1 month itraconazole 200 mg tid for 3 days, then 200 mg bid for 6–12 weeks is recommended.[4,33,35]

- In patients with severe acute pulmonary histoplasmosis, **amphotericin B** 0.7–1 mg/kg daily or a **lipid formulation of amphotericin B** 3–5 mg/kg daily for 1–2 weeks is recommended. This should be followed by itraconazole 200 mg tid for 3 days, then 200 mg bid for a total of 12 weeks.[4,33,35]
- Progressive disseminated histoplasmosis is likewise treated with amphotericin B followed by itraconazole.[35]
- A short course of **methylprednisolone** 0.5–1 mg/kg daily for 1–2 weeks may be useful in patients with ARDS.[4,33,35]
- Those with chronic cavitary pulmonary histoplasmosis should be treated with itraconazole 200 mg tid for 3 days, then 200 mg bid for 18–24 months with close monitoring for relapse.[33,35]

Complications

- In some cases, acute histoplasmosis infection may result in either granulomatous mediastinitis or fibrosing mediastinitis.
- In **granulomatous mediastinitis**, also known as mediastinal granuloma, patients develop persistently enlarged lymph nodes that sometimes coalesce into a large, caseating lesion. Patients are frequently asymptomatic, and the disease does not progress to fibrosing mediastinitis. Itraconazole 200 mg PO bid for 6–12 months is often used but its benefit has not been proven.[35]
- **Fibrosing mediastinitis** is a rare complication of acute histoplasmosis infection, caused by an exuberant fibrosing response to the infection. The fibrosis tissue can result in entrapment of the great vessels and bronchi, resulting in heart failure, pulmonary emboli, superior vena cava syndrome, dyspnea, cough, wheezing, and hemoptysis. It does not benefit from treatment with antifungal agents.

MUCORMYCOSIS

General Principles

- Mucormycosis is an invasive fungal infection that is caused by the family *Mucoraceae*, particularly by *Absidia*, *Mucor*, *Rhizomucor*, and *Rhizopus*.
- Mucormycosis is an uncommon infection that occurs **primarily in immunocompromised patients.**
- The fungi are commonly found on decaying organic material, such as fruit or bread, and are distributed worldwide.
- Inhalation of sporangiospores serves as the typical route of entry for the organism.
- Risk factors include diabetes, chronic renal failure, hematologic malignancies, bone marrow/stem cell and solid organ transplantation, iron overload/deferoxamine, neutropenia, graft versus host disease, corticosteroids, IV drug use, advanced HIV disease, and trauma.[37–42]
- Despite aggressive measures, the prognosis of mucormycosis is grave, with mortality ranging up to about 90%, depending on the site of infection and patient characteristics.[38]

Diagnosis

- Rhinocerebral mucormycosis is a fatal disease that involves the sinuses and frequently spreads to the orbits and brain. It is most commonly seen in diabetics, and patients present with high fevers, purulent nasal discharge, and sinus pain.

- Pulmonary mucormycosis is less common, and frequently presents with nonspecific symptoms, including cough, fever, and hemoptysis, which can be mistaken for IPA.
- Massive hemoptysis may occur as a result of invasion of the pulmonary artery.[42]

Diagnostic Testing

- Blood, sputum, and nasal swabs are usually of little diagnostic utility because the organisms are extremely difficult to isolate and culture.
- CXRs are rarely normal but the findings are variable. Infiltrates, consolidations, and cavitary lesions may all be seen, usually with upper lobe predominance.
- The diagnosis of pulmonary mucormycosis usually requires **tissue biopsy** with histopathologic examination. Silver or hematoxylin and eosin stains of infected tissues show broad, nonseptate hyphae branching at right angles.

Treatment

- IV **amphotericin B** is the mainstay of therapy for mucormycosis. Dosing ranges from 0.5 to 1.5 mg/kg daily, and is continued until resolution of all visible lesions, and throughout immunosuppression. Liposomal amphotericin B may be more effective.[4,38,42]
- **Posaconazole** 400 mg bid has also been shown to have in vitro activity and has been used with success in some patients.[4,38,42,43] Voriconazole is not active against *Mucorales.*
- In selected patients, aggressive **surgical debridement** of necrotic tissue may be of benefit but surgical therapy is frequently not possible due to the clinical condition of the patients.
- Glucose levels should be strictly monitored, and immunosuppressive therapies should be minimized as much as possible.

PNEUMOCYSTIS PNEUMONIA

General Principles

- *Pneumocystis jiroveci*, previously known as *Pneumocystis carinii*, is an opportunistic, ascomycetous, nonfilamentous fungal pathogen of the lungs that has a worldwide distribution. The cell wall of this organism lacks ergosterol and this explains its resistance to amphotericin B and azole antifungals. The true fungal nature of *Pneumocystis* was subsequently proven by ribosomal RNA sequencing.[44–46]
- The natural reservoir of the organism remains unknown but it has been found in the pulmonary system of many mammals, including humans.
- Most individuals are exposed to the organism at an early age, and clinically significant *Pneumocystis* **pneumonia is generally believed to represent reactivation of latent disease in a susceptible host**, although there has been recent evidence for airborne transmission.[44,46]
- Risk factors include HIV infection with CD4 count <200, hematologic and solid organ malignancy, use of immunosuppressive therapies, and transplantation.[45]
- Trimethoprim-sulfamethoxazole (TMP-SMX) is highly effective as **primary prophylaxis** against *P. jiroveci* and should be used in immunocompromised patients at risk of developing *Pneumocystis* pneumonia, including HIV-positive patients with CD4 counts <200 or there is a history of oral candidiasis, organ transplant recipients, patients on chemotherapeutic regimens, and patients on prolonged steroid regimens. Oral prophylaxis consists of one double-strength tablet (160 mg TMP with 800 mg SMX) daily or three times weekly.[44–46] Other possible prophylactic regimens include dapsone/pyrimethamine/leucovorin, pentamidine, and atovaquone.[45]

Diagnosis

- *Pneumocystis* pneumonia classically presents with fever, nonproductive cough, and dyspnea.
- Onset is insidious, with patients having symptoms for weeks to months before coming to medical attention.
- In a small percentage of patients, pleuritic chest pain with severe dyspnea is the presenting symptom due to spontaneous pneumothorax.
- On physical examination, lung auscultation is typically normal, and patients are often hypoxemic.

Diagnostic Testing

- Laboratory diagnostics are frequently nondiagnostic but may show an **elevated lactate dehydrogenase**.
- *Pneumocystis* remains difficult to reliably isolate in culture, so diagnosis continues to rely upon microscopic detection of the organism in a respiratory specimen, such as induced sputum or BAL fluid. The current gold standard technique uses **fluorescein-labeled monoclonal anti-*Pneumocystis* antibodies in histologic examination**. The sensitivity and specificity of BAL indirect fluorescence antibody staining are ~90–95% and are likely significantly less for induced sputum.[45,46]
- Newer techniques such as PCR testing are being explored.
- **CXR** classically shows bilateral, diffuse infiltrates, but may be normal in up to 40% of patients.
- **Chest CT** typically shows ground-glass opacities with patchy distribution that predominate the perihilar regions. Thin-walled cysts may be seen in 10–30% of patients, which predispose patients to developing pneumothoraces.[46]

Treatment

- Given its high mortality if untreated, **empiric treatment should be started once the diagnosis is considered**. Short courses of treatment <48 hours should not impair diagnosis.
- The treatment of choice remains **TMP-SMX** 15–20 mg/kg daily of the TMP component in oral or IV form divided into 3 or 4 doses. Treatment should be for 14 days in non–HIV-infected patients and 21 days in HIV-infected patients.[4,44–46]
- In those who are sulfa allergic or otherwise unable to tolerate TMP-SMX due to nephrotoxicity, Steven–Johnson syndrome, or bone marrow suppression, TMP plus dapsone, primaquine plus clindamycin, atovaquone, and pentamidine are alternative regimens.[4,44–46]
- In HIV-positive patients with arterial oxygen pressures ≤70 mm Hg or A–a gradients ≥35 mm Hg, **corticosteroids** are recommended; the regimen is prednisone 40 mg bid for 5 days, followed by 40 mg daily for 5 days, followed by prednisone 20 mg once daily for 11 days.[47]

SCEDOSPORIOSIS/PSEUDALLESCHERIASIS

General Principles

- The two primary pathogenic species of the *Scedosporium* genus are *S. apiospermum* and *S. prolificans*. The organisms are commonly found in the soil, sewage, manure, and stagnant or polluted water. Exposure occurs via inhalation or inoculation following trauma.[43,48–50]
- *S. apiospermum* is the asexual state of the ascomycete *Pseudallescheria boydii*.

- Infection with *P. boydii* produces two distinct diseases: **mycetoma and pseudallescheriasis (scedosporiosis)**.
- Disseminated fungemia occurs almost exclusively in immunosuppressed patients.
- Risk factors for developing disseminated disease include malignancy, cystic fibrosis, hematopoietic or solid organ transplantation, and near-drowning.[43,49,50]
- Outcomes in disseminated disease remain poor, with mortality exceeding 80%.[49]

Diagnosis

- **Mycetoma** is a rare, chronic, progressive granulomatous disease of the skin, SC tissue, and bone characterized by a triad of localized swelling, underlying sinus tracts, and production of pale grains or granules within the sinus tract. It most commonly occurs following **traumatic inoculation of fungal elements in otherwise healthy individuals.** Although the infection remains localized, it causes significant morbidity and disfigurement of the affected extremity.[48,50]
- **Pseudallescheriasis** encompasses all other infections caused by *P. boydii*, including **pneumonia, fungus balls, allergic bronchopulmonary disease, and disseminated disease.** Pneumonia occurs following inhalation of the organism into the lungs or sinuses. Patients present with fevers, chills, night sweats, weight loss, and hemoptysis. Fungus balls may occur in patients with prior cavitary lung disease.[48]
- Disseminated pseudallescheriasis disease has been described in patients with advanced HIV infection, recipients of solid organ transplantation, and patients with hematologic malignancy. Disseminated disease often involves the CNS as cerebral abscesses, although isolated CNS disease has been described in cases of near-drowning in contaminated water.

Diagnostic Testing

- Mycetoma is frequently a clinical diagnosis, although the organism may be visualized in the granules.
- Blood cultures, frequently remain negative in pseudallescheriasis, further complicating diagnosis.
- CXR findings in pseudallescheriasis are variable and nonspecific, and include pulmonary infiltrates, lobar consolidation, mass lesions, nodules with or without consolidation, necrotizing pneumonias, and pulmonary abscesses.
- Diagnosis of pseudallescheriasis relies upon **observation of the organism by histopathologic examination or isolation of the organism in culture**; molecular testing is not commercially available presently.[50]

Treatment

- Pseudallescheriasis is particularly difficult to treat due to its **resistance to multiple classes of antifungals.**[48]
- **Voriconazole** is the drug of choice but posaconazole has been used with success.[4,43,50]
- None of the other azoles, amphotericin B, nystatin, or flucytosine has shown appreciable in vitro activity.

REFERENCES

1. Zmeili OS, Soubani AO. Pulmonary aspergillosis: a clinical update. *Q J Med.* 2007;100:317–34.
2. Segal B. Aspergillosis. *N Engl J Med.* 2009;360(18):1870–84.
3. Denning DW. Chronic forms of pulmonary aspergillosis. *Clin Microbiol Infect.* 2001;7:25–31.
4. Limper AH, Knox KS, Sarosi GA, et al. An official American Thoracic Society statement: treatment of fungal infections in adult pulmonary and critical care patients. *Am J Respir Crit Care Med.* 2011;183:96–128.

5. Pfeiffer CE, Fine JP, Safdar N. Diagnosis of invasive aspergillosis using a galactomannan assay: a meta-analysis. *Clin Infect Dis.* 2006;42(10):1417–27.
6. Leeflang MM, Debets-Ossenkopp YJ, Visser CE, et al. Galactomannan detection for invasive aspergillosis in immunocompromized patients. *Cochrane Database Syst Rev.* 2008:CD007394.
7. D'Haese J, Theunissen K, Vermeulen E, et al. Detection of galactomannan in bronchoalveolar lavage fluid samples of patients at risk for invasive pulmonary aspergillosis: analytical and clinical validity. *J Clin Microbiol.* 2012;50:1258–63.
8. White PL, Wingard JR, Bretagne S, et al. Aspergillus polymerase chain reaction: systematic review of evidence for clinical use in comparison with antigen testing. *Clin Infect Dis.* 2015;61:1293–303.
9. Agarwal R. Allergic bronchopulmonary aspergillosis. *Chest.* 2009;135:805–26.
10. Schwartz HJ, Greenberger PA. The prevalence of allergic bronchopulmonary aspergillosis in patients with asthma, determined by serologic and radiologic criteria in patients at risk. *J Lab Clin Med.* 1991;117:138–42.
11. Saccente M, Woods GL. Clinical and laboratory update on blastomycosis. *Clin Microbiol Rev.* 2010;23:367–81.
12. McKinnell JA, Pappas PG. Blastomycosis: new insights into diagnosis, prevention, and treatment. *Clin Chest Med.* 2009;30(2):227–39.
13. Bradsher RW. Pulmonary blastomycosis. *Semin Respir Crit Care Med.* 2008;29(2):174–81.
14. Darouiche RO. Candida in the ICU. *Clin Chest Med.* 2009;30(2):287–93.
15. Cruciani M, Serpelloni G. Management of Candida infections in the adult intensive care unit. *Expert Opin Pharmacother.* 2008;9(2):175–91.
16. Haron E, Vartivarian S, Anaissie E, et al. Primary Candida pneumonia. Experience at a large cancer center and review of the literature. *Medicine (Baltimore).* 1993;72(3):137–42.
17. Azoulay E, Timsit JF, Tafflet M, et al. Candida colonization of the respiratory tract and subsequent pseudomonas ventilator-associated pneumonia. *Chest.* 2006;129:110–7.
18. Kontoyiannis DP, Reddy BT, Torres HA, et al. Pulmonary candidiasis in patients with cancer: an autopsy study. *Clin Infect Dis.* 2002;34:400–3.
19. Wood GC, Mueller EW, Croce MA, et al. Candida sp. isolated from bronchoalveolar lavage: clinical significance in critically ill trauma patients. *Intensive Care Med.* 2006;32:599–603.
20. Pappas PG, Kauffman CA, Andes D, et al. Clinical practice guidelines for the management of candidiasis: 2009 update by the Infectious Diseases Society of America. *Clin Infect Dis.* 2009;48: 503–35.
21. Galgiani JN, Ampel NM, Blair JE, et al. Coccidioidomycosis. *Clin Infect Dis.* 2005;41:1217–23.
22. Parish JM, Blair JE. Coccidioidomycosis. *Mayo Clin Proc.* 2008;83:343–9.
23. Spinello IM, Munoz A, Johnson RH. Pulmonary coccidioidomycosis. *Semin Respir Crit Care Med.* 2008;29:166–73.
24. Ampel NM. Coccidioidomycosis: a review of recent advances. *Clin Chest Med.* 2009;30:241–51.
25. Jarvis JN, Harrison TS. Pulmonary cryptococcosis. *Semin Respir Crit Care Med.* 2008;29:141–50.
26. Shirley RM, Baddley JW. Cryptococcal lung disease. *Curr Opin Pulm Med.* 2009;15:254–60.
27. Huston SM, Mody CH. Cryptococcosis: an emerging respiratory mycosis. *Clin Chest Med.* 2009;30:253–64.
28. Brizendine KD, Baddley JW, Papps PG. Pulmonary cryptococcosis. *Semin Respir Crit Care Med.* 2011;32:727–34.
29. Perfect JR, Dismukes WE, Dromer F, et al. Clinical practice guidelines for the management of cryptococcal disease: 2010 update by the Infectious Diseases Society of America. *Clin Infect Dis.* 2010;50:291–322.
30. Nucci M, Anaissie E. Fusarium infections in immunocompromised patients. *Clin Microbiol Rev.* 2007;20:695–704.
31. Ahearn DG, Zhang S, Stulting RD, et al. Fusarium keratitis and contact lens wear: facts and speculations. *Med Mycol.* 2008;46:397–410.
32. Nucci F, Nouér SA, Capone D, et al. Fusariosis. *Semin Respir Crit Care Med.* 2015;36:706–14.
33. McKinsay DS, McKinsey JP. Pulmonary histoplasmosis. *Semin Respir Crit Care Med.* 2011;32:735–44.
34. Kauffman CA. Histoplasmosis. *Clin Chest Med.* 2009;30:217–25.
35. Wheat LJ, Freifeld AG, Kleiman MB. Clinical practice guidelines for the management of patients with histoplasmosis: 2007 update by the Infectious Diseases Society of America. *Clin Infect Dis.* 2007;45:807–25.
36. Swartzentruber S, Rodes L, Kurkjian K, et al. Diagnosis of acute pulmonary histoplasmosis by antigen detection. *Clin Infect Dis.* 2009;49:1878–82.

37. Lee FYW, Mossad SB, Adal KA. Pulmonary mucormycosis: the last 30 years. *Arch Intern Med.* 1999;159:1301–9.
38. Sun HY, Singh N. Mucormycosis: its contemporary face and management strategies. *Lancet Infect Dis.* 2011;11:301–11.
39. Aboutanos MB, Joshi M, Scalea TM. Isolated pulmonary mucormycosis in a patient with multiple injuries: a case presentation and review of the literature. *J Trauma.* 2003;54:1016–19.
40. Pagano L, Offidani M, Fianchi L, et al. Mucormycosis in hematologic patients. *Haematologica.* 2004;89:207–14.
41. Lelievre L, Garcia-Hermoso D, Abdoul H, et al. Posttraumatic mucormycosis: a nationwide study in France and review of the literature. *Medicine (Baltimore).* 2014;93:395–404.
42. Pyrgos V, Shoham S, Walsh TJ. Pulmonary zygomycosis. *Semin Respir Crit Care Med.* 2008;29: 111–20.
43. Quan C, Spellberg B. Mucormycosis, pseudallescheriasis, and other uncommon mold infections. *Proc Am Thorac Soc.* 2010;7:210–5.
44. D'Avignon LC, Schofield CM, Hospenthal DR. Pneumocystis pneumonia. *Semin Respir Crit Care Med.* 2008;29:132–40.
45. Krajicek BJ, Thomas CF, Limper AH. Pneumocystis pneumonia: current concepts in pathogenesis, diagnosis, and treatment. *Clin Chest Med.* 2009;30:265–78.
46. Catherinot E, Lanternier F, Bougnoux ME, et al. Pneumocystis jirovecii pneumonia. *Infect Dis Clin N Am.* 2010;24:107–38.
47. Ewald H, Raatz H, Boscacci R, et al. Adjunctive corticosteroids for Pneumocystis jiroveci pneumonia in patients with HIV infection. *Cochrane Database Syst Rev.* 2015;4:CD006150.
48. Guarro J, Kantarcioglu AS, Horré R, et al. Scedosporium apiospermum: changing clinical spectrum of a therapy-refractory opportunist. *Med Mycol.* 2006;44:295–327.
49. Rodriguez-Tudela JL, Berenguer J, Guarro J, et al. Epidemiology and outcome of Scedosporium prolificans infection, a review of 162 cases. *Med Mycol.* 2009;47:359–70.
50. Cortez KJ, Roilides E, Quiroz-Telles F, et al. Infections caused by Scedosporium spp. *Clin Microbiol Rev.* 2008;21:157–97.

Viral Pulmonary Infections 16

Brian C. Keller and Steven L. Brody

GENERAL PRINCIPLES

- Viral respiratory infections account for nearly 50% of all acute respiratory illnesses. Most infections are self-limited.
- Approximately 200 antigenically distinct viruses cause multiple clinical syndromes ranging from common cold, pharyngitis, croup (i.e., laryngotracheobronchitis), tracheitis, bronchitis, bronchiolitis, and pneumonia.
- This chapter will introduce the major respiratory viruses encountered in clinical practice, assist in differentiating viral and bacterial respiratory infections, and guide antiviral therapy where specific therapy exists (Tables 16-1, 16-2, and 16-3).

Classification in the Normal Host

Upper Respiratory Tract Infections

- **Rhinosinusitis** is an upper respiratory tract infection (URTI) defined as inflammation of the mucosa of the nasal passage and paranasal sinuses lasting up to 4 weeks.
  - **The most common etiology is viral.** Bacteria can secondarily infect an inflamed sinus cavity, but this only accounts for 0.5–2% of cases.[1]
  - Since management of an **acute viral rhinosinusitis** (AVRS) is supportive, the main focus for the clinician should be in identifying those cases with **acute bacterial rhinosinusitis** (ABRS). Viral etiologies include rhinovirus, adenovirus, parainfluenza virus (PIV), influenza virus, human coronavirus (HCoV), and enterovirus.
  - The most common bacteria associated with ABRS are *Streptococcus pneumoniae, Haemophilus influenzae,* and *Moraxella catarrhalis.*
  - Significant complications of ABRS are rare and include orbital cellulitis, cavernous sinus thrombosis, osteomyelitis, meningitis, and brain abscess. These complications represent medical emergencies that require hospitalization.
  - **The diagnosis is clinical.** Acute rhinosinusitis of any etiology presents with three major symptoms: nasal congestion or blockage, purulent rhinorrhea, and facial pain or pressure.[2,3]
  - AVRS symptoms typically peak within 2–3 days of onset, decline gradually thereafter, and disappear within 10–14 days. Any pattern that deviates from the "classical" viral disease progression could suggest bacterial infection.
  - Three criteria may help distinguish ABRS from AVRS[4]:
    - Persistent signs and symptoms lasting for ≥10 days.
    - Severe symptoms for 3–4 consecutive days at the beginning of illness: high fever (≥39°C) and purulent rhinorrhea or facial pain.
    - Double-sickening: new onset of fever or increased nasal discharge following a typical viral URTI that lasted 5–6 days and was initially improving.
  - Imaging studies such as plain radiographs and CT scans are of little diagnostic value in uncomplicated acute rhinosinusitis and are not routinely recommended. An abnormal radiographic finding cannot distinguish a viral from bacterial etiology.[5]
  - Cultures obtained by sinus aspiration are not indicated for uncomplicated ABRS. They could be performed if the patient has failed to respond to initial empiric antimicrobial therapy.

TABLE 16-1 COMMON RESPIRATORY VIRUS INFECTIONS

Virus	Syndrome	Subtypes	Risk Factors	Incidence
Adenovirus	Keratoconjunctivitis, pharyngitis, croup, pharyngoconjunctival fever, tonsillitis, pneumonia	**Subgroup C** (AdV-1, 2, 5, 6), **subgroup B** (AdV-3, 7, 11, 16, 21), **subgroup E** (AdV-4)	Immunosuppressed, close quarters (barracks, daycares)	Year-round; peak in winter/spring
Coronavirus	URTI, pneumonia, ARDS	**SARS-CoV**, HCoV-OC43, HCoV-229E, HCoV-NL63, NCoV-HKU1	Household contacts, healthcare and laboratory workers	Late fall to early spring
CMV	Asymptomatic, mild URTI, pneumonia, systemic		Immunosuppressed, HIV	
Influenza virus	URTI, systemic symptoms, pneumonia, ARDS	A, B	Pregnant, elderly, young children	Late fall to early spring
hMPV	Common cold, bronchiolitis, pneumonia, otitis media (children)		Immunosuppressed, prematurity, cardiopulmonary disease, elderly	
PIV	Rhinitis, pharyngitis, croup, bronchitis, pneumonia	PIV1, PIV2, PIV3, PIV4	COPD, asthma	PIV1 biannual in fall; PIV3 annual in spring/summer
RSV	Rhinitis, conjunctivitis, otitis media, apnea (infants), bronchiolitis, pneumonia	A, B	Infant (<6 mo), cardiopulmonary disease, COPD, asthma, elderly, immunosuppressed	Late fall to early spring
Rhinovirus	Common cold, bronchitis, bronchiolitis, pneumonia	Many	COPD, asthma, cystic fibrosis	Year-round; peaks in fall and spring

URTI, upper respiratory tract infection; ARDS, acute respiratory distress syndrome; CMV, cytomegalovirus; HIV, human immunodeficiency virus; hMPV, human metapneumovirus; PIV, parainfluenza virus; COPD, chronic obstructive pulmonary disease; RSV, respiratory syncytial virus.

TABLE 16-2 DIAGNOSTIC STRATEGIES FOR VIRAL RESPIRATORY INFECTIONS

Diagnostic Test	Test Principle	Advantages	Disadvantages
PCR • Single • Multiplex	Amplification of a portion of the viral genome in a patient sample	High sensitivity High specificity Rapid Can detect multiple pathogens (multiplex) in single sample Can differentiate between viral strains/serotypes Can quantitate viral copies present in sample	Availability of equipment
Antibody-mediated • Direct or indirect antibody • ELISA	Antibody detection of viral protein in a patient sample or cell culture inoculated with the patient sample	Relatively good sensitivity Relatively good specificity	
Viral culture	Inoculation of cells with a patient sample and detection of virus by antibody or pathogenic change such as plaque formation	Specificity Confirms presence of live virus in sample	Sensitivity Incubation periods long Not all viruses culturable
Serology	Detection and titer of patient antibodies to a specific virus	Useful for epidemiologic surveys	Requires acute and convalescent sera Difficult to differentiate serotype
Cytopathology	Pathologic appearance of virus infection in patient cell sample	Can detect virus-induced cellular changes in absence of positive culture (e.g., CMV, RSV)	Requires tissue biopsy

PCR, polymerase chain reaction; ELISA, enzyme-linked immunosorbent assay; CMV, cytomegalovirus; RSV, respiratory syncytial virus.

TABLE 16-3 TARGETED ANTIVIRAL THERAPIES FOR VIRAL RESPIRATORY PATHOGENS

Virus	Vaccine	Antiviral Compound	Viral Target	Comment
Adenovirus	N	Cidofovir	DNA polymerase	For solid organ and bone marrow transplant patients
CMV	N	Ganciclovir	DNA polymerase	First-line therapy
		Cidofovir	DNA polymerase	
		Foscarnet	DNA polymerase	For ganciclovir resistance; nephrotoxic
HSV	N	Ganciclovir	DNA polymerase	First-line therapy
		Foscarnet	DNA polymerase	For ganciclovir resistance; nephrotoxic
Influenza	Y	Oseltamivir, zanamivir	Neuraminidase	Effective against influenza A and B; can be used for prophylaxis
		Amantadine, rimantadine	Ion channel	Second line due to viral resistance
PIV	N	Ribavirin	Purine RNA nucleotide	Infants, high-risk patients
RSV	N	Palivizumab	Fusion protein	Can be used for prophylaxis
		Ribavirin	Purine RNA nucleotide	Infants, high-risk patients
SARS	N	Nelfinavir, lopinavir, ritonavir	Protease	Randomized trials lacking
		Interferon		
		Convalescent plasma		
VZV	Y	Acyclovir	DNA polymerase	First-line therapy
		Foscarnet	DNA polymerase	For ganciclovir resistance; nephrotoxic

CMV, cytomegalovirus; HSV, herpes simplex virus; PIV, parainfluenza virus; RSV, respiratory syncytial virus; SARS, severe acute respiratory syndrome; VZV, varicella zoster virus.

- **Management of AVRS is supportive.**
  - Intranasal saline irrigation with either physiologic or hypertonic saline can be beneficial in symptomatic control, although the evidence supporting it is still very weak.[4]
  - Topical or systemic decongestants, antihistamines, and mucolytics are frequently used for symptom control. However, there are no significant data to support their use. Topical decongestants should not be used for more than 3 consecutive days to avoid rebound congestion and tachyphylaxis.
  - Intranasal corticosteroids have been shown to provide a modest relief in symptoms when compared to placebo and should certainly be strongly considered in patients with allergic rhinitis.[6]
  - Antibiotics may be beneficial for patients with a clinical diagnosis of ABRS and who have severe/persistent symptoms, temperature ≥39°C, or double-sickening. **Amoxicillin-clavulanate** is the drug of choice and doxycycline is an alternative. The infectious Disease Society of America (IDSA) recommends against trimethoprim-sulfamethoxazole and macrolides. High-dose amoxicillin-clavulanate is recommended where there is a ≥10% endemic rate of invasive penicillin-non-susceptible *S. pneumoniae,* severe infection (e.g., temperature ≥39°C, systemic toxicity, threat of suppurative complication), daycare attendance, age <2 or >65, recent hospitalization, antibiotic use during the past month, and immunocompromised state.[4]
- **Pharyngitis/tonsillitis**
  - The large majority of cases in adults are viral in etiology and do not require antibiotics. Antibiotics should be used in cases of Group A β-hemolytic streptococcal pharyngitis.
  - Symptoms strongly suggestive of a viral etiology include rhinorrhea, cough, oral ulcers, and hoarseness.[7]
  - The **modified Centor criteria** can be used to estimate the probability of streptococcal pharyngitis. One point each is given for the following: temperature >38°C, absence of cough, anterior cervical lymphadenopathy, and tonsillar swelling or exudate. The modification adds one point for age 3–14 and subtracts one point for age ≥45; age 15–44 has no effect on the score. The risk of streptococcal infection with ≤0 points is 1–2.5%; 1 point, 5–10%; 2 points, 11–17%; 3 points, 28–35%; and ≥4 points, 21–53%.[8–11]
  - Regardless, the IDSA recommends rapid strep testing whenever there is consideration of streptococcal pharyngitis, as **clinical features alone may cause under- and overdiagnosis.**[7]
  - Negative rapid strep tests should be confirmed with throat culture in children and adolescents due to a higher risk of developing acute rheumatic fever in these age groups. In adults, however, a backup culture is unnecessary because the pretest probability of rapid antigen detection testing is low to begin with.[7]
  - Common viral etiologies include rhinovirus, HCoV, adenovirus, herpes simplex virus (HSV), PIV, and influenza virus. Epstein–Barr virus (EBV), coxsackievirus, and acute HIV have also been identified.
  - Diagnostic testing of viral pharyngitis should be restricted to cases where symptoms fail to resolve within 1–2 weeks or for surveillance cultures during endemic virus outbreaks.
  - Treatment is mostly supportive with hydration, antipyretics, and analgesia. Topical anesthetics and lozenges alleviate throat pain.

Lower Respiratory Tract Infections

- **Bronchitis**
  - Bronchitis is classified as acute, which is essentially always infectious, or chronic.
    - Chronic bronchitis is a nonspecific clinical term with several meanings and is usually not due to infection.
    - In the general context of chronic obstructive pulmonary disease (COPD), it is defined as cough with sputum production for 3 months in each of the 2 prior years without other explanation—it may or may not be associated with demonstrable airflow obstruction on pulmonary function testing.

    - In an even broader context chronic bronchitis can imply a productive cough for >8–12 weeks. Chronic cough is discussed in detail in Chapter 8.
  - **Acute bronchitis is a self-limited infection** with cough as the predominant symptom usually lasting up to 3 weeks but can be as long as 6 weeks.[12] Significant rhinorrhea, fever, dyspnea, tachypnea, or hypoxemia suggests an alternative diagnosis.
  - **Ninety percent cases of acute bronchitis are viral** in nature, most commonly PIV, influenza, adenovirus, HCoV, human metapneumovirus (hMPV), PIV, respiratory syncytial virus (RSV), and rhinovirus.[13] When caused by bacteria, mostly the organisms are *M. pneumoniae, C. pneumoniae,* and *B. pertussis.* Superinfection with typical respiratory pathogens (i.e., *S. pneumoniae, H. influenzae,* and *M. catarrhalis*) is known to occur but are presumed to be very unusual.
  - Treatment is supportive with antitussives, expectorants, inhaled bronchodilators, and alternative therapies, despite a paucity of data to support their use.
  - **Routine use of antibiotics is discouraged.**[14–17] Likewise, there is limited value in treating smokers without COPD with antibiotics. An important exception is when *B. pertussis* is known or suspected in order to limit spread, particularly to unvaccinated infants. In this case, the treatment of choice is azithromycin. Unless started early, antibiotic treatment has little impact on the course of pertussis in typical, previously vaccinated adolescents and adults.[12]
  - Inhaled bronchodilators may be beneficial in patients who have airflow restriction and wheeze.[18]
- **Bronchiolitis**[19,20]
  - Bronchiolitis is an **almost exclusively viral** infection of the bronchioles and typically occurs in <2-year-old infants though it has been reported in adults.
  - Differentiated from bronchitis by respiratory symptoms, such as tachypnea and wheezing.
  - **RSV is the most common etiology**, but other viruses include rhinovirus, hMPV, and the more recently discovered human bocavirus (HBoV).
  - Treatment is primarily supportive with supplemental oxygen. Continuous positive airway pressure and high-flow nasal cannula therapy may provide effective ventilatory support and decrease the need for intubation.[21,22]
  - Several studies have evaluated the effectiveness of inhaled bronchodilators (epinephrine and albuterol), systemic corticosteroids, inhaled hypertonic saline, and heliox. None of these therapies demonstrated a consistent benefit on mortality or length of hospitalization.[23]
- **Pneumonia**[24]
  - Fifty percent to 70% of childhood pneumonia and up to 30% of adult pneumonia cases have been attributed to a viral etiology. Likely organisms include RSV, rhinovirus, influenza virus, hMPV, PIV, HBoV, and adenovirus.
  - Symptoms typically include fever, tachypnea, tachycardia, and clinical findings of lung involvement on examination. Other symptoms may include cough, rhinorrhea, sinus congestion, chills, and myalgias.
  - Physical examination and CXR may demonstrate consolidation due to alveolar or interstitial infiltrates in a lobar or multilobar distribution.
  - Viral pneumonia may be complicated by secondary bacterial pneumonia or concurrent viral and bacterial infection.
  - No specific clinical findings clearly differentiate viral from bacterial pneumonia. A high fever (>38.5°C), high respiratory rate, lobar consolidation on chest radiography and significantly elevated levels of C-reactive protein (CRP), white blood cell (WBC) count, and procalcitonin (PCT) suggest bacterial etiology.
  - Mild cases improve with supportive management on an outpatient basis, while severe cases may necessitate admission to an intensive care unit (ICU), respiratory support with mechanical ventilation or other aggressive measures.

- Empiric antibiotics should be given in cases of severe pneumonia while awaiting culture results. Once confirmatory diagnostic testing is completed, therapy should be narrowed to target the pathogen.[25]
- Specific antiviral therapies are discussed in more detail below.
- Systemic corticosteroid use for viral pneumonia is controversial and effects may vary depending on the particular viral etiology.

Respiratory Virus Infections in Chronic Airways Disease

- Viral lower respiratory tract infections in infants have been linked to later development of asthma in childhood, especially RSV and rhinovirus.
- Viral respiratory infections can lead to exacerbations of asthma and COPD and more severe respiratory infections and prolonged disease courses in these patients.
  - RSV, influenza virus, rhinovirus, and parainfluenza are common culprits.
  - Patients with acute COPD exacerbation are more likely to have viruses detected in airway samples than those with stable COPD.
- Influenza vaccinations of patients with asthma/COPD are recommended and may decrease the risk of exacerbations in some patients.

Respiratory Virus Infections in Special Adult Populations

- **Pregnancy**[26]
  - Susceptibility to virus infections is unchanged during pregnancy. However, the severity of viral respiratory infections can be worse in pregnancy, especially during the second and third trimesters.
  - Treatment is supportive with hydration, antipyretics, oxygen, blood pressure, and ventilatory support. Specific antiviral therapy should be used if available.
  - Antipyretics help to prevent fetal tachycardia and congenital abnormalities related to high maternal fevers.
  - Acyclovir is classified as category B but is recommended only for cases of serious infection and not for routine use in pregnancy.
  - **Ribavirin is a teratogen and is contraindicated in pregnancy.**
  - Controlled data on the safety of many other antiviral compounds in pregnancy are lacking. Most (oseltamivir, zanamivir, ganciclovir, cidofovir) are classified as category C by the U.S. Food and Drug Administration (FDA) and should be used only when the benefits of therapy outweigh the risks.
  - Killed or inactivated vaccines have been shown to be safe in pregnancy, especially during seasonal outbreaks when benefits outweigh small risks. **All pregnant females should be offered influenza vaccination.**
- **Immunocompromised**
  - Solid organ transplant recipients are at increased risk for developing cytomegalovirus (CMV), HSV-1, EBV, and varicella zoster virus (VZV), and more recently hMPV respiratory infections, especially in setting of prolonged respiratory failure in the ICU.
  - Adenovirus has also been documented in transplant recipients and may occur as a result of reactivation of latent virus.

Prevention

- **Vaccination**, when available, remains the best means of preventing viral respiratory illness, but few vaccines are available.
- **Influenza** vaccine
  - Vaccine strains may change yearly, so influenza vaccines must be administered annually.
  - Influenza virus vaccines are manufactured as an inactivated (killed virus) vaccine injection or as a live attenuated vaccine nasal spray.

  - High-dose influenza vaccination may be considered in adults ≥65 years old, though this is not expressly recommended by Centers for Disease Control (CDC) Advisory Committee on Immunization Practices.[27]
- **Varicella Zoster Virus** vaccine
  - A live, attenuated vaccine given in two doses. Dose #1 is generally administered to infants between 12 and 15 months. Dose #2 is given to children at 4–6 years.
  - In adults the vaccine is administered as a 2-dose regimen 4–8 weeks apart.
  - Contraindicated in pregnant women, immunosuppressed patients, and patients who have other active illnesses.
- All vaccines are contraindicated in patients who are allergic to specific vaccine components (e.g., eggs in the case of most influenza virus vaccines) or who have had a severe allergic reaction to a previous dose of the particular vaccine. Flublok is a recently approved egg-free, trivalent, recombinant hemagglutinin (HA), injectable influenza vaccine.
- Additional information regarding specific vaccines is available on the CDC website, www.cdc.gov/vaccines. Accessed 9/10/15.

Diagnosis

- Diagnosis may be possible, based on clinical grounds alone and particularly during seasonal outbreaks (Table 16-2).
- Radiographic findings are not pathognomonic for specific viral etiologies.
- Diagnostic specimens can be collected from nasopharyngeal or oral swabs, nasal washings, induced sputum, nasopharyngeal or tracheal aspirates, bronchial washings, bronchoalveolar lavage (BAL), endobronchial brush biopsy, or lung biopsy (transbronchial vs. percutaneous needle biopsy), depending on the examination findings and severity of disease.
  - In children, nasopharyngeal swabs and washings have similar sensitivities for detection of respiratory viruses by polymerase chain reaction (PCR).
  - In adults, nasopharyngeal swab is more sensitive than throat swab.
- Viral culture remains the gold standard for diagnosing many viral infections. However, prolonged incubation times required to grow the virus in the laboratory preclude the utility of viral culture in many cases.
- Multiplex PCR testing is becoming more common, due to its high sensitivity, specificity, and rapidity.
- Direct and indirect fluorescence antibody-based assays and enzyme-linked immunosorbent assays (ELISA) are also useful for detection of certain viral pathogens.
- Cytopathology may also aid diagnosis by demonstrating cytopathologic effect (adenovirus), giant cells (CMV) or syncytial formation (RSV) in tissue specimens.

Treatment

Supportive Care

- Supportive care with adequate hydration and symptom control are mainstays of treatment.
  - Nasal steroids, antipyretics, antihistamines, decongestants, analgesics, and bronchodilators are sometimes helpful in appropriate patients.
  - Steroids may be useful for significant wheezing.
  - Nebulized epinephrine can be used in cases of stridor.
- In severe cases, transfer to an ICU and ventilatory support with noninvasive or invasive mechanical ventilation may be necessary.

Specific Antiviral Therapies

- Targeted antiviral therapies exist for some viral respiratory illnesses such as influenza, CMV, HSV, RSV, adenovirus, and severe acute respiratory syndrome coronavirus (SARS-CoV). Others are currently in development.

- These drugs target specific viral proteins including DNA polymerases, proteases, ion channels, and neuraminidase (NA) (in the case of influenza virus).
- Newer therapies such as palivizumab are monoclonal antibodies directed against viral proteins (RSV).
- Table 16-3 lists common viral respiratory pathogens, directed antiviral therapies and vaccines, if available.

SPECIAL CONSIDERATIONS: SPECIFIC VIRAL PATHOGENS

Adenovirus

- **Virology:** Adenovirus is a nonenveloped, double-stranded DNA virus. There are 51 different serotypes with 6 subgroups, A through F. Adenoviruses of subgroup C primarily infect the upper respiratory tract while viruses in subgroups B and E cause disease of the lower respiratory tract. They can integrate into the host genome leading to latent infection.[28]
- **Epidemiology**
  - Adenoviruses have a worldwide distribution, and infections are more frequent in winter and spring.
  - Up to 5% of acute respiratory infections in children are attributed to adenoviruses so that by age 10 most individuals have serologic evidence of adenoviral infection.
  - Adenovirus is commonly encountered in households and daycare centers where young children are found.
  - Epidemics of adenovirus acute respiratory disease (ARD) have been reported among military recruits, immunocompromised patients, and in daycare settings.
  - Transmission occurs via fomites, aerosolized particles, and the fecal–oral route. Adenoviruses can cause persistent infections, and the virus may be shed in the feces for months.
  - Adenoviral infections have been transmitted to kidney and liver transplant recipients, suggesting that reactivation of latent virus (possibly in the transplanted organ) may be another important mode of transmission.
  - Vertical transmission has been reported in infants who were exposed to infected cervical secretions.
- **Clinical presentation**
  - The presentation depends on the age and immune status of the infected host.
  - Adenovirus can cause upper respiratory tract illnesses such as coryza, pharyngitis, and croup but can also cause lower respiratory tract disease—that is, laryngotracheobronchitis, bronchiolitis, and pneumonia.
  - **Pharyngoconjunctival fever** is an adenovirus syndrome presenting with pharyngitis, conjunctival injection, fever, and cervical lymphadenopathy.
  - **Keratoconjunctivitis** presenting as pink eye without purulent discharge is caused by adenovirus serotypes 8, 19, and 37.
  - Gastrointestinal (GI) symptoms are caused by other adenovirus serotypes.
  - Adenovirus is **the most common cause of tonsillitis in infants**. Exudative tonsillitis and palpable cervical adenopathy may be seen, making differentiation from strep throat in older children difficult.
  - Pneumonia is most common in infants but rare in immunocompetent adults.
  - Complications include bronchiectasis in children and **ARD** in young adults. ARD is especially common in close-quarter dwellings. Patients with ARD develop fever, pharyngitis, cough, hoarseness, and conjunctivitis.
  - Bone marrow transplant patients may develop a wide range of respiratory clinical syndromes, including pneumonia. Solid organ transplant recipients may develop asymptomatic shedding, all manner of respiratory syndromes, and even fatal

disseminated disease. Adenoviral pneumonia is a well-known early complication of lung transplantation.

- **Diagnosis**
  - The diagnosis is difficult to make on clinical grounds alone. PCR-based assays are the test of choice.
  - Viral culture is the historical gold standard. All adenoviruses except serotypes 40 and 41 cause a characteristic cytopathic effect in culture. Samples for culture can be obtained from nasopharyngeal swabs or aspirates, throat washings or swabs, rectal swabs, urine, CSF, or tissue biopsies. Cultures may take up to a week for completion and may not detect adenovirus in cases where there may be a low viral load (e.g., immunocompromised hosts). Because prolonged shedding may be seen in immunocompromised patients without overt disease, culture positivity should be interpreted with respect to the clinical situation.
  - Histopathology may provide definitive diagnosis of adenovirus in tissue biopsies and can be supplemented by other detection techniques (PCR, immunohistochemistry).
- **Treatment**
  - Treatment is supportive.
  - In case reports and small series of solid organ transplant and bone marrow transplant patients, cidofovir has shown the most promise in treating adenoviral infections, especially when therapy is initiated early.[28]
  - Randomized, controlled trials of antiviral agents are presently lacking, and data on other antiviral agents including ribavirin and vidarabine are conflicting.

Coronavirus and SARS Virus

- **Virology**
  - HCoV are positive-sense, single-stranded RNA viruses encased in a crown-like envelope with a diameter of 80–160 nm.
  - HCoV-OC43, HCoV-229E, and the recently identified HCoV-NL63 and HCoV-HKU1 strains cause community-acquired respiratory infections.
  - HCoV also include SARS-CoV, the causative agent of the SARS epidemic.
  - Primary sites of replication include the lungs and intestinal tract.
- **Epidemiology**
  - HCoV were initially discovered in the 1960s and are responsible for 10–20% of cases of the common cold.
  - Respiratory infections are spread in a manner similar to that of rhinoviruses, via direct contact with infected secretions or via large aerosol droplets.
  - In temperate climates, they cause disease in late fall, winter, and early spring and are associated with outbreaks every 2–4 years.
  - In late 2002 and into 2003, an outbreak of SARS-CoV originated in China and Hong Kong and then spread globally causing more than 8000 cases with a case fatality rate of 9.6%.[29] China, Taiwan, Hong Kong, Singapore, and Canada experienced the highest number of cases. Initial human cases of SARS-CoV appeared to be acquired from infected civets, although more recent data suggest that bats may be the natural reservoir for the virus. Those at increased risk include wildlife handlers, household contacts, healthcare workers, and laboratory workers.[30]
  - HCoV are stable at room temperature for 7 days but can be inactivated by common hospital disinfectants.
- **Clinical presentation**
  - In adults, HCoV causes an acute URTI that is **very similar to rhinovirus infection**. HCoV are also implicated as important causes of acute otitis media in children and triggers of asthma exacerbations.

- Newer strains have been shown to cause LRTI, including severe pneumonia. Much of the pathogenesis is believed to derive from a significant host response to infection rather than from direct damage by the virus itself.
- Potential complications include secondary bacterial infection, acute respiratory distress syndrome (ARDS), and acute respiratory failure requiring mechanical ventilation.

- **Diagnosis**
  - RT-PCR is the standard diagnostic test for HCoV.
  - Other diagnostic tests include serologic detection and antigen detection but these are less useful clinically.
  - For SARS-CoV, the diagnosis should be considered in patients at risk for SARS exposure (wildlife handlers from Southeast Asia, close family contacts, healthcare workers, and laboratory personnel) who present with a rapidly progressive pneumonia.
- **Treatment**
  - Patients with suspected HCoV, including SARS, should be placed on contact, droplet, and airborne precautions. This is especially important as up to one-third of SARS cases occurred in healthcare workers.
  - **Treatment is primarily supportive** with symptom management, hydration, and ventilatory support. One study showed that early noninvasive ventilation in patients with severe SARS-CoV disease reduced the need for intubation and improved mortality.
  - There are no randomized controlled trials of antiviral therapies in HCoV infection. Data from retrospective studies and case series during the SARS epidemic are inconclusive in regard to effective therapies.[31]
    - Promising treatments have included viral protease inhibitors (lopinavir/ritonavir or nelfinavir), interferon, and convalescent plasma. NO may also improve outcome in severe respiratory failure.
    - Combination therapy with ribavirin and/or corticosteroids may also be beneficial. Further studies are needed for confirmation.
    - Newer directed therapies including monoclonal antibodies targeting the SARS-CoV S protein or its receptor, angiotensin-converting enzyme 2 (ACE2) are in development.

Cytomegalovirus

- **Virology:** CMV, a member of the *Herpesviridae* family, is a large, enveloped double-stranded DNA virus with a diameter of 120–200 nm.
- **Epidemiology**
  - **Active CMV is often found in immunocompromised patients.** It can affect multiple organ systems but the lung, GI tract, and kidney are most common.
  - CMV can also be a source of severe viral pneumonia, even in immunocompetent individuals.
  - Seroprevalence increases with age and number of sexual partners.
- **Clinical presentation**
  - Primary CMV infection usually is asymptomatic or mild URTI in immunocompetent hosts, after which the virus becomes latent. CMV community-acquired pneumonia, however, has been reported in immunocompetent hosts and may be severe.[32]
  - Severe disease tends to occur in immunocompromised patients. Solid organ and bone marrow transplantation patients are at highest risk of infection during the first 100 days after transplantation.
  - CMV can also involve the liver, spleen, GI tract, central nervous system, or bone marrow.
  - CMV has been shown in multiple studies to infect alveolar epithelial cells, and the main pulmonary manifestation is CMV pneumonitis, which may occur in up to 15% of transplant populations. The disease is usually severe with hypoxemia, a high incidence of respiratory failure and a mortality rate exceeding 80%. Patients may present with focal infiltrates, bilateral patchy infiltrates, or diffuse interstitial infiltrates.

  - CMV may reactivate in the chronically ventilated ICU patient.
  - Pulmonary manifestations are also seen in HIV patients but have become less prevalent with the advent of highly active antiretroviral therapy. CMV is often identified in patients presenting with *Pneumocystis jiroveci* pneumonia, although the virus may not contribute to the severity of disease or symptoms.
  - Clinical laboratory features of CMV include elevation of serum transaminases, relative lymphopenia, atypical lymphocytes, and thrombocytopenia and suggest CMV over other viral infections.
- **Diagnosis**
  - PCR has a high sensitivity and specificity for detecting viremia and is useful for monitoring resolution, although serology demonstrating an elevated CMV IgM level or fourfold increase in IgG levels is still the most common diagnostic test.
  - Isolation of CMV from sputum culture, bronchial washings, and BAL fluid is diagnostic, but CMV grows very slowly and confirmation can take several days and up to 3 weeks.
  - CMV pneumonitis is confirmed histologically (obtained by bronchoscopy or surgery) as giant CMV-infected pneumocyte inclusions. Immunohistochemical stains for CMV have also been developed.
- **Treatment**[33]
  - First line: **ganciclovir** (5 mg/kg IV q12h).
  - Oral **valganciclovir** (900 mg PO q12h) can also be used in some cases, or as an extension following induction therapy with IV ganciclovir. Therapy typically lasts 21 days.
  - Other agents effective against CMV include foscarnet, cidofovir, and CMV immune globulin (cytogam).
    - Foscarnet is nephrotoxic and usually reserved for cases of ganciclovir-resistant CMV.
    - Cytogam is reserved for cases of life-threatening CMV infection (e.g., transplant patients with severe disease). See Chapter 29, for more information on diagnosis and treatment of CMV infection in this patient population.

Herpesviruses: HSV-1, EBV, VZV

- The *Herpesviridae* family includes HSV-1, HSV-2, VZV, EBV, and human herpesvirus-8 (HHV-8, the causative agent of Kaposi sarcoma).
- In certain ICU populations (immunocompromised, ARDS, chronically ventilated, postsurgical, or burn), HSV-1 is an important cause of upper (and possibly lower) respiratory tract infection.
- EBV infection has been implicated in the development of posttransplant lymphoproliferative disease (see Chapter 29).
- VZV manifests with chickenpox on primary exposure and as zoster with reactivation. Primary pneumonias are rare but have a high mortality rate. Immunocompromised patients are at greatest risk of VZV pulmonary infection. Infections are treated with IV acyclovir. Preventative measures in immunocompromised patients may include vaccination of seronegative patients before transplantation, administration of varicella zoster immune globulin to exposed patients, or the use of prophylactic acyclovir.

Influenza Virus

- **Virology**
  - Influenza is an acute respiratory illness caused by type A or type B influenza virus infection.
  - They are negative-strand, segmented RNA virus in the *Orthomyxoviridae* family, subdivided into antigenic subgroups based on the properties of the HA and NA glycoproteins.
  - Influenza viruses circulate in humans, birds, and swine. New influenza strains can arise from reassortment of viral gene products in coinfected organisms (e.g., a pig coinfected with an avian strain and a swine strain).

- **Epidemiology**
  - Influenza traditionally occurs in a seasonal, epidemic form in the winter months.
  - Pandemic influenza arises periodically with strains more highly pathogenic than the seasonal variants (e.g., 1918 H1N1 Spanish influenza pandemic that resulted in 20–40 million deaths worldwide, 1957 H2N2 Asian influenza, 1968 H3N2 Hong Kong influenza, and 2009 H1N1 influenza).[34–36]
- **Clinical presentation**
  - Most cases of influenza are mild, self-limited upper respiratory infections. The incubation period ranges from 1 to 3 days.
  - Typical symptoms include fever, myalgias, fatigue, and headache, with respiratory symptoms such as rhinorrhea, sore throat, and cough. GI symptoms, including vomiting, and diarrhea, may also occur, especially in children.
  - Severe cases may present with dyspnea, hemoptysis, purulent sputum, rapidly progressive hypoxemia, primary and secondary pneumonia, respiratory failure, ARDS, multiorgan failure, and even death.
  - Pneumonia may be primary (viral pneumonitis) or secondary to bacterial coinfection, notably *Staphylococcus aureus, S. pneumoniae, S. pyogenes,* and *H. influenzae.* Patients with primary influenza pneumonia usually have persistent or worsening symptoms, very high fevers, and dyspnea with or without cyanosis, whereas patients with secondary bacterial pneumonias may show some improvement in their influenza-related symptoms before developing worsening fever and respiratory complaints.
  - Postinfluenza asthenia refers to weakness and fatigue after an influenza infection that may last several weeks.
- **Diagnosis**
  - Clinical symptoms during seasonal epidemics provide a high degree of clinical suspicion.
  - Common radiographic findings include bilateral patchy, interstitial, and alveolar infiltrates, predominantly in the lower lobes. Ground-glass opacities may also be present.
  - Rapid detection of influenza can be made by RT-PCR. Multiple testing of samples from various sites (nasopharyngeal swab, tracheal aspirate, and bronchial lavage) can improve diagnostic yield.
  - Viral culture may take up to a week for positive identification and is thus not as useful.
- **Treatment**
  - Treatment is largely supportive.
  - Acetaminophen is recommended over salicylates (to avoid Reye syndrome in patients <18 years old.) Antitussives may also be used, and adequate hydration is essential.
  - Antibiotics are reserved for bacterial superinfections, including pneumonia, otitis media, and sinusitis.
  - NA inhibitors are most effective if prescribed with 48 hours of symptom onset.
    - **Oseltamivir** (75 mg bid × 5 days) has activity against both type A and type B influenza viruses and can reduce viral shedding, symptom duration, length of hospitalization, and even mortality in severe cases. Treatment is generally 5 days in length. Higher doses (150 mg bid) and longer durations can be used in more severe disease.[37–39]
    - **Zanamivir** (10 mg inhaled bid for 5 days) can be used to treat influenza in patients over 7 years old. It can cause bronchospasm and should be avoided in patients with chronic pulmonary disease.[39]
  - Amantadine (100 mg PO bid for 5 days) and rimantadine (100 mg PO bid for 5 days) are active only against influenza A, are less effective (75–100%), and recommended as second-line agents. These medications act against the viral M2 protein.
- **Prevention**
  - **Immunization is the most effective prevention for influenza.** Options include injectable inactivated split-virus injected (recommended for all people >6 months old) and

live attenuated virus inhaled (for healthy, nonpregnant people aged 2–49). Live vaccines should be avoided in patients who are immunosuppressed. As previously noted, flublok is a recently approved egg-free, trivalent, recombinant HA, injectable influenza vaccine.
  - Flu vaccines are recommended, especially in pregnant women, children <5 years old, adults >50 years old, people with chronic medical conditions (e.g., chronic respiratory disease, cardiovascular disease, diabetes, obesity, renal disease, immunosuppression), healthcare workers, residents of long-term care facilities, and people who live with or care for patients at high risk for severe influenza (including children under 6 months of age who cannot be vaccinated).[40]
  - Flu vaccines are not recommended for patients with serious documented allergies to eggs or egg components (excepting flublok), previous reaction to an influenza vaccine, children younger than 6 months old, and patients who are acutely ill.
  - **Chemoprophylaxis** can be used with both oseltamivir (in patients ≥1 year old) and zanamivir (in patients >5 years old). Dosing is once daily for 7 days. In long-term care facilities and hospitals, chemoprophylaxis should be provided for a minimum of 2 weeks and up to 1 week after the date of the last diagnosed case.[41]

Metapneumovirus

- **Virology:** hMPV is a member of the *Paramyxoviridae* (like RSV and PIV).
- **Epidemiology:** It was discovered in 2001 and is now recognized as a cause of upper and lower respiratory tract infections, primarily in children of whom 90–100% have evidence of infection by age 10. hMPV has been implicated in 10% of all hospitalized cases of respiratory viral infections.
- **Clinical presentation** ranges from the cold-like symptoms to bronchiolitis and severe pneumonia. Risk factors for severe disease include immunosuppression, elderly, and prematurity and underlying cardiopulmonary disease in children. hMPV can also trigger exacerbations of asthma and other chronic cardiopulmonary diseases.
- **Diagnosis** is by RT-PCR, direct immunofluorescence, and/or viral culture.
- **Treatment:** There are no approved targeted therapies, although studies of ribavirin and neutralizing monoclonal antibodies are in progress.[42]

Nipah Virus

- Nipah virus (NiV), like hMPV, is a newly emergent member of the *Paramyxoviridae* family and *Henipavirus* genus. Hendra virus and Cedar virus are also a member of this genus.
- The original outbreak of NiV in Malaysia and Singapore in 1999 had a case fatality rate of nearly 40%. More recent outbreaks in Bangladesh and India have been more severe with case fatality rates reaching 90%. There is concern NiV could be spread due to the global nature of today's transportation systems.[43,44]
- Transmission is likely through infected secretions, foodborne and fomite transmissions.
- Clinical presentation is rapidly progressive encephalitis and/or severe respiratory illness.
- Currently there is no treatment or vaccine for NiV. Reports from the original outbreaks suggested that patients treated with ribavirin had lower mortality but further study is warranted.

Parainfluenza Virus

- **Virology:** PIV is another member of *Paramyxoviridae* with four major serotypes: PIV1, PIV2, PIV3, and PIV4. PIV3 is the most prevalent serotype, with 90–100% of children being seropositive by age 5.
- **Epidemiology**
  - PIV causes ~20% of acute respiratory tract infections in hospitalized children, ranking as the second most common etiology for lower respiratory tract infections in this

patient population. Up to 10% of acute lower respiratory tract infections in hospitalized adults can be attributed to PIV.
  - Spread of the virus occurs through large droplet inhalation, and the virus is easily spread by person-to-person contact.
  - PIV1 causes epidemics every 2 years during the fall, while PIV3 occurs in annual spring and summer epidemics. PIV2 and PIV4 occur in less predictable patterns. However, studies in adults suggest year-round circulation of all four serotypes.[45]
- **Clinical presentation**
  - PIV causes upper and lower respiratory infections in adults and children. Primarily infects nasal and oropharyngeal epithelial cells, with subsequent distal spread to the large and small airways. The incubation period is typically 2–8 days.
  - **PIV1 and PIV2 are the primary causes of childhood croup** (fever, rhinitis, pharyngitis, with a barking cough). Symptoms last up to 4 days. Stridor, dyspnea, and respiratory distress can develop in severe cases.
  - PIV3 is associated with bronchiolitis and pneumonia and is often mistaken for RSV infection.
  - In adults, PIV usually causes a mild URTI but lower respiratory disease is possible, especially in the setting of chronic lung disease.
  - PIV has been associated with COPD and asthma exacerbations.
  - Immunocompromised hosts are susceptible to serious PIV infections, including pneumonia or even disseminated infections. Bone marrow, stem cell, and less commonly solid organ transplantation recipients may have PIV infections and a relatively high mortality.[45–47]
  - Complications may include secondary bacterial pneumonia, sinusitis, otitis media, meningitis, pericarditis, myocarditis, and Guillain–Barré syndrome. The last three complications are very rare.
- **Diagnosis** is often made clinically, although RT-PCR has become more common. As with other respiratory viruses, viral culture is the gold standard but clinically not useful.
- **Treatment**
  - Treatment is largely supportive.
  - There are no antiviral agents with specific activity against PIV. Ribavirin has been used to treat bone marrow transplant recipients but few data exist on its efficacy. Combination therapy with ribavirin and immunoglobulin has not altered the duration of illness or mortality in clinical studies.[48]
  - **Steroids** (dexamethasone 0.6 mg/kg PO or IV) recommended in children with severe croup can decrease length of hospitalization, need for additional therapies, and need for intubation. Nebulized epinephrine can be added if stridor or respiratory distress is present.[49]

Respiratory Syncytial Virus

- **Virology**
  - RSV is an enveloped, single-stranded, negative-sense RNA virus of the *Paramyxoviridae* family.
  - RSV can be divided into two distinct antigenic groups (RSV-A and RSV-B), both of which are present during outbreaks.
  - RSV primarily infects airway epithelial cells. Following cellular entry and replication, the virus is transmitted from cell to cell through fusion of neighboring cells into large multinucleated syncytia.
- **Epidemiology**
  - RSV is the most common cause of LRIs in infants and young children. Highest rates of illness are seen in infants aged 1–6 months, with peak rates occurring at 3 months. Risk factors include preterm birth, male sex, immunodeficiency, lack of breastfeeding, and overcrowding.[50]

- In adults, RSV is an underrecognized cause of LRI with >5% of adult LRIs attributable to RSV, especially elderly and immunocompromised patients.[51]
- Outbreaks occur in late fall through early spring.
- RSV transmission occurs by contact with respiratory secretions or large respiratory droplets and fomites.
- Previous infection with RSV does not confer complete protection against reinfection. Humoral immunity, however, may reduce the severity of subsequent RSV infections. Elderly patients who have lower antibody titers are more likely to develop symptomatic disease.

- **Clinical Presentation**
  - RSV URTIs present with cough, coryza, rhinorrhea, conjunctivitis, and otitis media.
  - Apneic episodes may be seen in infants admitted with RSV infections but the exact mechanism remains unclear and may precipitate sudden infant death syndrome. Prevalence estimates for apnea vary widely.[20]
  - **LRIs present with bronchospasm, bronchiolitis**, pneumonia, and in severe cases, respiratory failure. Patients at risk for lower respiratory tract disease include infants (<6 months of age), children with underlying structural lung and heart disease, patients of any age group with significant asthma or COPD, institutionalized elderly patients, and immunocompromised patients.
  - RSV has been associated with the development of asthma in children.[51]
- **Diagnosis**
  - RT-PCR is the diagnostic test of choice because of its rapidity, sensitivity, and specificity.
  - Viral culture from nasal or throat swabs, tracheal aspirates, bronchial washings, or BAL specimens remains the gold standard for diagnosis. Culture may take days to weeks before identification of virus by immunofluorescence staining.
  - Diagnostic serology is unhelpful because individuals may have high levels of antibodies in circulation from previous RSV infections.
- **Treatment**
  - Treatment is supportive with oxygen supplementation and fluid resuscitation.[20]
  - Bronchodilators may be used in adults with underlying asthma/COPD. Nebulized epinephrine may improve airway obstruction in RSV bronchiolitis. Neither is recommended for infants and children with bronchiolitis.[20]
  - Mechanical ventilation may be required in some patient with severe disease.
  - The evidence for steroids is not compelling but may still be used in cases of significant wheezing.[20,23]
  - **Ribavirin**, a synthetic nucleoside analog, may be considered in:
    - Infants with structural heart or lung disease, immunosuppressed, or with mechanical ventilation.
    - In bone marrow and stem cell transplantation recipients, the early use of ribavirin has been shown to reduce morbidity and mortality compared to historic controls.[52–54]
    - Ribavirin has no proven efficacy in immunocompetent adults but use may be considered in severe cases of respiratory failure.
    - Ribavirin is contraindicated in pregnancy.
  - **Palivizumab**, an RSV-specific humanized monoclonal antibody, is primarily used for infants.
    - In immunocompromised adults, studies of combined therapy of palivizumab and ribavirin suggest improved outcome.[55–57]
    - Motavizumab, a second-generation RSV-specific monoclonal antibody, is currently in trials.[58]
    - Preventive palivizumab is recommended during the first year of life for infants with hemodynamically significant heart disease or chronic lung disease of prematurity.[20]

- Other therapies currently in development include RSV fusion protein inhibitors, RSV polymerase inhibitors, small interfering RNA (siRNA), leukotriene antagonists, and surfactant.
- RSV IV immunoglobulin (IVIG) is probably not helpful and is no longer available.[59]

Rhinovirus

- **Virology**
  - Rhinoviruses are nonenveloped, single-stranded RNA viruses in the *Picornaviridae* family.
  - They preferentially grow at 33–35°C, the temperature in the nasal passages and upper airways.
  - There are 100 different serotypes in RV-A and RV-B. A third lineage, RV-C, discovered in 2006 includes over 50 strains. No one strain predominantly circulates at any one time.
- **Epidemiology**
  - **Rhinoviruses are responsible for about half of common colds.**
  - Infection rates are highest among young children and infants, with an average of six infections per year. Infection rates decrease with advancing age except in the 20s, when another peak is seen. Risks for infections include contact with small children aged <6 years.
  - Rhinovirus infections peak in autumn and spring in North America and Europe. They are more active during the rainy season in tropical regions of the world.
  - Transmission is via direct contact with infected secretions. Subsequent self-inoculation of the nasal or conjunctival mucosa leads to infection. Transmission by fomites and aerosolized virus may also occur.
  - Despite any anecdotal evidence and popular beliefs, cold temperature exposure, fatigue, and sleep deprivation have not been associated with increased rates of transmission.
  - **Diligent hand washing** can effectively prevent the spread of rhinoviruses.
- **Clinical presentation**
  - Incubation period is 1–2 days.
  - Symptoms may include rhinorrhea and sneezing (50–70%), sore throat (50%), malaise, mild headaches, and otitis media in some cases. Symptoms generally last about a week to 10 days but minor symptomatology can linger longer and viral shedding may occur up to 3 weeks following infection.[60]
  - Hoarseness and cough are less common but can occur due to upper airway irritation or concurrently with sinusitis and bronchitis. Fever, chills, and myalgias are unusual and should prompt the clinician to search for other potential causes, such as influenza.
  - The nasal mucosa becomes edematous and hyperemic and produces a mucoid discharge. The nasal turbinates often become engorged, which can lead to sinus cavity obstruction and occasionally bacterial superinfection.
  - Rhinovirus may also infect the lower respiratory tract, although causation is hard to discern as coinfection with other viruses is fairly common.
  - Rhinovirus infections are associated with exacerbations of asthma, COPD, and cystic fibrosis.[60]
- **Diagnosis:** Rhinovirus infection is usually diagnosed clinically as a common cold, although with poor specificity. Viral diagnosis can be confirmed by RT-PCR from nasal swab or nasal washing but generally unnecessary.
- **Treatment** is supportive and symptom based.

Complications

- **Postviral cough**
  - Cough is a common symptom during acute viral upper and lower respiratory tract infection.

- **Many cases of subacute cough (persisting for 3–8 weeks) are due to postviral cough**, which may not respond well to common antitussive therapy.[61]
- Although postviral cough is the most common etiology for subacute cough, other potential causes including postnasal drip, gastroesophageal reflux disease, eosinophilic airway inflammation, angiotensin-converting enzyme (ACE) inhibitor, and *Bordetella pertussis* should be evaluated and ruled out, particularly if the cough persists beyond 8 weeks.
- In patients with asthma or COPD, cough may be a manifestation of prolonged exacerbation. In these patients, spirometry can guide therapy.

- **Postviral wheeze/asthma**
  - Postviral wheezing/asthma is more common in children and may continue up to 1 year after resolution of the infection.
  - For most patients wheezing will spontaneously resolve over time.
  - Multiple studies have implicated infantile rhinovirus and RSV infections in the subsequent development of asthma in children and teens.[62]

REFERENCES

1. Gwaltney JM Jr. Acute community-acquired sinusitis. *Clin Infect Dis.* 1996;23:1209–23.
2. Rosenfeld RM, Andes D, Bhattacharyya N, et al. Clinical practice guideline: adult sinusitis. *Otolaryngol Head Neck Surg.* 2007;137:S1–31.
3. Meltzer EO, Hamilos DL. Rhinosinusitis diagnosis and management for the clinician: a synopsis of recent consensus guidelines. *Mayo Clin Proc.* 2011;86:427–43.
4. Chow AW, Benninger MS, Brook I, et al. IDSA clinical practice guideline for acute bacterial rhinosinusitis in children and adults. *Clin Infect Dis.* 2012;54:e72–112.
5. Gwaltney JM Jr, Phillips D, Miller D, et al. Computed tomographic study of the common cold. *N Engl J Med.* 1994;330:25–30.
6. Zalmanovici Trestioreanu A, Yaphe J. Intranasal steroids for acute sinusitis. *Cochrane Database Syst Rev.* 2013;12:CD005149.
7. Shulman ST, Bisno AL, Clegg HW, et al. Clinical practice guideline for the diagnosis and management of group A streptococcal pharyngitis: 2012 update by the Infectious Diseases Society of America. *Clin Infect Dis.* 2012;55:1279–82.
8. Centor RM, Witherspoon JM, Dalton HP, et al. The diagnosis of strep throat in adults in the emergency room. *Med Decis Making.* 1981;1:239–46.
9. McIsaac WJ, White D, Tannenbaum D, et al. A clinical score to reduce unnecessary antibiotic use in patients with sore throat. *CMAJ.* 1998;158:75–83.
10. McIsaac WJ, Goel V, To T, et al. The validity of a sore throat score in family practice. *CMAJ.* 2000;163:811–5.
11. McIsaac WJ, Kellner JD, Aufricht P, et al. Empirical validation of guidelines for the management of pharyngitis in children and adults. *JAMA.* 2004;291:1587–95.
12. Tiwari T, Murphy TV, Moran J. Recommended antimicrobial agents for the treatment and postexposure prophylaxis of pertussis: 2005 CDC guidelines. *MMWR Recomm Rep.* 2005;54 (RR-14):1–16.
13. Wenzel RP, Fowler AA 3rd. Clinical practice. Acute bronchitis. *N Engl J Med.* 2006;355:2125–30.
14. Snow V, Mottur-Pilson C, Gonzales R. Principles of appropriate antibiotic use for treatment of acute bronchitis in adults. *Ann Intern Med.* 2001;134:518–20.
15. Gonzales R, Bartlett JG, Besser RE, et al. Principles of appropriate antibiotic use for treatment of uncomplicated acute bronchitis: background. *Ann Intern Med.* 2001;134:521–9.
16. Braman SS. Chronic cough due to acute bronchitis: ACCP evidence-based clinical practice guidelines. *Chest.* 2006;129:95S–103S.
17. Smith SM, Fahey T, Smucny J, et al. Antibiotics for acute bronchitis. *Cochrane Database Syst Rev.* 2014;3:CD000245.
18. Becker LA, Hom J, Villasis-Keever M, et al. Beta2-agonists for acute cough or a clinical diagnosis of acute bronchitis. *Cochrane Database Syst Rev.* 2015;9:CD001726.
19. Schuh S. Update on management of bronchiolitis. *Curr Opin Pediatr.* 2011;23:110–4.
20. Ralston SL, Lieberthal AS, Meissner HC, et al. Clinical practice guideline: the diagnosis, management, and prevention of bronchiolitis. *Pediatrics.* 2014;134:e1474–502.

21. Donlan M, Fontela PS, Puligandla PS. Use of continuous positive airway pressure (CPAP) in acute viral bronchiolitis: a systematic review. *Pediatr Pulmonol.* 2011;46:736–46.
22. Wing R, James C, Maranda LS, et al. Use of high-flow nasal cannula support in the emergency department reduces the need for intubation in pediatric acute respiratory insufficiency. *Pediatr Emerg Care.* 2012;28:1117–23.
23. Fernandes RM, Bialy LM, Vandermeer B, et al. Glucocorticoids for acute viral bronchiolitis in infants and young children. *Cochrane Database Syst Rev.* 2010;CD004878.
24. Ruuskanen O, Lahti E, Jennings LC, et al. Viral pneumonia. *The Lancet.* 2011;377:1264–75.
25. Mandell LA, Wunderink RG, Anzueto A, et al. Infectious Diseases Society of America/American Thoracic Society consensus guidelines on the management of community-acquired pneumonia in adults. *Clin Infect Dis.* 2007;44:S27–72.
26. Longman RE, Johnson TRB. Viral respiratory disease in pregnancy. *Curr Opin Obstet Gynecol.* 2007;19:120–5.
27. DiazGrenados CA, Dunning AJ, Kimmel M, et al. Efficacy of high-dose versus standard-dose influenza vaccine in older adults. *N Engl J Med.* 2014;371:635–45.
28. Lynch JP III, Fishbein M, Echavarria M. Adenovirus. *Semin Resp Crit Care Med.* 2011;32:494–511.
29. Centers for Disease Control and Prevention (CDC). Revised U.S. surveillance case definition for severe acute respiratory syndrome (SARS) and update on SARS cases—United States and worldwide, December 2003. *MMWR Morb Mortal Wkly Rep.* 2003;52:1202–6.
30. Centers for Disease Control and Prevention (CDC). Severe acute respiratory syndrome (SARS). Available at http://www.cdc.gov/sars/. Accessed 11/4/15.
31. Wong SSY, Yuen KY. The management of coronavirus infections with particular reference to SARS. *J Antimicrob Chemother.* 2008;62:437–41.
32. Cunha BA. Cytomegalovirus pneumonia: community-acquired pneumonia in immunocompetent hosts. *Infect Dis Clin N Am.* 2010;24:147–58.
33. Kotton CN, Kumar D, Caliendo AM, et al. Updated international consensus guidelines on the management of cytomegalovirus in solid-organ transplantation. *Transplantation.* 2013;96:333–60.
34. Centers for Disease Control and Prevention. CDC estimates of 2009 H1N1 influenza cases, hospitalizations and deaths in the United States, April 2009–March 13, 2010. Available at http://www.cdc.gov/h1n1flu/estimates/April_March_13.htm. Accessed 11/4/15.
35. Bautista E, Chotpitayasunondh T, Gao Z, et al. Clinical aspects of pandemic 2009 influenza A (H1N1) virus infection. *N Engl J Med.* 2010;362:1708–19.
36. Ramsey C, Kumar A. H1N1: viral pneumonia as a cause of acute respiratory distress syndrome. *Curr Opin Crit Care.* 2011;17:64–71.
37. Dobson J, Whitley RJ, Pocock S, et al. Oseltamivir treatment for influenza in adults: a meta-analysis of randomised controlled trials. *Lancet.* 2015;385:1729–37.
38. Kumar A. Early versus late oseltamivir treatment in severely ill patients with 2009 pandemic influenza A (H1N1): speed is life. *J Antimicrob Chemother.* 2011;66:959–63.
39. Heneghan CJ, Onakpoya I, Thompson M, et al. Zanamivir for influenza in adults and children: systematic review of clinical study reports and summary of regulatory comments. *BMJ.* 2014; 348:g2547.
40. Centers for Disease Control and Prevention. Influenza (flu). Preventing seasonal flu with vaccination. Available at http://www.cdc.gov/flu/protect/vaccine/index.htm. Accessed 11/4/15.
41. Fiore AE, Fry A, Shay D, et al. Antiviral agents for the treatment and chemoprophylaxis of influenza—recommendations of the Advisory Committee on Immunization Practices (ACIP). *MMWR Recomm Rep.* 2011;60:1–24.
42. Feuillet F, Lina B, Rosa-Calatrava M, et al. Ten years of human metapneumovirus research. *J Clin Virol.* 2012;53:97–105.
43. Lo MK, Rota PA. The emergence of Nipah virus, a highly pathogenic paramyxovirus. *J Clin Virol.* 2008;43:396–400.
44. Luby SP, Gurley ES. Epidemiology of henipavirus disease in humans. *Curr Top Microbiol Immunol.* 2012;359:25–40.
45. Hall CB. Respiratory syncytial virus and parainfluenza virus. *N Engl J Med.* 2001;344:1917–28.
46. Vilchez RA, Dauber J, McCurry K, et al. Parainfluenza virus infection in adult lung transplant recipients: an emergent clinical syndrome with implications on allograft function. *Am J Transplant.* 2003;3:116–20.
47. Chemaly RF, Hanmod SS, Rathod DB, et al. The characteristics and outcomes of parainfluenza virus infections in 200 patients with leukemia or recipients of hematopoietic stem cell transplantation. *Blood.* 2012;119:2738–45.

48. Nichols WG, Corey L, Gooley T, et al. Parainfluenza virus infections after hematopoietic stem cell transplantation: risk factors, response to antiviral therapy, and effect on transplant outcome. *Blood.* 2001;98:573–8.
49. Russell KF, Liang Y, O'Gorman K, et al. Glucocorticoids for croup. *Cochrane Database Syst Rev.* 2011:CD001955.
50. Sommer C, Resch B, Simões EA. Risk factors for severe respiratory syncytial virus lower respiratory tract infection. *Open Microbiol J.* 2011;5:144–54.
51. Falsey AR, Hennessey PA, Formica MA, et al. Respiratory syncytial virus infection in elderly and high-risk adults. *N Engl J Med.* 2005;352:1749–59.
52. McColl MD, Corser RB, Bremner J, et al. Respiratory syncytial virus infection in adult BMT recipients: effective therapy with short duration nebulised ribavirin. *Bone Marrow Transplant.* 1998;21:423–5.
53. Small TN, Casson A, Malak SF, et al. Respiratory syncytial virus infection following hematopoietic stem cell transplantation. *Bone Marrow Transplant.* 2002;29:321–7.
54. Waghmeare A, Campbell AP, Xie H, et al. Respiratory syncytial virus lower respiratory disease in hematopoietic cell transplant recipients: viral RNA detection in blood, antiviral treatment, and clinical outcomes. *Clin Infect Dis.* 2013;57:1731–41.
55. Boeckh M, Berrey MM, Bowden RA, et al. Phase 1 evaluation of the respiratory syncytial virus-specific monoclonal antibody palivizumab in recipients of hematopoietic stem cell transplants. *J Infect Dis.* 2011;184:350–4.
56. Walsh EE. Respiratory syncytial virus infection in adults. *Semin Respir Crit Care Med.* 2011;32: 423–32.
57. Shah JN, Chemaly RF. Management of RSV infections in adult recipients of hematopoietic stem cell transplantation. *Blood.* 2011;117:2755–63.
58. Carbonell-Estrany X, Simões EA, Dagan R, et al. Motavizumab for prophylaxis of respiratory syncytial virus in high-risk children: a noninferiority trial. *Pediatrics.* 2010;125:e35–51.
59. Fuller H, Del Mar C. Immunoglobulin treatment for respiratory syncytial virus infection. *Cochrane Database Syst Rev.* 2006:CD004883.
60. Anzueto A, Niederman MS. Diagnosis and treatment of rhinovirus respiratory infections. *Chest.* 2003;123:1664–72.
61. Braman SS. Postinfectious cough: ACCP evidence-based clinical practice guidelines. *Chest.* 2006;129:138S–46S.
62. Feldman AS, He Y, Moore ML, et al. Toward primary prevention of asthma. Reviewing the evidence for early-life respiratory viral infections as modifiable risk factors to prevent childhood asthma. *Am J Respir Crit Care Med.* 2015;191:34–44.

Cystic Fibrosis

17

Robert Guzy and Daniel B. Rosenbluth

GENERAL PRINCIPLES

Definition

Cystic fibrosis (CF) is an **autosomal recessive** disorder caused by mutations in the **cystic fibrosis transmembrane conductance regulator gene** (CFTR), resulting in dysfunction in numerous exocrine organs.

Epidemiology

- CF is the most common lethal inherited disease affecting the white population.
- The incidence is ~1 in 3300 white births but all races are affected. The incidence in nonwhite populations is estimated to be 1:9200 Hispanic births, 1:10,900 Native American births, 1:15,000 African American births, and 1:30,000 Asian births. Approximately 1000 new cases are diagnosed annually in the United States and the overall prevalence is just under 30,000 patients.[1–3]
- Since newborn screening has been adopted by all states the proportion of new cases identified via newborn screening is increasing (62% in 2013).[2] Early asymptomatic diagnosis may have better pulmonary function during early childhood.[3,4]
- Aside from newborn screening most cases are identified in babies born with meconium ileus or young children who present with respiratory symptoms, most commonly recurrent pulmonary infections.
- Up to 10% of patients are diagnosed at age 10 or older.[2,5] These patients are more likely to present with nonclassic CF symptoms including bronchiectasis without pancreatic insufficiency, recurrent or chronic pancreatitis, or infertility (azoospermia with congenital absence of the vas deferens).
- The median age of survival in the United States is 40.7 years (95% confidence interval 37.7–44.1).[2]

Pathophysiology

- **CF is a multisystem disease, with highly variable disease presentation.**
- Progressive lung disease and chronic respiratory tract infection, however, is the major cause of morbidity and mortality.[3]
  - Pulmonary disease is related to abnormal electrolyte transport in airways, resulting in decreased airway surface liquid and impaired mucociliary clearance. Infection, inflammation, and chronic airway obstruction ultimately result in bronchiectasis, chronic infection, and premature death.[6,7]
  - Thickened secretions in the pancreatic and biliary ducts result in malabsorption, maldigestion, diabetes, and occasionally liver disease.
- A genetic mutation in the CFTR gene leading to an abnormal protein is the basic molecular defect responsible for CF.
  - The CFTR gene is located on chromosome 7.
  - CFTR is a cyclic AMP-regulated chloride ion channel on the apical surface of epithelial cells that primarily plays a role in chloride transport.

- In CF, this protein is missing or malfunctioning, leading to abnormal chloride transport.
- Abnormal function leads to **decreased chloride secretion** and increased sodium absorption on the apical surface of epithelial cells. This results in **thickened secretions** in airways, sinuses, pancreatic ducts, biliary ducts, intestines, sweat ducts, and reproductive tract.[6,7]
- CFTR also plays a role in the regulation of other ion channels that may be important in the pathogenesis of CF.
- Many of the specific mechanisms by which the molecular defect of CF leads to clinical disease remain unclear and are the subject of current investigations.
- CFTR mutations can be divided into five classes, based on the effect of the mutation on CFTR protein production and function.[2]
  - Class I mutations lead to defective protein production. These are often nonsense, frameshift, or splicing mutations leading to complete absence of CFTR protein.
    - G542X, W1282X, R533X are examples.
    - Class I accounts for 2–5% of all CF cases.[2]
  - Class II mutations lead to defective protein processing. The CFTR protein is produced but is prevented from trafficking properly.
    - F508del, N1303K are examples.
    - **The most common CFTR mutation is F508del**, which is a deletion of three nucleotides which encode phenylalanine (F) at amino acid 508. This mutation is **found in over 80% of patients with CF in the United States** (46.5% homozygotes and 39.9% heterozygotes).[2]
  - Class III mutations lead to defective regulation of the CFTR protein. CFTR is present on the membrane; however, channel activity is diminished. G551D is the most common example.
  - Class IV mutations lead to defective conduction of the CFTR protein. CFTR is produced, localized, and regulated normally; however, ion conductance and channel opening are reduced. R117H is the most common example.
  - Class V mutations cause decreased numbers of normally functioning CFTR protein.
  - Information about specific mutations and reported phenotypes can be found at http://www.cftr2.org. Accessed 27/10/15.

DIAGNOSIS

Clinical Presentation

Pulmonary

- Nearly all patients have **chronic sinusitis** on radiographic studies. Nasal polyposis is common.
- **Chronic lower airway infections** are characteristics of this disease.
  - Chronic infection causes inflammation, increased mucus secretion and obstruction, and direct destruction of pulmonary parenchyma.
  - Pulmonary infections with *Haemophilus influenzae* and *Staphylococcus aureus* are common early in the disease process.
  - Later, ***Pseudomonas aeruginosa*** **becomes the dominant lung pathogen in a majority of CF patients.** Progressive inflammation, lung damage, decline in lung function, and progressive dyspnea are most closely correlated with this organism.
  - Infection with other gram-negative organisms such as *Burkholderia cepacia* can lead to a fulminant course with a high mortality rate.
  - Colonization with *Aspergillus fumigatus* is common but invasive disease from this organism is relatively rare.
  - CF patients are at higher risk for infection with nontuberculous mycobacteria, with prevalence ranging from 4% to 19%. The most common strains identified are *Mycobacterium avium* complex and *Mycobacterium abscessus*.[8,9]

- **Acute exacerbation of CF** is a common presentation of pulmonary disease.
  - The typical exacerbation presents with some combination of symptoms, including increased cough, changing sputum, increased shortness of breath, decreased exercise tolerance, and weight loss. Low-grade fever is common but not universal.
  - The specific factors causing exacerbations are unclear but viral infections have been implicated in some studies.[10]
  - Occasionally, a reduction in pulmonary function on spirometry may be the only abnormality noted.
  - CXRs are often unchanged during exacerbations but are useful to exclude other pulmonary complications of CF.
- **Pneumothorax** is a relatively common pulmonary complication that presents in CF.
  - The incidence of pneumothorax rises with increasing age secondary to worsening lung disease. Approximately 3.4% of CF patients will experience pneumothorax (1 in 167 patients per year).[11]
  - Patients typically present with chest pain and dyspnea (but may present atypically) because of decreased compliance in the CF lung.
- A second pulmonary complication is minor **hemoptysis** (<240 mL), which is common (9.1% of patients) and often occurs with acute exacerbations of this disease.[12]
  - Approximately 4% of CF patients will experience massive, life-threatening hemoptysis (>500 mL/24 hr) during their lifetime (1 in 115 patients per year).[13]
  - Hypertrophic bronchial arteries from chronic inflammation are the typical source of bleeding.
  - Patients presenting with hemoptysis should be treated with antibiotics.
- **Respiratory failure** is the most concerning pulmonary presentation of CF. Unless reversible etiologies are responsible, this complication often indicates end-stage lung disease and carries a poor prognosis for recovery.

Gastrointestinal

- Approximately 90% of CF patients exhibit **exocrine pancreatic insufficiency.**
  - Patients with pancreatic insufficiency have **significantly lower life expectancies** than those with pancreatic sufficiency.
  - Pancreatic sufficiency is more common in patients who present later in life.[5]
  - Pancreatic exocrine insufficiency can lead to steatorrhea, chronic malnutrition, edema secondary to hypoalbuminemia, and various vitamin deficiencies.
  - Fat-soluble vitamins A, D, E, and K are most commonly affected. Vitamin A deficiency can lead to visual deficiencies such as night blindness, and in severe cases xerophthalmia, keratomalacia, and complete blindness. Vitamin D deficiency can lead to poor bone mineralization. Vitamin E deficiency can lead to ataxia and absent deep tendon reflexes.
- **Gastroesophageal reflux disease** is more common in CF patients than healthy control subjects and is possibly linked to worsening lung disease.[14]
- Another presentation of GI disease is the **distal intestinal obstruction syndrome** (DIOS), which can be considered an adult equivalent of meconium ileus.
  - Colicky abdominal pain with a palpable mass is a typical presentation.
  - Radiographic patterns consistent with partial or complete obstruction can be seen on obstructive series.
  - Caution must be exercised, however, because these signs and symptoms are present in other abdominal conditions that present in CF patients. Empiric treatment of DIOS while evaluation is underway for other conditions is recommended.
- Volvulus, intussusception, and rectal prolapse can occur.
- Cholelithiasis and cholecystitis are seen.
- CF can be associated with an asymptomatic increase in alkaline phosphatase and a mild transaminitis in up to one-third of patients, whereas biliary cirrhosis is much less common.

- A small percentage of patients do have significant **liver disease** with about 3% of deaths in CF patients attributed to liver disease.[2]

Endocrine and Reproductive

- **Men are usually infertile** secondary to obstructive azoospermia. Patients that are diagnosed at older ages may present with **congenital absence of the vas deferens**.
- **Women have reduced fertility** because of thick cervical mucus as well as other, less understood factors.
- Puberty is often late in onset owing to malnutrition.
- **Osteoporosis** occurs in approximately one-third of adult CF patients.
- **Diabetes mellitus** is common in CF, affecting more than 20% of adults.[2]
  - Diabetes in CF is primarily due to deficient insulin production, although insulin resistance may play a role as well.
  - CF patients may be dependent on insulin for glucose control but diabetic ketoacidosis is rare.

Diagnostic Criteria

- The diagnosis of CF is based on **clinical presentation** coupled with confirmatory testing.
- At least one criterion from each set of features is required to diagnose CF[15]:
  - Compatible clinical feature of CF (persistent colonization/infection with typical organisms, chronic cough and sputum production, persistent CXR abnormalities, airway obstruction, sinus abnormalities/polyps, clubbing, meconium ileus, DIOS, rectal prolapse, pancreatic insufficiency/pancreatitis, jaundice/biliary cirrhosis, malnutrition, acute salt depletion, chronic metabolic alkalosis, obstructive azoospermia) **OR**
  - Positive family history **OR**
  - Positive newborn screening test

  AND
  - Elevated sweat chloride >60 mmol/L on two occasions **OR**
  - Presence of two disease-causing mutations in CFTR **OR**
  - Abnormal nasal transepithelial potential difference test

Differential Diagnosis

- Primary ciliary dyskinesia: bronchiectasis, sinusitis, and infertility are common. Gastrointestinal (GI) symptoms are limited and sweat chloride levels are normal. Dextrocardia or situs inversus totalis can be seen.
- Shwachman–Diamond syndrome: pancreatic insufficiency, cyclic neutropenia, and short stature are seen. Sweat chloride levels are normal.
- Young syndrome: bronchiectasis, sinusitis, and azoospermia. Respiratory symptoms are mild, and there is a lack of GI symptoms. Sweat chloride testing is normal.
- Immunoglobulin deficiency leads to recurrent sinus and pulmonary infections and can cause bronchiectasis. GI symptoms are absent and sweat chloride testing is normal.
- Idiopathic bronchiectasis.
- Chronic rhinosinusitis.
- Chronic idiopathic pancreatitis.

Diagnostic Testing

- Diagnosis of CF is usually made during childhood. Approximately 10% of patients are diagnosed after age 10.[5] In 2013, over 60% of new diagnoses were made from newborn screening, which has increased the frequency of early diagnosis.[2]
- **Pilocarpine iontophoresis**, or **sweat testing**, is the most common confirmatory test and is **the gold standard** for CF diagnosis.[15]
  - A quantitative test with a **chloride value of >60 mmol/L** on two occasions is consistent with CF.

- Other conditions produce abnormal sweat tests but can usually be differentiated from CF based on their clinical presentation.
- Borderline or nondiagnostic results should prompt repeat or additional testing depending on clinical suspicion.

- **Transepithelial potential difference** can be used as confirmatory testing in the rare instance in which CF is suspected clinically but sweat testing is inconclusive. This testing is only available at specialized centers, and should be repeated on two separate days. Voltage across epithelial lining of the nose is measured at rest, after sodium channel inhibition, and after CFTR stimulation.
- Genetic testing for CF is available but usually is not used as the initial diagnostic test. There are >1800 known mutations and a number of unknown mutations that can lead to CF disease.
  - **Two mutations on different alleles must be present to diagnose CF.**
  - Commercially available probes, while identifying >90% of abnormal genes in the white Northern European population, test for a minority of known CF mutations.
  - Full gene sequencing is available but interpretation may be complex.
- Other diagnostic evaluation can support the presence of CF but is generally neither specific nor sensitive for the diagnosis.
- **Pulmonary function tests** show an obstructive pattern early in the disease and tend to change to a mixed obstructive and restrictive pattern later when more fibrosis is present.
- Early in the disease, radiographic testing tends to show hyperinflated lungs. Bronchiectasis with cyst formation and mucus plugging is a later finding.
- **Sputum cultures** are typically positive for multiple organisms, including *P. aeruginosa, S. aureus,* nontypeable *H. influenzae, Stenotrophomonas maltophilia, B. cepacia,* and mucoid variants of *P. aeruginosa.* Use of special culture media to identify fastidious organisms is recommended. Nontuberculous mycobacteria are frequently isolated and may be pathogenic.[8,9]
- Testing for pancreatic insufficiency and malabsorption is not commonly done, as the diagnosis based on history, vitamin deficiency, and response to pancreatic enzyme supplementation is often sufficient for diagnosis. Seventy-two-hour stool collections for fecal fat or measurement of fecal elastase levels can be helpful in situations where the diagnosis is not clear.

TREATMENT

- The overall goals of CF therapy are to improve quality of life, decrease number and frequency of exacerbations and hospitalizations, reduce the rate of decline in lung function, and prolong life expectancy.
- **Comprehensive care at an accredited CF care center is recommended.**

Pulmonary

- Management of the acute pulmonary exacerbation is probably the most common reason for the hospital admission of CF patients.
- **Immunizations** should be kept up to date in an attempt to prevent exacerbations. **Yearly influenza vaccination** decreases the frequency of infection.[2]
- **Pulmonary rehabilitation,** when performed with exercise rehabilitation may improve functional status and assist with airway clearance.[16–18]
- **Inhaled bronchodilators** (e.g., albuterol, salmeterol, formoterol) are recommended for all CF patients, particularly in association with chest physiotherapy or other nebulized agents. Bronchodilators facilitate clearance of airway secretions and limit bronchial constriction seen in response to certain inhaled agents, such as hypertonic saline and dornase ALFA.

- **Respiratory therapy**, including chest percussion and postural drainage, has long been known to be efficacious in exacerbations.[19,20] Other techniques including percussors, pneumatic compression vests, and oscillating positive expiratory pressure devices such as the Flutter and Acapella are available to assist in airway clearance.[21–25]
- **Hypertonic saline** (7%) is administered as an inhalation, and functions to improve mucociliary clearance of airway secretions.[26]
  - Hypertonic saline increases water content of secretions by creating a high osmotic gradient.
  - Mucus clearance is improved, with mild improvements in lung function and decreased incidence of respiratory exacerbations.
  - Albuterol should be administered prior to hypertonic saline to reduce bronchospasm. Patients with FEV_1 <40% should be given a test dose under observation before initiating therapy at home.
- **Inhaled recombinant DNase** (dornase ALFA) digests extracellular DNA and reduces the viscosity of CF sputum.[27,28]
  - Shown to be effective in reducing sputum viscosity and improving pulmonary function.
  - In patients with normal pulmonary function, dornase ALFA has been shown to slow the rate of decline in lung function.
  - Dornase ALFA decreases the incidence of respiratory tract infections requiring parenteral antibiotics.
  - Side effects include pharyngitis, laryngitis, rash, chest pain, and conjunctivitis.
- **Antibiotics** are the main treatment for acute exacerbations.[29]
  - Antibiotic use in CF patients differs from that in other patients. Higher doses of antibiotics are needed because of increased clearance and volumes of distribution. Longer courses of antibiotics are required. Fourteen- to twenty-one-day courses are typical of effective regimens.
  - Sputum culture results should guide antibiotic choice.
  - In general, antibiotics are selected based on respiratory tract cultures and susceptibilities, however:
    - The utility of in vitro susceptibility testing has been questioned, since there appears to be discordance between susceptibility testing and clinical response to antibiotics.
    - In a study published in 2003, treatment outcomes of patients experiencing a CF exacerbation with IV tobramycin or IV ceftazidime did not correlate with MIC values of *P. aeruginosa* obtained from sputum cultures.[30]
  - Oral antibiotics are appropriate for mild exacerbations. The main barrier to using oral antibiotics is the limited number of agents active against *Pseudomonas.* **Ciprofloxacin** (750 mg PO bid) is the antibiotic of choice against *Pseudomonas.* Use of this drug should be limited to 3-week courses given the rapid rise of resistant organisms when longer courses are used.
  - For moderate to severe exacerbations or failed oral treatment courses, IV regimens are the standard of care.[29]
    - A typical two-drug regimen consists of an **aminoglycoside** (gentamicin/tobramycin, 3 mg/kg IV q8h or 10 mg/kg q24h following peak and trough levels) plus an **extended-spectrum penicillin** (piperacillin/tazobactam, 4.5 g IV q6h) or **cephalosporin** (cefepime, 2 g IV q8h).
    - Measurement of aminoglycoside peaks and troughs or other evaluations of aminoglycoside pharmacokinetics should be employed to optimize aminoglycoside dosing and prevent toxicity. Once-daily dosing is preferred.
    - Occasionally, **methicillin-resistant *S. aureus*** is isolated from the sputum and requires **IV vancomycin** (15 mg/kg adjusted to maintain a trough of ~10–15) for adequate coverage.

- ◦ **Inhaled tobramycin** in patients with chronic airways infection with *P. aeruginosa* used in 28-day cycles was shown to improve pulmonary function and decrease the rate of hospitalization.[31]
  - ◦ **Inhaled aztreonam** in patients with chronic airways infection with *P. aeruginosa* has been shown to improve pulmonary function and increase the time until subsequent antibiotic treatment.[32,33]
  - ◦ There is some evidence that home IV treatment can be as effective as hospital treatment.[29,34,35] However, the decision of inpatient versus outpatient treatment must be made on an individual basis. Resources available in the hospital such as intensive monitoring and extensive chest physical therapy are generally unavailable at home.
- Inflammation in CF is an additional target for CF therapeutics.
  - ◦ Chronic treatment with **azithromycin** (500 mg three times a week) in patients chronically infected with *P. aeruginosa* has been shown to improve lung function and reduce days in the hospital for treatment of acute exacerbations.[36] Its use should be limited to patients with multiple cultures negative for nontuberculous mycobacterial infection.
  - ◦ One trial compared prednisone therapy 1 mg/kg versus 2 mg/kg versus placebo on alternate days. The prednisone group had a higher percentage of predicted forced vital capacity.[37] However, complications of steroid therapy, such as growth retardation and glycemic control, have limited the use of this therapy, and long-term use should be avoided.
  - ◦ High-dose ibuprofen has been used with some success in young patients with mild disease but is again limited by side effects including renal failure and peptic ulcer disease.[38,39]
- Treatment for chronic respiratory failure is usually supportive.
  - ◦ Oxygen therapy should be provided based on standard rest and exercise oxygen assessments.
  - ◦ Noninvasive ventilation or even intubation has been used as a bridge to lung transplantation.
  - ◦ **Bilateral lung transplantation** is the treatment of choice.[40] The challenges of lung transplantation for this population are formidable given the incidence of pre-existing infections and poor nutrition. However, success rates compare favorably to other indications for transplantation.
- Chronic sinusitis is common, and many patients benefit from nasal steroids. Nasal saline washes are helpful. Some patients may require functional endoscopic sinus surgery and nasal polypectomy.

Gastrointestinal

- Achieving **adequate nutrition** in CF patients affects both pulmonary status and overall mortality.
  - ◦ **Replacement of pancreatic enzymes** as supplements is important for this goal.[41]
  - ◦ The usual starting dose is 500 lipase units/kg/meal PO, which can be increased to maximum dose of 2500 units/kg/meal. Dosing is adjusted to achieve one to two semisolid stools per day and maintain adequate nutrition.
  - ◦ Acid suppression may be necessary in some patients as enzymes may be inactivated in an acidic environment, though supporting data are limited.[42]
  - ◦ Adequate proportions of fat and protein calories need to be ingested, which usually require increased caloric intake.
  - ◦ Dietary goals should aim for a body mass index of ≥50th percentile or in adult males ≥22 and females ≥23. Better lung function is associated with a higher BMI. More severe disease and worse pancreatic function result in greater caloric deficits and intake recommendations should be tailored to the individual patient. Nutritional supplementation should be provided when appropriate.[2,41]
  - ◦ Fat-soluble vitamins should be provided in supplements.

- The preferred treatments for other GI complications are less clear.
  - Ursodeoxycholic acid probably has a role in the management of CF-induced cholestasis.
  - Management of end-stage liver disease and the resulting complications of portal hypertension are the same as in other etiologies of end-stage liver disease.
  - **DIOS** may be managed by oral administration of laxative electrolyte solutions such as magnesium citrate or polyethylene glycol. With the presence of complete obstruction, diatrizoate meglumine and diatrizoate sodium (hypaque) enemas can be used as both a diagnostic and a therapeutic maneuver.[43] Surgery is rarely required.

Endocrine and Reproductive

- Glucose intolerance as well as **diabetes mellitus** is more common in CF patients. Screening with a 2-hour 75-g glucose tolerance test should be done yearly.[44] Management of CF-related diabetes mellitus generally relies on insulin therapy.
- **Osteopenia** should be managed with calcium and vitamin D supplementation. Bisphosphonate therapy is effective for **osteoporosis** in adult CF patients.[45]
- Most males are **infertile** secondary to obstructive azoospermia. Microsurgical epididymal sperm aspiration with intracytoplasmic sperm injection into the ova may be used to overcome male infertility. Likewise, intrauterine insemination has overcome many of the factors that decrease fertility rates for female CF patients.

Lung Transplantation

- CF remains one of the most common indications for bilateral lung transplantation.
- In general, transplantation improves life expectancy in patients who have an estimated 5-year survival of 30% or less.[40]
- Criteria for referral to a lung transplantation center include[46,47]:
  - FEV_1 <30% predicted or a rapid decline in FEV_1 or 6-minute walk distance <400 m. Other criteria should be met in addition to a decline in FEV_1 prior to referral to a lung transplantation center.
  - Increasing frequency of exacerbations.
  - Refractory/recurrent pneumothorax.
  - Recurrent hemoptysis.
  - Hypoxemia or hypercapnia.
  - Pulmonary hypertension.
- Many transplant centers consider respiratory tract infection with *B. cepacia* complex to be a contraindication for lung transplantation in CF patients.

Emerging Therapies

- **Aggressive treatment of pulmonary infections and inflammation**, as well as attention to the **nutritional issues**, involved in CF has largely been responsible for the significant improvement in mortality over the past five decades.
- New understanding of the genetic and molecular basis of CF holds the promise for similar advances in the decades ahead.
- New therapies can be divided into those that attempt to improve the function of the mutant CFTR protein, manipulate the function of alternative ion channels, and those that attempt to treat the genetic defect directly.
- Since the isolation of the CF gene in 1989, there has been interest in applying the principles of **gene therapy** to CF. The theoretical promise of this approach is still great but there are many technical difficulties to overcome before this becomes a common approach to CF therapy.
- **CFTR modulators**
  - **Ivacaftor** (150 mg PO bid), which was approved by the U.S. Food and Drug Administration (FDA) for use in CF in January 2012, is the first agent that restores function by activating mutant CFTR.[48]

    - Approved for use in patients with the G551D mutation who are >6 years old, which is present in ~5% of patients with CF and causes a class III mutation.
    - Developed using large-scale chemical screen for agents that increase chloride ion efflux in cells expressing a G551D CFTR mutant.
    - A phase III randomized, placebo-controlled trial demonstrated an increase in FEV_1 by 10.4% with ivacaftor compared to an FEV_1 decline of 0.2% in placebo controls after 24 weeks of treatment. Sweat chloride levels, frequency of CF exacerbations, and adverse events were all significantly lower in patients treated with ivacaftor. Weight gain was common in subjects receiving ivacaftor.
    - Ivacaftor is best absorbed when combined with fat- and enzyme-containing meals, and the channel modulating effects may decrease rapidly with missed doses. Reinforcement of proper use is crucial for optimal outcomes.
  - **Ataluren** (PTC124) is an agent that causes ribosomes to read through premature stop codons, without affecting their ability to recognize normal stop codons. Early clinical trials have shown significant improvements in nasal potential differences in children, but a phase 3 clinical trial has not definitively substantiated its efficacy.[49,50]
  - Oral agents intended to correct the abnormal CFTR trafficking that characterizes the F508del mutation are in various phases of preclinical and clinical development. These agents may be administered with ivacaftor in an attempt to increase their efficacy.[51]

SPECIAL CONSIDERATIONS

- Corresponding with the increasing life expectancy are increasing rates of pregnancy in CF patients.
- Women with good lung function and good nutritional status generally do well during pregnancy.[52,53]
  - Prepregnancy FEV_1 <50% of predicted is associated with poorer outcomes. For example, in a UK study by Edenborough, women with FEV_1 <60% delivered more preterm infants and had a greater decrease in lung function during the pregnancy compared to those with milder disease.[54]
  - Women should be encouraged to reach 90% of their ideal weight before their pregnancy. Nocturnal tube feeds can be used in those patients having difficulty gaining weight.
  - Exacerbations should be treated aggressively. Cephalosporins and synthetic penicillins are generally safe. Aminoglycosides potentially cause fetal ototoxicity but may be necessary.
- Families should be counseled on the genetic risk of CF. All children of a parent with CF carry a single CF mutation; their chances of having CF disease depend on the genetics of the affected parent's partner.

COMPLICATIONS

- **Pneumothorax** is an indication for hospital admission.[55]
  - If small (<20% of the hemithorax volume), pneumothoraces can be managed conservatively with serial CXRs.
  - BiPAP treatment should be withheld until the pneumothorax has resolved. Airplane travel, weight lifting, and spirometry should be avoided for 2 weeks after the pneumothorax has resolved.
  - In general, airway clearance measures utilizing positive expiratory pressure (flutter valve), intrapulmonary percussive ventilation, and exercise should be avoided in most instances of large pneumothorax.
  - If the pneumothorax enlarges or is symptomatic, a chest tube should be placed.
  - Obliterative procedures such as pleurodesis should be considered for persistent and recurrent pneumothoraces.
  - Surgical pleurodesis is preferred over chemical pleurodesis.

- **Hemoptysis** is usually minor and responds to conservative treatment with IV antibiotics.[55]
  - Moderate to massive hemoptysis usually requires a more interventional approach.
  - Basic treatment involves correction of coagulation parameters, withholding chest physiotherapy, and stopping inhaled antibiotics.
  - Bronchial artery embolization plays an important role in massive or recurrent hemoptysis. A small study showed decreased bleeding and pulmonary exacerbations as well as increased quality of life when early bronchial artery embolization was used.[56] Bronchoscopy is not recommended prior to bronchial artery embolization.
  - Repeated embolization in the setting of recurrent hemoptysis is frequently successful, and atypical sources of neovascularization should be considered in patients with prior embolization and persistent bleeding.
  - Surgery is the last option if bronchial artery embolization fails to control the bleeding.

REFERENCES

1. Hamosh A, FitzSimmons SC, Macek M Jr, et al. Comparison of the clinical manifestations of cystic fibrosis in black and white patients. *J Pediatr.* 1998;132:255–9.
2. Cystic Fibrosis Foundation. *Patient Registry Annual Data Report to the Center Directors, 2013.* Bethesda, MD: Cystic Fibrosis Foundation; 2014. Available at https://ωωω.cff.org/Our-Research/CF-Patient-Registry/. Accessed 28/10/15.
3. Strausbaugh SD, Davis PB. Cystic fibrosis: a review of epidemiology and pathobiology. *Clin Chest Med.* 2007;28:279–88.
4. Wang SS, O'Leary LA, FitzSimmons SC, et al. The impact of early cystic fibrosis diagnosis on pulmonary function in children. *J Pediatr.* 2002;141:804–10.
5. Gilljam M, Ellis L, Corey M, et al. Clinical manifestations of cystic fibrosis among patients with diagnosis in adulthood. *Chest.* 2004;126:1215–24.
6. Donaldson SH, Boucher RC. Update on pathogenesis of cystic fibrosis lung disease. *Curr Opin Pulm Med.* 2003;9:486–91.
7. Rowe SM, Miller S, Sorscher EJ. Cystic fibrosis. *N Engl J Med.* 2005;352:1992–2001.
8. Whittaker LA, Teneback C. Atypical mycobacterial and fungal infections in cystic fibrosis. *Semin Respir Crit Care Med.* 2009;30:539–46.
9. Olivier KN, Weber DJ, Wallace RJ Jr, et al. Nontuberculous mycobacteria. I: multicenter prevalence study in cystic fibrosis. *Am J Respir Crit Care Med.* 2003;167:828–34.
10. Collinson J, Nicholson KG, Cancio E, et al. Effects of upper respiratory tract infections in patients with cystic fibrosis. *Thorax.* 1996;51:1115–22.
11. Flume PA, Strange C, Ye X, et al. Pneumothorax in cystic fibrosis. *Chest.* 2005;128:720–8.
12. Efrati O, Harash O, Rivlin J, et al. Hemoptysis in Israeli CF patients—prevalence, treatment, and clinical characteristics. *J Cyst Fibros.* 2008;7:301–6.
13. Flume PA, Yankaskas JR, Ebeling M, et al. Massive hemoptysis in cystic fibrosis. *Chest.* 2005;128:729–38.
14. Robinson NB, DiMango E. Prevalence of gastroesophageal reflux in cystic fibrosis and implications for lung disease. *Ann Am Thorac Soc.* 2014;11:964–8.
15. Farrell PM, Rosenstein BJ, White TB, et al. Guidelines for diagnosis of cystic fibrosis in newborns through older adults: Cystic Fibrosis Foundation consensus report. *J Pediatr.* 2008;153:S4–14.
16. Orenstein DM, Hovell MF, Mulvihill M, et al. Strength vs aerobic training in children with cystic fibrosis: a randomized controlled trial. *Chest.* 2004;126:1204–14.
17. Blau H, Mussaffi-Georgy H, Fink G, et al. Effects of an intensive 4-week summer camp on cystic fibrosis: pulmonary function, exercise tolerance, and nutrition. *Chest.* 2002;121:1117–22.
18. Schneiderman-Walker J, Pollock SL, Corey M, et al. A randomized controlled trial of a 3-year home exercise program in cystic fibrosis. *J Pediatr.* 2000;136:304–10.
19. Flume PA, Robinson KA, O'Sullivan BP, et al. Clinical practice guidelines for Pulmonary Therapies Committee. Cystic fibrosis pulmonary guidelines: airway clearance therapies. *Respir Care.* 2009;54:522–37.
20. Warnock L, Gates A, van der Schans CP. Chest physiotherapy compared to no chest physiotherapy for cystic fibrosis. *Cochrane Database Syst Rev.* 2013;9:CD001401.

21. McIlwaine M, Wong L, Peacock D, et al. Long-term comparative trial of conventional postural drainage and percussion versus positive expiratory pressure physiotherapy in the treatment of cystic fibrosis. *J Pediatr.* 1997;131:570–4.
22. McKoy NA, Saldanha IJ, Odelola OA, et al. Active cycle of breathing technique for cystic fibrosis. *Cochrane Database Syst Rev.* 2012;12:CD007862.
23. Moran F, Bradley JM, Piper AJ. Non-invasive ventilation for cystic fibrosis. *Cochrane Database Syst Rev.* 2013;4:CD002769.
24. Morrison L, Agnew J. Oscillating devices for airway clearance in people with cystic fibrosis. *Cochrane Database Syst Rev.* 2014;7:CD006842.
25. McIlwaine M, Button B, Dwan K. Positive expiratory pressure physiotherapy for airway clearance in people with cystic fibrosis. *Cochrane Database Syst Rev.* 2015;6:CD003147.
26. Elkins MR, Robinson M, Rose BR, et al. A controlled trial of long-term inhaled hypertonic saline in patients with cystic fibrosis. *N Engl J Med.* 2006;354:229–40.
27. Fuchs HJ, Borowitz DS, Christiansen DH, et al. Effect of aerosolized recombinant human DNase on exacerbations of respiratory symptoms and on pulmonary function in patients with cystic fibrosis. The Pulmozyme Study Group. *N Engl J Med.* 1994;331:637–42.
28. Hubbard RC, McElvaney NG, Birrer P, et al. A preliminary study of aerosolized recombinant human deoxyribonuclease I in the treatment of cystic fibrosis. *N Engl J Med.* 1992;326:812–5.
29. Flume PA, Mogayzel PJ, Robinson KA, et al. Cystic fibrosis pulmonary guidelines: treatment of pulmonary exacerbations. *Am J Respir Crit Care Med.* 2009;180:802–8.
30. Smith AL, Fiel SB, Mayer-Hamblett N, et al. Susceptibility testing of Pseudomonas aeruginosa isolates and clinical response to parenteral antibiotic administration: lack of association in cystic fibrosis. *Chest.* 2003;123:1495–502.
31. Ramsey B, Pepe MS, Quan JM, et al. Intermittent administration of inhaled tobramycin in patients with cystic fibrosis. *N Engl J Med.* 1999;340:23–30.
32. McCoy KS, Quittner AL, Oermann CM, et al. Inhaled aztreonam lysine for chronic airway Pseudomonas aeruginosa in cystic fibrosis. *Am J Respir Crit Care Med.* 2008;178:921–8.
33. Retsch-Bogart GZ, Quittner AL, Gibson RL, et al. Efficacy and safety of inhaled aztreonam lysine for airway pseudomonas in cystic fibrosis. *Chest.* 2009;135:1223–32.
34. Pond MN, Newport M, Joanes D, et al. Home versus hospital intravenous antibiotic therapy in the treatment of young adults with cystic fibrosis. *Eur Respir J.* 1994;7:1640–4.
35. Collaco JM, Green DM, Cutting GR, et al. Location and duration of treatment of cystic fibrosis respiratory exacerbations do not affect outcomes. *Am J Respir Crit Care Med.* 2010;182:1137–43.
36. Southern KW, Barker PM, Solis-Moya A, et al. Macrolide antibiotics for cystic fibrosis. *Cochrane Database Syst Rev.* 2012;11:CD002203.
37. Eigen H, Rosenstein B, FitzSimmons S, et al. A multicenter study of alternate-day prednisone therapy in patients with cystic fibrosis. *J Pediatr.* 1995;126:515–23.
38. Konstan MW, Byard PJ, Hoppel CL, et al. Effect of high-dose ibuprofen in patients with cystic fibrosis. *N Engl J Med.* 1995;332:848–54.
39. Lands LC, Stanojevic S. Oral non-steroidal anti-inflammatory drug therapy for lung disease in cystic fibrosis. *Cochrane Database Syst Rev.* 2013;6:CD001505.
40. Liou TG, Adler FR, Cahill BC, et al. Survival effect of lung transplantation among patients with cystic fibrosis. *JAMA.* 2001;286:2683–9.
41. Stallings VA, Stark LJ, Robinson KA, et al. Evidence-based practice recommendations for nutrition-related management of children and adults with cystic fibrosis and pancreatic insufficiency: results of a systematic review. *J Am Diet Assoc.* 2008;108:832–9.
42. Ng SM, Franchini AJ. Drug therapies for reducing gastric acidity in people with cystic fibrosis. *Cochrane Database Syst Rev.* 2014;7:CD003424.
43. Colombo C, Ellemunter H, Houwen R, et al. Guidelines for the diagnosis and management of distal intestinal obstruction syndrome in cystic fibrosis patients. *J Cyst Fibros.* 2011;10:S24–8.
44. Moran A, Brunzell C, Cohen RC, et al. CFRD Guidelines Committee. Clinical care guidelines for cystic fibrosis-related diabetes: a position statement of the American Diabetes Association and a clinical practice guideline of the Cystic Fibrosis Foundation, endorsed by the Pediatric Endocrine Society. *Diabetes Care.* 2010;33:2697–708.
45. Conwell LS, Chang AB. Bisphosphonates for osteoporosis in people with cystic fibrosis. *Cochrane Database Syst Rev.* 2012;4:CD002010.
46. Weill D, Benden C, Corris PA, et al. A consensus document for the selection of lung transplant candidates: 2014—an update from the Pulmonary Transplantation Council of the International Society for Heart and Lung Transplantation. *J Heart Lung Transplant.* 2015;34:1–15.

47. Braun AT, Merlo CA. Cystic fibrosis lung transplantation. *Curr Opin Pulm Med.* 2011;17:467–72.
48. Ramsey BW, Davies J, McElvaney NG, et al. A CFTR potentiator in patients with cystic fibrosis and the G551D mutation. *N Engl J Med.* 2011;365:1663–72.
49. Wilschanski M, Miller LL, Shoseyov D, et al. Chronic ataluren (PTC124) treatment of nonsense mutation cystic fibrosis. *Eur Respir J.* 2011;38:59–69.
50. Kerem E, Konstan MW, De Boeck K, et al. Ataluren for the treatment of nonsense-mutation cystic fibrosis: a randomised, double-blind, placebo-controlled phase 3 trial. *Lancet Respir Med.* 2014;2:539–47.
51. Boyle MP, Bell SC, Konstan MW, et al. A CFTR corrector (lumacaftor) and a CFTR potentiator (ivacaftor) for treatment of patients with cystic fibrosis who have a phe508del CFTR mutation: a phase 2 randomised controlled trial. *Lancet Respir Med.* 2014;2:527–38.
52. Hilman B, Aitken M, Constantinescu M. Pregnancy in patients with cystic fibrosis. *Clin Obstet Gynecol.* 1996;39:70–86.
53. Edenborough FP, Borgo G, Knoop C, et al. European Cystic Fibrosis Society. Guidelines for the management of pregnancy in women with cystic fibrosis. *J Cyst Fibros.* 2008;7:S2–32.
54. Edenborough FP, Stableforth DE, Webb AK, et al. Outcome of pregnancy in women with cystic fibrosis. *Thorax.* 1995;50:170–4.
55. Flume PA, Mogayzel PJ, Robinson KA, et al. Cystic fibrosis pulmonary guidelines: pulmonary complications: hemoptysis and pneumothorax. *Am J Respir Crit Care Med.* 2010;182:298–306.
56. Antonelli M, Midulla F, Tancredi G, et al. Bronchial artery embolization for the management of nonmassive hemoptysis in cystic fibrosis. *Chest.* 2002;121:796–801.

Hemoptysis

18

Daniel R. Crouch and Tonya D. Russell

GENERAL PRINCIPLES

Definition

- **Hemoptysis** refers to the expectoration of blood originating from the lower airway or lung.
- **Massive hemoptysis** is defined as the expectoration of large amounts of blood.
  - There is no consensus on the volume of blood needed to be classified as massive but definitions range from 100 to > 600 mL over a 24-hour period.
  - Massive hemoptysis can be life threatening and should be considered a medical emergency. Death is usually from asphyxiation or exsanguination with flooding of the alveoli resulting in refractory hypoxemia.
  - Massive hemoptysis accounts for about 1–5% of all patients presenting with hemoptysis.
- **The most common causes of hemoptysis in the United States are bronchitis, bronchiectasis, bronchogenic carcinoma, TB, and pneumonia.**
- The pulmonary circulation consists of dual blood supplies: the pulmonary and bronchial artery systems.
  - The pulmonary artery system is a low-pressure system with pressures of 15–20/5–10 mm Hg. It delivers blood from the right ventricle to the pulmonary capillary beds for oxygenation and returns it to the left atrium via the pulmonary veins.
  - The bronchial arteries arise from the aorta and thus exhibit systemic pressures. There are one or two bronchial arteries per lung and these arteries are the main source of nutrients and oxygenation of the lung tissue and hilar lymph nodes.
- In patients with normal pulmonary artery pressures, bleeding from the pulmonary arterial system only accounts for ~5% of massive hemoptysis cases.
- **Mortality risk factors** identified for in-hospital mortality include mechanical ventilation, pulmonary artery bleeding, cancer, aspergillosis, chronic alcoholism, and an admission CXR with infiltrates in more than two quadrants.[1]

DIAGNOSIS

- A thorough history, physical examination, and laboratory evaluation can help determine the correct etiology of the hemoptysis and clarify the best diagnostic procedure.
- Processes that could be confused with hemoptysis, such as hematemesis or bleeding from the upper airway, must first be eliminated.

Clinical Presentation

- Important historical points to cover include prior lung, cardiac, or renal disease, history of smoking cigarettes, prior hemoptysis, pulmonary symptoms, infectious symptoms, family history of hemoptysis or brain aneurysms (hereditary hemorrhagic telangiectasia), chemical exposures (asbestos, organic chemicals), travel history, TB exposures, bleeding disorders, use of anticoagulants or antiplatelet agents, and gastrointestinal or upper airway complaints.

- Signs that may aid in diagnosis include telangiectasias (hereditary hemorrhagic telangiectasia), skin rashes (vasculitis, rheumatologic diseases, infective endocarditis), splinter hemorrhages (endocarditis, vasculitis), clubbing (chronic lung disease, carcinoma), bruits that increase with inspiration (large arteriovenous [AV] malformations), cardiac murmurs (endocarditis, mitral stenosis, congenital heart disease), and lower extremity edema (deep vein thrombosis).

Differential Diagnosis

The differential diagnosis of hemoptysis is presented in Table 18-1 (also see Chapter 19).

Diagnostic Testing

Laboratories

- Complete blood count: to assess the magnitude and acuity of bleeding and for thrombocytopenia.
- Renal function and urinalysis: to look for evidence of pulmonary-renal syndromes.

TABLE 18-1 CAUSES OF HEMOPTYSIS

Infection
Bronchitis
Endocarditis
Lung abscess
Mycetoma
Pneumonia (viral, tuberculous, fungal, necrotizing)

Malignancy
Primary bronchogenic carcinoma
Kaposi sarcoma
Lung metastases

Pulmonary
Bronchiectasis
Bullous emphysema
Cystic fibrosis

Trauma/foreign body
Broncholithiasis
Direct lung trauma
Foreign body
Tracheovascular fistula

Cardiac/pulmonary vascular
Arteriovenous malformation
Endocarditis
Mitral stenosis
Pulmonary artery rupture
Pulmonary embolism/infarction

Miscellaneous
Amyloidosis
Cryptogenic
Endometriosis

Alveolar hemorrhage
Vasculitis
- Behçet syndrome
- Goodpasture syndrome
- Granulomatosis with polyangiitis (Wegener granulomatosis)
- Henoch–Schönlein purpura
- Microscopic polyangiitis

Rheumatologic
- Rheumatoid arthritis
- Systemic sclerosis
- Systemic lupus erythematosus

Hematologic
- Antiphospholipid antibody syndrome
- Autologous or allogeneic stem cell transplant
- Coagulopathy

Medication/drugs/toxin exposure (penicillamine, cytotoxics, nitrofurantoin, amiodarone, retinoic acid, crack cocaine, solvents)

Idiopathic pulmonary hemosiderosis

- Coagulation profile: to assess for the presence of a coagulopathy.
- Pulse oximetry and an arterial blood gas: to assess oxygenation.

Imaging

- The three traditional methods of evaluating the etiology of hemoptysis include CXR, CT scan, and bronchoscopy.
- Performing a **CXR** first is reasonable for the majority of patients. Findings may lead to at least localization of the site of bleeding.
  - A negative CXR may not be very helpful, depending on the clinical picture. For example, a nonsmoking young patient with a relatively small amount of transient hemoptysis in the setting of acute bronchitis and a normal CXR likely does not require further evaluation.
  - In other patients a normal CXR does not eliminate the possibility of a serious cause, including malignancy.[2]
  - Further imaging (usually CT scan) is appropriate in patients with hemoptysis >30 mL **or** >40 years old **and** >30 pack-years of smoking, persistent/recurrent hemoptysis <30 mL and >40 years old **or** >30 pack-years of smoking, and in patients with massive hemoptysis (>300–400 mL).[2–6]
- **High-resolution CT**
  - The sensitivity of high-resolution CT (HRCT) scanning is better than CXR, particularly for certain diagnoses, such as bronchiectasis.[7–9]
  - HRCT has better diagnostic yield (i.e., abnormal finding leading to a specific diagnosis) when compared to bronchoscopy alone in some studies.[2,9–11]

Diagnostic Procedures

- **Bronchoscopy**
  - The overall diagnostic yield of bronchoscopy specifically for hemoptysis is difficult to say with precision, likely depends on patient population, and may be fairly low. In a study by Gong et al., flexible bronchoscopy in the acute setting versus delayed has been shown to be more likely to visualize active bleeding (41% vs. 8%) or the site of bleeding (34% vs. 11%).[12]
  - In patients with abnormal, but nonlocalizing CXRs, the diagnostic yield reported by Hirshburg et al. was 34–55%. In the patients with moderate to severe hemoptysis, bronchoscopy was able to localize the site of bleeding in ~65% of patients. Bronchoscopy combined with CT scanning had a diagnostic yield of 93%.[7]
  - In patients with localizing CXR, the yield of bronchoscopy has been as high as 82%.[13]
- **Flexible bronchoscopy versus rigid bronchoscopy** in the setting of massive hemoptysis.
  - Flexible bronchoscopy has the advantage of better visualization of airways, ability to navigate into small subsegments, and can be performed at the bedside. However, suctioning blood is inferior with flexible bronchoscopy compared to that with rigid bronchoscopy.
  - Rigid bronchoscopy usually requires operating room resources, only allows direct visualization of larger airways, but bleeding can be better controlled and therapeutic interventions can be performed.

TREATMENT

- **Nonmassive hemoptysis:** treat the underlying cause (i.e., antibiotics for an infection, radiation therapy or laser therapy for an endobronchial tumor).
- **Massive hemoptysis:** management of massive hemoptysis should focus on **airway protection and stabilization, localization of bleeding, and bleeding control.** A patient with massive hemoptysis should be observed in the intensive care unit (ICU,) even if not intubated.

- **Airway protection and stabilization**
  - If the location is known, the patient should be placed in the **lateral decubitus position** with the affected side down.
  - The patient with massive hemoptysis often requires intubation. The patient can be selectively (right or left) intubated on the nonbleeding side.
  - **Selective intubation** can be performed using a double-lumen endotracheal (ET) tube, selective mainstem intubation using a standard ET tube into the nonbleeding lung, or a standard ET tube in the trachea with a Fogarty catheter placed around the ET tube into the bleeding lung.
    - If bleeding occurs in the left lung, it is not advised to place a standard ET tube into the right mainstem bronchus due to the proximal position of the right upper lobe bronchus takeoff and high risk of right upper lobe collapse. Instead, a double-lumen ET tube or an ET tube in the trachea with placement of a Fogarty catheter are preferable. Placement of a Fogarty catheter is often done using a bronchoscope.
    - Both positioning and selective intubation are used to prevent aspiration of blood into the nonbleeding lung.
  - It is important to remember that blood clots in the large bronchi can be life threatening even without large decreases in hematocrit.
  - The use of strong cough suppressants (e.g., opiates) can also be helpful.
  - Large-bore IV access should be obtained and fluid resuscitation should be started.
- **Localization of the bleeding**
  - Localization is very important in the management of massive hemoptysis.
  - Localization can be attempted using the imaging and diagnostic procedures listed in the previous section in addition to a careful pulmonary examination.
  - The presence of rhonchi or wheezes on examination might suggest the site of bleeding.
- **Control of bleeding**
  - First, the patient's medication list should be reviewed for anticoagulants (e.g., warfarin, dabigatran, etc.) or platelet inhibitors (e.g., aspirin, clopidogrel), and these medications should be held at least until bleeding is controlled.
  - If a coagulopathy is present, it should be corrected with the use of appropriate factor replacement and platelet transfusions.
  - In patients with a history of renal failure, consider desmopressin for possible platelet dysfunction.
  - Once bronchoscopy has been performed to localize the site of bleeding, therapeutic options can be performed through the bronchoscope, including iced saline lavage, topical epinephrine, endobronchial tamponade, and laser photocoagulation.
- **Pulmonary angiography and bronchial artery embolization** by interventional radiology may also be attempted.
  - It is frequently used to try to stop massive hemoptysis or recurrent hemoptysis (from sources such as mycetomas). The short-term success rate of bronchial artery embolization is between about 65% and 95% but rebleeding can recur in a minority of patients.[14–17]
  - Bronchial artery embolization is contraindicated if the anterior spinal artery arises from the bronchial artery, as this could lead to spinal cord ischemia. The overall risk of spinal cord ischemic injury is <1%. Bronchoscopy prior to angiography is helpful in directing the radiologist to the affected area of lung and can allow for embolization of potential culprit vessels in the setting of a negative angiogram.
- **Surgery**
  - Surgery is a potential option for patient who can sustain a lobectomy or even pneumonectomy.
  - Mortality rates that have been reported vary between 1% and 50%.

- Thoracic surgery consultation and evaluation should be obtained early in an unstable hemoptysis patient.
- Operative complications include recurrence and spinal cord injury/ischemia due to disruption of the anterior spinal arteries.

REFERENCES

1. Fartoukh M, Khoshnood B, Parrot A, et al. Early prediction of in-hospital mortality of patients with hemoptysis: an approach to defining severe hemoptysis. *Respiration.* 2012;83:106–14.
2. Thirumaran M, Sundar R, Sutcliffe IM, et al. Is investigation of patients with haemoptysis and normal chest radiograph justified. *Thorax.* 2009;64:854–6.
3. Poe RH, Israel RH, Marin MG, et al. Utility of fiberoptic bronchoscopy in patients with hemoptysis and a nonlocalizing chest roentgenogram. *Chest.* 1988;93:70–5.
4. O'Neil KM, Lazarus AA. Hemoptysis: indications for bronchoscopy. *Arch Intern Med.* 1991;151:171–4.
5. Herth F, Ernst A, Becker HD. Long-term outcome and lung cancer incidence in patients with hemoptysis of unknown origin. *Chest.* 2001;120:1592–4.
6. Ketai LH, Mohammed TL, Kirsch J, et al. ACR appropriateness criteria hemoptysis. *J Thorac Imaging.* 2014;29:W19–22.
7. Hirshberg B, Biran I, Glazer M, et al. Hemoptysis: etiology, evaluation and outcomes in a tertiary hospital. *Chest.* 1997;112:440–4.
8. Tasker AD, Flower CD. Imaging the airways. Hemoptysis, bronchiectasis, and small airways disease. *Clin Chest Med.* 1999;20:761–73.
9. Revel MP, Fournier LS, Hennebicque AS, et al. Can CT replace bronchoscopy in the detection of the site and cause of bleeding in patients with large or massive hemoptysis. *AJR Am J Roentgenol.* 2002;179:1217–24.
10. Set PA, Flower DC, Smith IE, et al. Hemoptysis: comparative study of the role of CT and fiberoptic bronchoscopy. *Radiology.* 1993;189:677–80.
11. Laroche C, Fairbairn I, Moss H, et al. Role of computed tomographic scanning of the thorax prior to bronchoscopy in the investigation of suspected lung cancer. *Thorax.* 2000;55:359–63.
12. Gong H Jr, Salvatierra C. Clinical efficacy of early and delayed fiberoptic bronchoscopy in patients with hemoptysis. *Am Rev Respir Dis.* 1981;124:221–5.
13. Hsiao EI, Kirsch DM, Kagawa FT, et al. Utility of fiberoptic bronchoscopy before bronchial artery embolization for massive hemoptysis. *AJR Am J Roentgenol.* 2001;177:861–7.
14. Cremaschi P, Nascimbene C, Vitulo P, et al. Therapeutic embolization of bronchial artery: a successful treatment in 209 cases of relapse hemoptysis. *Angiology.* 1993;44:295–9.
15. Jean-Baptiste E. Clinical assessment and management of massive hemoptysis. *Crit Care Med.* 2000;28:1642–7.
16. Woo S, Yoon CJ, Chung JW, et al. Bronchial artery embolization to control hemoptysis: comparison of N-butyl-2-cyanoacrylate and polyvinyl alcohol particles. *Radiology.* 2013;269:594–602.
17. Larici AR, Franchi P, Occhipinti M, et al. Diagnosis and management of hemoptysis. *Diagn Interv Radiol.* 2014;20:299–309.

Diffuse Alveolar Hemorrhage

19

Amber A. Afshar and Richard D. Brasington

GENERAL PRINCIPLES

- Diffuse alveolar hemorrhage (DAH) encompasses a heterogeneous group of pulmonary and nonpulmonary disorders characterized by widespread intra-alveolar bleeding.
- DAH is a medical emergency that can result in acute respiratory failure and death.
- The exact incidence and prevalence of DAH are unknown owing to the variety of underlying etiologies but the most common cause of DAH appears to be systemic vasculitis, in particular granulomatosis with polyangiitis (GPA) (Fig. 19-1).[1,2]
- The pathogenesis of DAH is thought to be secondary to direct effects of autoantibodies on the alveolar capillary endothelium.
- Differentiation from localized etiologies (Table 19-1) of pulmonary hemorrhage is difficult to ascertain on history and physical examination alone; diagnostic procedures such as CXR and fiberoptic bronchoscopy are often needed.

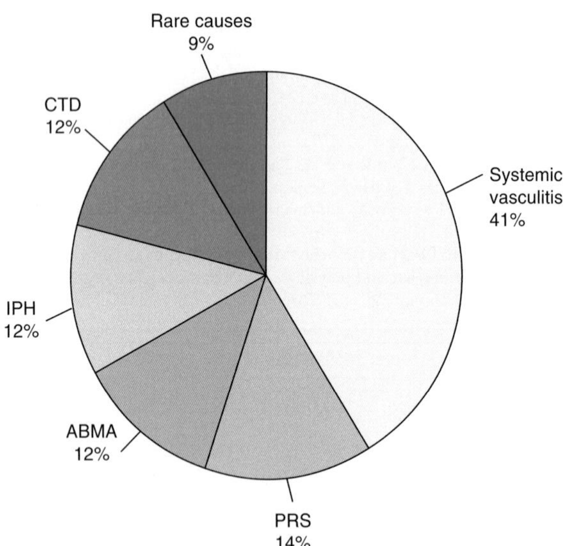

FIGURE 19-1. Causes of diffuse alveolar hemorrhage. ABMA, antibasement membrane antibody–mediated disease; CTD, connective tissue disease; IPH, idiopathic pulmonary hemorrhage; PRS, pulmonary renal syndromes. (Data from Travis WD, Colby TV, Lombard C, et al. A clinicopathologic study of 34 cases of diffuse pulmonary hemorrhage with lung biopsy confirmation. *Am J Surg Pathol.* 1990;14:1112–25.)

TABLE 19-1 CAUSES OF LOCALIZED PULMONARY HEMORRHAGE
Upper airway or gastrointestinal bleeding with resultant aspiration—that is, epistaxis or hematemesis (may be difficult to distinguish from diffuse alveolar hemorrhage)
Neoplasm (primary bronchogenic, Kaposi sarcoma)
Cavitary lung disease (secondary to TB, aspergillosis)
Pulmonary infarction
Bronchitis
Bronchiectasis
Broncholithiasis
Necrotizing bronchopneumonia
Arteriovenous malformations

DIAGNOSIS

- Appropriate diagnosis of DAH requires high clinical suspicion and a thorough history and physical examination.
- **Rapid diagnosis of DAH is mandatory** given the potential for excessive morbidity (renal failure, restrictive and obstructive lung disease) and mortality rates approaching 70–80% in untreated subsets of patients.

Clinical Presentation

- DAH should be suspected whenever a patient presents with **hemoptysis, dyspnea, and a predisposing condition**, such as an underlying connective tissue disorder, systemic vasculitis, or certain drug or occupational exposures.
- Hemoptysis, a presumed cardinal symptom of DAH, may be absent in up to one-third of cases despite pronounced and life-threatening alveolar hemorrhage.
- A **detailed history of past and present medications** (prescribed, over-the-counter, and recreational) and **occupational exposures** should be obtained.
  - Amiodarone, retinoic acid, sirolimus, penicillamine, and crack cocaine have all been implicated as causative agents of DAH.[3]
  - Inhalation of trimellitic anhydride, a chemical found in paints, varnishes, and plastics, has also been reported as a cause of DAH.
- **Physical examination findings are nonspecific** and may include fever, hypoxemia, tachypnea, and diffuse crackles.
- Signs suggesting an underlying systemic disorder should be sought. These signs may include sinusitis, iritis, oral ulcers, arthritis, synovitis, palpable purpura, neuropathy, and cardiac murmurs.

Differential Diagnosis

DAH is infrequently the initial presentation of an underlying systemic disorder (Table 19-2 and Fig. 19-1).[1–14] Twenty percent of patients with systemic lupus erythematosus (SLE) and 5–10% of patients with Goodpasture syndrome present with DAH as the initial or sole manifestation. Therefore, emphasis should be placed on the rheumatologic, renal, pulmonary, and cardiac review of systems.

Diagnostic Testing

Laboratories

- Laboratory evaluation is crucial for the diagnosis of DAH.
- Complete blood count

TABLE 19-2 CAUSES OF DIFFUSE ALVEOLAR HEMORRHAGE

Rheumatologic	**Hematologic**
Systemic lupus erythematosus[5]	Autologous or allogeneic stem cell transplant[7]
Rheumatoid arthritis[6]	Thrombotic thrombocytopenic purpura[8]
Mixed connective tissue disorder[6]	Idiopathic thrombocytopenic purpura
Systemic sclerosis	Disseminated intravascular coagulation
Juvenile rheumatoid arthritis	Cryoglobulinemia
Polymyositis	Antiphospholipid antibody syndrome[9]
	Multiple myeloma
Vasculitis	**Gastrointestinal**
Behçet disease	Ulcerative colitis
Cryoglobulinemia	**Medication/drugs**
Goodpasture syndrome	Abciximab[10]
Granulomatosis with polyangiitis (Wegener granulomatosis)	Amiodarone[11]
Henoch–Schönlein purpura	Crack cocaine[3]
Microscopic polyangiitis	Nitrofurantoin
Pulmonary	Penicillamine
Isolated pauci-immune pulmonary capillaritis	Propylthiouracil
Idiopathic pulmonary fibrosis	Phenytoin
Idiopathic pulmonary hemosiderosis	Retinoic acid[12]
Acute lung transplant rejection	Sirolimus[13]
Pulmonary venoocclusive disease	Tirofiban[10]
Pulmonary capillary hemangiomatosis	Warfarin[14]
Renal	**Occupational exposures**
IgA nephropathy	Trimellitic anhydride
Idiopathic glomerulonephritis	Radiation exposure
Poststreptococcal glomerulonephritis	Asbestosis
Cardiac	Welder pneumoconiosis
Mitral stenosis	
Bacterial endocarditis	

  - Anemia is commonly found, and repeated bouts of DAH may lead to an iron-deficiency anemia.
  - Thrombocytopenia or elevated coagulation parameters should raise the possibility of hemorrhage secondary to an acquired coagulopathy or antiphospholipid antibody syndrome.
- Coagulation parameters
- Basic metabolic profile. If creatinine is abnormal, urine microscopy should be assessed for dysmorphic red blood cells or casts.
- Urinalysis
- Drug screen should be obtained on all patients to rule out cocaine use.[3]
- **Serologic markers** should also be obtained and their selection guided by the differential diagnosis.

- **Antineutrophil cytoplasmic antibodies** (ANCA) (see Chapter 20)
  - Commonly found in GPA (Wegener granulomatosis), microscopic polyangiitis (MPA), Churg–Strauss syndrome (CSS), and isolated pauci-immune capillaritis. ANCAs are occasionally seen in other disease states.[15]
  - Cytoplasmic ANCA (c-ANCA) screens for the definitive antibody test, antiproteinase 3 (PR3), and likewise for perinuclear ANCA (p-ANCA) and antimyeloperoxidase (MPO). The level of c-ANCA may sometimes be useful in following disease activity but this is not consistently the case. In a literature review by Rao et al., the sensitivity of c-ANCA in active GPA was 91% versus 63% in inactive disease. The specificity was equivalent in both situations and approached 99%.[16]
  - p-ANCA, antibodies directed against MPO, is less specific and may be associated with many clinical syndromes. p-ANCA is found in 80% of patients with MPA. p-ANCA has also been identified in 15–20% of patients with GPA and up to 20–30% of patients with Goodpasture syndrome.
- **Antiglomerular basement membrane (Anti-GBM) antibodies**
  - Diagnostic for Goodpasture syndrome, characterized by antibodies (predominantly IgG) directed against the noncollagenous domain of type IV collagen, alpha 3.[17]
  - The sensitivity and specificity of anti-GBM approaches 98%. Two percent to 3% of patients with renal biopsy-proven Goodpasture syndrome may have negative serum anti-GBM, making renal (and not lung) biopsy the gold standard for diagnosis.[17,18]
- Other serologic markers help to assess for SLE.
  - Antinuclear antibody (ANA)
  - Antidouble-stranded DNA (anti-dsDNA)
  - Complement levels (C3 and C4)

Imaging

- Chest X-rays
  - Standard PA/LAT CXRs in DAH are nonspecific for any of the underlying etiologies and often reveal bilateral alveolar infiltrates during the acute episode.
  - Pulmonary fibrosis or severe obstructive lung disease may develop in chronic, recurrent bouts of DAH. Accordingly, persistent interstitial infiltrates or hyperinflation may be evident on successive CXRs.
- Chest CT
  - Generally not specifically indicated in DAH, as it adds little information to the CXR.
  - However, chest CT may help in the differential diagnosis for hemoptysis or better localize parenchymal findings such as cavitary lung disease, malignancy, or fibrosis.

Diagnostic Procedures

- **Pulmonary function testing** (PFTs)
  - PFTs are unnecessary in the diagnostic assessment but may demonstrate restriction and gas exchange abnormalities, in chronic cases.
  - In acute DAH, an increase in the diffusing capacity for carbon monoxide (DLCO) is often present, attributed to the increased binding of carbon monoxide to intra-alveolar hemoglobin.
  - Varying degrees of hypoxemia result from the ventilation–perfusion abnormalities produced by the alveolar hemorrhage.
- **Fiberoptic bronchoscopy**
  - Bronchoscopy with **bronchoalveolar lavage** (BAL) is the diagnostic gold standard for DAH and helps to rule out infectious causes.
    - Criteria for DAH include progressively bloodier returns from sequential BAL performed in three separate subsegmental bronchi or >20% hemosiderin-laden macrophages.[19]

    - False-positive results can occur in smokers (so-called smokers' macrophages, the most common cause of hemosiderin-laden macrophages) and with distal bronchiolar sources of hemorrhage.[20]
    - A false negative may occur if bronchoscopy is performed too early or too late. On average, 48–72 hours are necessary for hemosiderin-laden macrophages to be seen in alveoli and interstitial spaces. After 2–4 weeks, hemosiderin-laden macrophages generally clear.
  - The role of **bronchoscopic biopsies** is less significant for the differential diagnosis of DAH.
    - Only 17.6% of directed endobronchial biopsies were diagnostic of Wegener granulomatosis in the setting of observed ulcerating tracheobronchitis.[21]
    - Transbronchial biopsies may be of low yield (see Microscopic findings below).
- **Surgical lung biopsy** is reserved for rare occasions where the diagnosis is not clear from history, physical examination, and serologic markers.
  - Methods are video-assisted thoracoscopy (VATS) and open lung biopsy.
  - **Microscopic findings**[1,4,20]
    - Typically one of three light microscopic patterns: pulmonary capillaritis, diffuse alveolar damage, or bland pulmonary hemorrhage.
    - The most common histologic finding in DAH is pulmonary capillaritis: fibrin thrombi occluding capillaries, fibrinoid necrosis of capillary walls, neutrophils and nuclear dust in the interstitium and surrounding alveoli, and interstitial red blood cells and hemosiderin. In one series of 34 patients with biopsy-proven DAH, 88% of patients displayed pulmonary capillaritis.[2]
    - Diffuse alveolar damage is a stereotypic response to lung injury, characterized by interstitial edema, intra-alveolar hyaline membranes, and type 2 alveolar cell hyperplasia in the acute phase.
    - Bland pulmonary hemorrhage is characterized by blood cells in the alveolar spaces without inflammation, necrosis, or destruction of the alveolar walls. Causes can include bleeding disorders, anticoagulation, and heart failure.
    - None of these patterns is pathognomonic for any specific disease and multiple histologic findings can be associated with the same disease process.

TREATMENT

- Treatment of DAH depends primarily on the underlying disorder.
- Therapies ranging from watchful waiting (in idiopathic pulmonary hemosiderosis) to high-dose corticosteroids and cytotoxic therapy (in ANCA-associated vasculitides).[1,22,23]
- Typical regimens for life-threatening alveolar hemorrhage include:
  - Cyclophosphamide, 1–2 mg/kg/d initially, and subsequent prolonged maintenance therapy with cyclophosphamide.
  - Methylprednisolone, 1 g/d IV for 3 days, followed by prednisone (1 mg/kg/d for 3 months followed by a 3-month taper).
  - Plasmapheresis is indicated in certain cases such as Goodpasture syndrome.[24–27]
  - Also see Chapter 20.

REFERENCES

1. Lara AR, Schwarz MI. Diffuse alveolar hemorrhage. *Chest.* 2010;137:1164–71.
2. Travis WD, Colby TV, Lombard C, et al. A clinicopathologic study of 34 cases of diffuse pulmonary hemorrhage with lung biopsy confirmation. *Am J Surg Pathol.* 1990;14:1112–25.
3. Haim DY, Lippmann ML, Goldberg SK, et al. The pulmonary complications of crack cocaine. A comprehensive review. *Chest.* 1995;107:233–40.

4. Green RJ, Ruoss SJ, Kraft SA, et al. Pulmonary capillaritis and alveolar hemorrhage. Update on diagnosis and management. *Chest.* 1996;110:1305–16.
5. Zamora MR, Warner ML, Tuder R, et al. Diffuse alveolar hemorrhage and systemic lupus erythematosus: clinical presentation, histology, survival, and outcome. *Medicine.* 1997;76:192–202.
6. Schwarz MI, Zamora MR, Hodges TN, et al. Isolated pulmonary capillaritis and diffuse alveolar hemorrhage in rheumatoid arthritis and mixed connective tissue disease. *Chest.* 1998;113:1609–15.
7. Afessa B, Tefferi A, Litzow MR, et al. Diffuse alveolar hemorrhage in hematopoietic stem cell transplant recipients. *Am J Respir Crit Care Med.* 2002;166:641–5.
8. Martinez AJ, Maltby JD, Hurst DJ. Thrombotic thrombocytopenic purpura seen as pulmonary hemorrhage. *Arch Intern Med.* 1983;143:1818–20.
9. Crausman RS, Achenbach GA, Pluss WT, et al. Pulmonary capillaritis and alveolar hemorrhage associated with the antiphospholipid antibody syndrome. *J Rheumatol.* 1995;22:554–6.
10. Ali A, Patil S, Grady KJ, et al. Diffuse alveolar hemorrhage following administration of tirofiban or abciximab: a nemesis of platelet glycoprotein IIb/IIIa inhibitors. *Cathet Cardiovasc Interv.* 2000; 49:181–4.
11. Vizioli LD, Cho S. Amiodarone-associated hemoptysis. *Chest.* 1994;105:305–6.
12. Nicolls MR, Terada LS, Tuder RM, et al. Diffuse alveolar hemorrhage with underlying pulmonary capillaritis in the retinoic acid syndrome. *Am J Respir Crit Care Med.* 1998;158:1302–5.
13. Vlahakis NE, Rickman OB, Morgenthaler T. Sirolimus-associated DAH. *Mayo Clin Proc.* 2004; 79:541–5.
14. Barnett VT, Bergmann F, Humphrey H, et al. Diffuse alveolar hemorrhage secondary to superwarfarin ingestion. *Chest.* 1992;102:1301–2.
15. Gal AA, Velasquez A. Antineutrophil cytoplasmic autoantibody in the absence of Wegener's granulomatosis or microscopic polyangiitis: implications for the surgical pathologist. *Mod Pathol.* 2002;15:197–204.
16. Rao JK, Weinberger M, Oddone EZ, et al. The role of antineutrophil cytoplasmic antibody testing in the diagnosis of Wegener's granulomatosis. A literature review and meta-analysis. *Ann Intern Med.* 1995;123:925–32.
17. Hudson BG, Tryggvason K, Sundaramoorthy M, et al. Alport's syndrome, Goodpasture's syndrome, and type IV collagen. *N Engl J Med.* 2003;348:2543–56.
18. Salama AD, Dougan T, Levy JB, et al. Goodpasture's disease in the absence of circulating anti-glomerular basement membrane antibodies as detected by standard techniques. *Am J Kidney Dis.* 2002;39:1162–7.
19. De Lassence A, Fleury-Feith J, Escudier E, et al. Alveolar hemorrhage. Diagnostic criteria and results in 194 immunocompromised hosts. *Am J Respir Crit Care Med.* 1995;151:157–63.
20. Colby TV, Fukuoka J, Ewaskow SP, et al. Pathologic approach to pulmonary hemorrhage. *Ann Diagn Pathol.* 2001;5:309–19.
21. Daum TE, Specks U, Colby TV, et al. Tracheobronchial involvement in Wegener's granulomatosis. *Am J Respir Crit Care Med.* 1995;151:522–6.
22. Jantz MA, Sahn SA. Corticosteroids in acute respiratory failure. *Am J Respir Crit Care Med.* 1999; 160:1079–100.
23. Metcalf JP, Rennard SI, Reed EC, et al. Corticosteroids as adjunctive therapy for diffuse alveolar hemorrhage associated with bone marrow transplantation. *Am J Med.* 1994;96:327–34.
24. Gallagher H, Kwan JT, Jayne DR. Pulmonary renal syndrome: a 4-year, single-center experience. *Am J Kidney Dis.* 2002;39:42–7.
25. Klemmer PJ, Chalermskulrat W, Reif MS, et al. Plasmapheresis therapy for diffuse alveolar hemorrhage in patients with small-vessel vasculitis. *Am J Kidney Dis.* 2003;42:1149–53.
26. Jayne DR, Gaskin G, Rasmussen N, et al. Randomized trial of plasma exchange or high-dosage methylprednisolone as adjunctive therapy for severe renal vasculitis. *J Am Soc Nephrol.* 2007; 18:2180–8.
27. Walsh M, Catapano F, Szpirt W, et al. Plasma exchange for renal vasculitis and idiopathic rapidly progressive glomerulonephritis: a meta-analysis. *Am J Kidney Dis.* 2011;57:566–74.

Pulmonary Vasculitis

20

Amit Patel and Alfred H. J. Kim

Vasculitis Overview

GENERAL PRINCIPLES

- This chapter discusses the pulmonary features of systemic vasculitides, primarily focusing on the antineutrophil cytoplasmic antibody (ANCA)-associated small-vessel vasculitides **granulomatosis with polyangiitis** (GPA) (formally known as Wegener granulomatosis), **microscopic polyangiitis** (MPA), and **Churg–Strauss syndrome** (CSS). Each of these vasculitides will be considered in separate sections in this chapter.
- Other vasculitides with pulmonary manifestations will be described under special considerations.

Definition

- Systemic vasculitides feature inflammatory leukocytes damaging the walls of blood vessels. This damage can lead to **vessel wall inflammation and downstream tissue ischemia.**
- **Vasculitis is a pathologic finding, not a diagnosis.** Clinicians must determine the cause of the vasculitic condition.

Classification

- Vasculitides may be classified as **primary versus secondary processes.** Primary vasculitides are further classified by the size and type of involved blood vessels.
- **Primary vasculitis** occurs in the absence of an underlying illness and without identifiable etiology.
  - Several classification schemes have been described, but the most commonly utilized one is derived from the 1993 **Chapel Hill Consensus Conference**, so-called "CHC criteria".[1]
  - While vasculitis may often affect vessels of more than one size, the CHC criteria organized the vasculitides based on the **size of the vessels primarily affected** (Table 20-1).[1] The small-vessel vasculitides are further subdivided into ANCA positive or ANCA negative.
- **Secondary vasculitis** occurs in the presence of an underlying condition, such as the capillaritis seen in systemic lupus erythematosus (SLE) or virus-induced vasculitis.

Epidemiology

- Although the primary systemic vasculitides are rare and epidemiologic studies have been difficult in the setting of evolving classification systems and nomenclature, the **frequency of vasculitic diagnoses has been increasing**, possibly because vasculitic syndromes are more readily recognized.
- At an annual incidence of 13 cases/million adults, **giant-cell arteritis (GCA) represents the most common vasculitis.** GCA is followed in annual incidence by rheumatoid arthritis (RA)-associated vasculitis (12.5 cases/million), GPA (8.5 cases/million), MPA (2.4 cases/million), CSS (2.4 cases/million), and Henoch–Schönlein purpura (1.2 cases/million).[2]

TABLE 20-1 CLASSIFICATION OF VASCULITIS

Large Vessel
- Takayasu arteritis
- Giant-cell arteritis

Medium Vessel
- Polyarteritis nodosa
- Kawasaki disease
- Primary angiitis of the central nervous system

Small Vessel
- **Immune complex related**
  - Hypersensitivity vasculitis[a]
  - Henoch–Schönlein purpura
  - Cryoglobulinemic vasculitis[b]
  - Connective tissue disease-associated vasculitis[c]
- **Pauci-immune**
  - ANCA-associated granulomatous vasculitis[d]
  - Churg–Strauss syndrome
  - Microscopic polyangiitis

[a]Most often cause by medications, infections, and malignancies.

[b]Most often associated with hepatitis B and C, Epstein–Barr virus, plasma cell dyscrasias, chronic inflammatory/autoimmune disorders, and lymphoproliferative malignancies.

[c]Most often associated with rheumatoid arthritis, systemic lupus erythematosus, and Sjögren syndrome.

[d]Also known as Wegener granulomatosis.

Adapted from Jennette JC, Falk RJ, Andrassy K, et al. Nomenclature of systemic vasculitides. Proposal of an international consensus conference. *Arthritis Rheum.* 1994;37:187–92.

DIAGNOSIS

- Clinicians should consider a diagnosis of vasculitis in patients whose clinical presentation includes **systemic symptoms** (e.g., fatigue, weakness, fever) as well as **evidence of organ dysfunction** (e.g., renal, neurologic, pulmonary). As the clinical manifestations of the vasculitides are quite variable and overlap with many other disorders, a thorough history and physical examination is essential to aid in the diagnosis of vasculitis. The clinical presentation of the small-vessel ANCA-associated vasculitides will be discussed in each of their respective sections found below.
- **Pulmonary manifestations** of the systemic vasculitides may range from shortness of breath due to mild upper respiratory tract symptoms to pulmonary failure resulting from devastating alveolar hemorrhage. While the lungs may not represent the only involved organ system for many cases of vasculitis, respiratory symptoms often motivate these patients to seek medical attention.[3]
- Basic laboratory tests for the vasculitides should include serum creatinine, liver function tests, complete blood count, muscle enzyme tests, erythrocyte sedimentation rate (ESR), C-reactive protein (CRP), viral hepatitis and HIV serologies, urinalysis, and urine toxicology screen. More specific tests may include **antinuclear antibody** (ANA, for lupus), **serum complement levels** (depressed in mixed cryoglobulinemia and lupus), and **ANCA** (often directed against proteinase 3 in GPA and against myeloperoxidase (MPO) in MPA).

- Certain procedures are often crucial for the diagnosis of vasculitides. Specifically, **tissue biopsy** can definitively establish the presence of vasculitis. **Arteriography** is useful for vasculitides affecting large- and medium-sized blood vessels, as in arch angiography for Takayasu arteritis. Similarly, mesenteric or renal artery angiography can assist in patients suspected of having polyarteritis nodosa (PAN).

TREATMENT

While the treatments for ANCA-associated vasculitis will be discussed in their respective sections, management of most vasculitides generally involves **corticosteroids, typically in combination with other immunosuppressive agents.** Other considerations in management specific to a particular vasculitis will be discussed with that particular syndrome.

SPECIAL CONSIDERATIONS

- **Primary large-vessel vasculitides**
  - **GCA or temporal arteritis** represents the most common vasculitis among Caucasians, predominantly affects the elderly, and classically involving the **extracranial branches of the carotid artery.**
    - Respiratory symptoms such as cough, hoarseness, or throat pain represent the initial complaint in up to one-quarter of patients, although CXRs and pulmonary function testing may be normal.
    - In a patient with suspected GCA, fulfilling three of the following five criteria is associated with >90% sensitivity and specificity for the diagnosis of GCA: **age ≥50 years at disease onset, new-onset localized headache, tenderness or decreased pulse of temporal artery, ESR >50, and a biopsy with necrotizing arteritis with a predominance of mononuclear cells or a granulomatous process with multinucleated giant cells.**[4]
    - A common variant of GCA is **large-vessel GCA,** which manifests as **arm claudication**, pulselessness, aortic aneurysms, or aortic insufficiency.
    - Treatment: **long-term prednisone treatment** (9–12 months) usually leads to symptom resolution in GCA.[5] Optimal steroid dosing is not precisely known.
  - **Takayasu arteritis** affects the **aorta and its major branches**, and is classically described in young Asian females.
    - Manifestations can include mild pulmonary hypertension, fistula formation between branches of the pulmonary artery and bronchial arteries, and/or nonspecific inflammatory interstitial lung disease.
    - CT or MRI angiography demonstrates **pulmonary artery stenoses and occlusion** in nearly half of patients.
    - Diagnostic criteria: 3 of 6 is associated with a sensitivity of 90% and specificity of 98% for the diagnosis of Takayasu arteritis: **age ≤40 years at disease onset, extremity claudication, decreased pulsation of at least one brachial artery, systolic blood pressure difference ≥10 mm Hg between the arms, bruit over a subclavian artery or abdominal aorta, and arteriographic narrowing or occlusion of the aorta or its major branches not due to other causes.**[6]
    - Treatment: Glucocorticoids and immunosuppression are used for initial treatment, while methotrexate or vascular bypass are options for severe or refractory cases.
- **Primary medium-vessel vasculitides**
  - PAN is a necrotizing systemic vasculitis affecting both **medium and small muscular arteries.**
    - Associated with **hepatitis B infection.**
    - Can present with skin nodules, mononeuritis multiplex, orchitis, and mesenteric artery involvement, but does not typically cause glomerulonephritis or vasculitis of the arterioles, capillaries, or venules.

    - Although pulmonary involvement is extremely rare in PAN, it can occur as alveolar hemorrhage or diffuse alveolar damage, manifesting as diffuse interstitial or patchy alveolar infiltrates, even when hepatitis B virus related.[7]
    - Treatment: high-dose corticosteroids and, if necessary, additional immunosuppressants.
  - **Kawasaki disease** (KD), while primarily a medium-vessel vasculitis, can also affect large and small blood vessels.
    - Usually seen in **children**, this vasculitis has a predilection for the **coronary arteries**, and may be associated with a mucocutaneous lymph node syndrome.
    - While pulmonary symptoms are not among the criteria for diagnosis, pulmonary involvement can occasionally occur in KD, and may be misinterpreted as **atypical pneumonia or unresolving pneumonia**, with findings ranging from subclinical interstitial micronodular infiltrates to larger inflammatory pulmonary nodules.
    - Treatment: typically **aspirin and IV immunoglobulin.**
- **Behçet disease**
  - Behçet disease is a relapsing multisystem disorder characterized by **recurrent oral ulcerations** and at least two of the following findings: **genital ulcers, uveitis, cutaneous nodules or pustules, and positive pathergy test.**[8] A more recent scoring system provides better sensitivity for the diagnosis.[9]
  - Vessels of all sizes in both the arterial and venous systems may be affected, although it is most common to have **arterial small vessel or venous involvement.**
  - While cough, dyspnea, or chest pain may represent initial respiratory symptoms, massive hemoptysis may be the most significant complication. Credited as the underlying mechanism in Behçet disease, **immune complex deposition** can lead to lung findings such as **pulmonary artery aneurysms** due to destruction of the elastic lamina or arterial–bronchial fistulae due to erosion of the bronchi.[10] Resultant massive hemoptysis carries an associated mortality of nearly 40%. Pulmonary angiography has given way to CT and magnetic resonance angiography in the diagnosis of Behçet disease.
  - Treatment
    - **Prednisone with azathioprine or cyclophosphamide** produces the best outcomes for pulmonary artery aneurysms, although chlorambucil, colchicine, cyclosporine, and methotrexate in combination with prednisone have been used.
    - Aspirin at 81 mg/d should be considered for the prevention of recurrent venous thrombosis but should be avoided in any patient with known pulmonary involvement, given the risk of hemoptysis.
- **Secondary vasculitides**
  - Both **RA and SLE** are associated with a secondary vasculitis thought to be immune complex mediated. Complications include **rheumatoid nodules in the lungs in RA** and **pulmonary hypertension and alveolar hemorrhage in SLE**. While the mortality associated with alveolar hemorrhage in SLE is considerable, treatment with the combination of plasmapheresis and pulse-dose cyclophosphamide has limited success.
  - **Necrotizing sarcoid granulomatosis** is distinguished from sarcoidosis by its **extensive vasculitis and necrosis**, lack of extrapulmonary involvement, and radiographic findings of pulmonary masses, nodules, and pleural involvement (all less commonly seen in sarcoidosis). The vasculitis may be epithelioid granulomatous (with histiocytes and multinucleated giant cells reminiscent of GCA) or lymphocytic without granuloma formation. Necrotizing sarcoid granulomatosis often features a subacute clinical onset and may include nonspecific respiratory symptoms such as cough, dyspnea, or wheezing. While prognosis is good (with spontaneous resolution seen in some cases), further therapy can include oral corticosteroids (similar to chronic pulmonary sarcoidosis).

Granulomatosis with Polyangiitis

GENERAL PRINCIPLES

- GPA, formerly known as Wegener granulomatosis, is a multisystem disease primarily involving small- and occasionally medium-sized blood vessels. While GPA was originally described as a variant of PAN, the findings of a **progressive granulomatous process that involved the upper and lower respiratory tract** led the German pathologist Frederick Wegener to believe that he had discovered a unique vasculitic syndrome. Recently, concerns have been raised about Wegener's association with the Nazi regime. In 2011, the American College of Rheumatology (ACR), the American Society of Nephrology, and the European League Against Rheumatism formally changed the name to GPA.[11]
- The Chapel Hill Consensus Conference defined GPA as "**granulomatous inflammation involving the respiratory tract, and necrotizing vasculitis affecting small- to medium-sized vessels.**"[1]
- In terms of classification, GPA can be divided into limited and generalized disease.
  - **Limited** GPA includes cases **without kidney involvement** (generally, limited to the upper respiratory tract or the lungs) and reflects pathology mainly due to necrotizing granulomas and not active vasculitis.
  - **Generalized** GPA features pathology characterized by vasculitis and/or with any evidence of end-organ disease or impending organ failure.
- While GPA can occur at any age, ANCA-associated vasculitis typically affects middle-aged and older adults. GPA affects men and women equally but has a predilection for Caucasians.

DIAGNOSIS

Clinical Presentation

- The **initial presentation** of GPA may be insidious, with generalized complaints such as malaise, fatigue, weight loss, hearing loss, and upper respiratory symptoms. Soon after, patients may develop symptoms that involve multiple organ systems. Limited GPA tends to feature constitutional symptoms (and may progress to generalized GPA if left untreated), while generalized GPA can involve end-organ disease.
  - **Ear, nose, and throat involvement** is present in up to 99% of cases of GPA, and may include chronic rhinitis and/or sinusitis, sinus pain, epistaxis, and nasal crusting. Destruction of the nasal cartilage can lead to nasal septal perforation or the saddle-nose deformity. Other manifestations include ulcerations of the oropharynx, gingival hyperplasia, and the rare **strawberry gingival hyperplasia** pathognomonic of GPA.[12]
  - Patients can also develop symptoms that can be confused with asthma from tracheobronchial ulcerations, intraluminal inflammatory pseudotumor, and bronchomalacia. Scarring from these lesions can lead to significant **airway obstruction**.
  - The primary pulmonary manifestations of GPA include **necrotizing granulomas, cavitary lesions, and scattered nodules**. Capillaritis in the lung can lead to diffuse alveolar hemorrhage with an associated mortality of nearly 50%. This clinical presentation may be indistinguishable from Goodpasture syndrome or MPA.
  - **Dermatologic** findings in GPA span papules, vesicles, palpable purpura, ulcers, or SC nodules. **Leukocytoclastic vasculitis** represents the most common manifestation, present in almost one-half of cases of GPA. Other skin lesions such as pyoderma gangrenosum and granulomatous skin lesions have been reported.
  - **Nervous system** involvement is thought to be secondary to vasculitis of the vasa nervorum. Most commonly, patients may have **mononeuritis multiplex**, typically a sensorimotor polyneuropathy with asymmetric involvement (i.e., foot or wrist drop).

TABLE 20-2 AMERICAN COLLEGE OF RHEUMATOLOGY 1990 CRITERIA FOR DIAGNOSIS OF GRANULOMATOSIS WITH POLYANGIITIS

The presence of at least 2 of the following 4 are required:

- Nasal or oral inflammation (painful or painless ulcers, purulent or bloody nasal discharge)
- Abnormal CXR (nodules, fixed infiltrates or cavities)
- Hematuria or red blood cell casts in urine sediment
- Pathologic evidence of granulomas, leukocytoclastic vasculitis, and necrosis

Adapted from Leavitt RY, Fauci AS, Bloch DA, et al. The American College of Rheumatology 1990 criteria for the classification of Wegener's granulomatosis. *Arthritis Rheum.* 1990;33:1101–7.

Less commonly, patients may have cranial neuritis, cerebral vasculitis, or granulomatous infiltration.

- ○ **Renal** involvement in GPA due to capillaritis leads to a **pauci-immune crescentic glomerulonephritis.** If left untreated, the renal disease may lead to end-stage renal failure.

Diagnostic Criteria

- Although the **classic "Wegener triad"** includes necrotizing granulomatous inflammation of the respiratory tract, generalized necrotizing vasculitis of the small arteries and veins, and necrotizing glomerulonephritis, fewer than one-half of the originally described cases fulfilled these criteria.
- The original 1990 ACR classification criteria, which did not have a separate classification for MPA, included: **nasal or oral inflammation, abnormal CXR (with nodules, fixed infiltrates, or cavitations), abnormal urinary sediment (microscopic hematuria), and granulomatous inflammation on biopsy** (Table 20-2).[13]
- The Chapel Hill Consensus Conference classified GPA, as noted above, as a granulomatous inflammation affecting the respiratory tract and necrotizing vasculitis affecting small- and medium-sized blood vessels.[1]
- More recent algorithms have added ANCA as a diagnostic criterion and proposed surrogate markers suggestive of granulomatous involvement of the upper or lower airway as well as glomerulonephritis to facilitate the diagnosis of GPA without biopsy.
  - ○ **Upper airway:** bloody nasal discharge and crusting for >1 month or nasal ulceration; chronic sinusitis, otitis media, or mastoiditis for >3 months; retro-orbital mass or inflammation (pseudotumor); subglottic stenosis; saddle-nose disease and/or destructive sinonasal disease.
  - ○ **Lower airway:** chest radiographic evidence of fixed pulmonary infiltrates, nodules, or cavitations present for >1 month; bronchial stenosis.
  - ○ **Renal vasculitis (glomerulonephritis):** hematuria associated with red blood cell (RBC) casts or >10% dysmorphic erythrocytes; a 2+ proteinuria on urinalysis.

Diagnostic Testing

Laboratories

- Initial laboratory data may reveal a leukocytosis, anemia, and/or an active urinary sediment with dysmorphic RBC and RBC casts in small-vessel vasculitis. Limited GPA often shows modest increases in inflammatory markers such as ESR and CRP, while generalized GPA can show marked elevations in ESR and CRP.
- **Cytoplasmic ANCA** (c-ANCA, or PR3-ANCA) is most commonly directed against serine proteinase 3, and c-ANCA positivity is prevalent in 70–95% of generalized GPA

and 40–50% of limited GPA (with a specificity as high as 80–100% in all GPA patients). However, serial measurements of c-ANCA have not been shown to reliably assess disease course or predict relapse.[14]
- **Perinuclear ANCA** (p-ANCA) positivity, while quite prevalent in MPA and to a lesser extent, CSS, is only present in 0–10% of cases of GPA. A definitive positive ANCA test must possess **c-ANCA specificity to PR3** and **p-ANCA specificity to MPO by ELISA.** The absence of this result renders this test negative.

Imaging
- **CXR** may reveal lung nodules with or without cavitation, and/or patchy or diffuse opacities. Less commonly, pleural effusions, hilar lymphadenopathy, or diffuse bilateral opacities may be seen.
- **High-resolution CT scanning** of the chest has increased the sensitivity for diagnosis of GPA. CT findings in GPA may include the aforementioned nodules with or without cavitations (and so-called feeding blood vessels leading to these nodules), patchy or diffuse ground-glass or consolidative opacities, pulmonary microinfarction, irregular and enlarged peripheral pulmonary arteries, or even tracheal or bronchial stenosis.[15]

Diagnostic Procedures
- The histopathologic hallmarks of GPA include **vasculitis, necrosis, and granulomatous inflammation of small- and medium-sized vessels.** While the lung and upper respiratory tract offer the highest sensitivity and specificity for biopsy sampling, the size of the biopsy specimen as well as any concurrent immunosuppressive therapy may affect the diagnostic value of the biopsy.
- Flexible **fiberoptic bronchoscopy** can aid diagnosis by providing direct visual inspection and to obtain tissue biopsies. Ulcerating tracheobronchitis and mucosalcobblestoning may be seen, and healing can lead to secondary scarring complicated by airway stenosis, obstruction, bronchomalacia, and postobstructive pneumonia. While only 20% of bronchoscopic biopsy samples may be diagnostic of GPA, bronchoscopic findings in combination with the appropriate clinical presentation and laboratory data may save patients from an open lung biopsy.
- **Renal biopsy** typically reveals a focal segmental necrotizing glomerulonephritis that may be indistinguishable from that found in MPA, Goodpasture syndrome, or SLE. Immunofluorescence microscopy can differentiate GPA and MPA (**pauci-immune crescentic glomerulonephritis**) from the linear fluorescence staining seen in Goodpasture syndrome and the granular pattern of immune deposits found in SLE.

TREATMENT

- Before current therapy, the mortality associated with untreated GPA was nearly universal, with a mean survival of ~5 months.
- Therapy for GPA is managed according to disease activity (limited vs. generalized) and can also be divided into **induction and maintenance therapy.**
  - For generalized GPA, induction includes **cyclophosphamide and prednisone (1 mg/kg/d) or methylprednisolone (1 g/d) for 3 days.**
  - Once a therapeutic response is achieved, the prednisone may be tapered over 2–3 months and then discontinued if remission persists. The cyclophosphamide may be continued for 3 months, and is then followed by maintenance therapy. A **complete remission rate of about 75–90%** can be achieved with this protocol, typically at 2–6 months.
  - For relapse of disease, this protocol should be reinitiated. Apart from the toxicities associated with glucocorticoid administration, the treatment-associated toxicity of cyclophosphamide therapy (which up to one-half of patients may suffer from) includes amenorrhea, hemorrhagic cystitis, bladder cancer, and myelodysplasia. In cases of

alveolar hemorrhage, progressive glomerulonephritis, or other severe disease, **plasmapheresis** may improve clinical outcomes.[16–19]
  - In patients who cannot tolerate cyclophosphamide, the RAVE trial demonstrated that **rituximab** is not inferior to cyclophosphamide for induction.[20]
  - For limited GPA, **methotrexate** is the drug of choice with a small side effect profile and limited toxicity. For these patients, the NORAM trial suggested that methotrexate is as effective as cyclophosphamide for the induction of remission, but may be associated with a higher relapse rate after termination of treatment.[21]
- Maintenance therapy in GPA remains somewhat unclear. **Azathioprine or methotrexate** is the most promising in patients (no standard regimen or duration of treatment exists). The CYCAZAREM trial demonstrated that the substitution of azathioprine for cyclophosphamide after the achievement of remission did not increase the rate of relapse.[22] Other agents such as mycophenolate mofetil and leflunomide are undergoing investigation.
- Given that the combination of glucocorticoid and additional immunosuppressive therapy has been shown to increase the risk of *Pneumocystis jiroveci* pneumonia, prophylaxis with trimethoprim-sulfamethoxazole now standard.

Microscopic Polyangiitis

GENERAL PRINCIPLES

- MPA is a necrotizing vasculitis that primarily affects small blood vessels. GPA and MPA are virtually the same disease, except that MPA has **no granulomatous pathology**.
- The Chapel Hill Consensus Conference defined MPA as a "**necrotizing vasculitis with few or no immune deposits affecting small vessels**. Necrotizing arteritis of small- and medium-sized arteries may be present. Necrotizing glomerulonephritis is very common, and pulmonary capillaritis often occurs." Notably, granulomatous inflammation is not present in MPA.[1]
- Similar to GPA, MPA can present at nearly any age but has a mean age of onset of 50 years. Men and women are probably affected equally, though some studies have suggested a female predominance.

DIAGNOSIS

Clinical Presentation

- The clinical presentation of MPA can be similar to that described above for GPA. The exception is the ear, nose, and throat manifestations, which are seen almost exclusively in GPA.
- **Renal and pulmonary involvement** are the main clinical features of MPA. Pulmonary symptoms can range from mild hemoptysis with transient pulmonary infiltrates seen on CXR to massive hemoptysis with diffuse alveolar hemorrhage.
- **Pulmonary–renal failure** may the initial clinical presentation in fulminant MPA, and hemodynamic, respiratory, and/or renal replacement support may be needed.
- Other typical features of small-vessel vasculitis such as cutaneous, peripheral nerve, and even gastrointestinal manifestations may also be present.

Diagnostic Criteria

- While the original ACR classification criteria did not distinguish between MPA and GPA, the Chapel Hill Consensus Conference differentiated MPA from the other small-vessel ANCA-associated vasculitides GPA and CSS by the **absence of granulomatous inflammation**.[1]

- More recently developed classification algorithms allow for the diagnosis of MPA once GPA and CSS have been excluded. While significant overlap exists in the clinical presentation and ANCA serologies between GPA and MPA, **the finding of granulomatous changes on biopsy in GPA represents the key pathologic distinction.**

Diagnostic Testing

- The initial laboratory work-up for MPA is similar to that for GPA. As noted above, while GPA is associated with c-ANCA positivity, MPA is associated with **p-ANCA** positivity, which is present in up to 80% of patients with MPA. The p-ANCA staining needs to be confirmed by ELISA for reactivity to **MPO.**
- Findings on chest imaging (both CXR and CT) can be similar to that of GPA.
- Biopsy of affected areas demonstrates necrotizing vasculitis and the typical histology of MPA is **pulmonary capillaritis.** Renal biopsy usually reveals a necrotizing glomerulonephritis indistinguishable from that caused by GPA. However, a key distinction between GPA and MPA is the presence of granulomatous changes on biopsy in GPA.

TREATMENT

- As in GPA, **remission induction begins with oral steroids and cyclophosphamide.** However, **relapses are common in MPA.** While cyclophosphamide is effective for treating active disease, it has not been shown to prevent disease relapse. Rituximab may be used in those intolerant to cyclophosphamide.[20]
- Many patients with MPA may experience disease relapse during the tapering of remission maintenance or after therapy is discontinued. Relapses, however, are generally milder than the initial presentation, though some may include end-organ damage.
- Mild relapse is often managed with increases in dosage of oral steroids, while major relapse often requires the reintroduction of initial therapy. In **treatment failure,** plasma exchange may be considered.[16–18] IV immunoglobulin has been used in refractory cases with limited success.

Churg–Strauss Syndrome

GENERAL PRINCIPLES

- CSS, also known as allergic granulomatosis and angiitis and eosinophilic GPA, is a small- to medium-artery vasculitis characterized by **asthma, hypereosinophilia, and necrotizing vasculitis.**
- The Chapel Hill Consensus Conference defined CSS as an "**eosinophil-rich and granulomatous inflammation involving the respiratory tract and necrotizing vasculitis affecting small- to medium-sized vessels, and associated with asthma and blood eosinophilia.**"[1]
- Like GPA and MPA, CSS can present at any age and affects men and women equally.

DIAGNOSIS

Clinical Presentation

- The clinical course of CSS classically includes **three phases.** While the phases do not have to proceed in order, the ACR has found them to be 95% sensitive and specific for CSS when coupled with histopathologic evidence of vasculitis.[23,24]
  - The **first, or prodromal, phase** consists of asthma and rhinosinusitis, and can last up to 20 years.

  - The **second, or eosinophilic, phase** is characterized by peripheral and tissue eosinophilia.
  - The **third, or vasculitic, phase** is marked by an extensive vasculitis that most commonly involves the **lungs**, but can also affect the dermatologic, nervous, cardiovascular, gastrointestinal, and renal organ systems.
- The hallmark pulmonary manifestation of CSS is the **prodromal asthma** present in >95% of patients but **allergic rhinitis, sinusitis, and nasal polyps** are also common. Because many patients have been treated with steroids for asthma-type symptoms, the diagnosis of CSS can be delayed.
- Extrapulmonary manifestations of CSS
  - **Mononeuritis multiplex**, which affects up to three-quarters of patients with CSS, represents the most common extrapulmonary finding.
  - **Dermatologic** findings are also quite common (found in up to two-thirds of patients with CSS) and may include purpura, livedo reticularis, and SC nodules.
  - **Cardiovascular** involvement accounts for a significant fraction of the morbidity and mortality of CSS, and findings may include ECG abnormalities, heart failure, eosinophilic myocarditis, coronary vasculitis, or pericardial effusions.
  - **Renal** involvement, present in one-quarter of CSS patients and seen far less commonly than in GPA or MPA, typically manifests as a focal segmental necrotizing glomerulonephritis but does not usually result in fulminant renal failure.
  - Eosinophilic or vasculitic involvement of the **gastrointestinal tract** can result in abdominal pain, and other gastrointestinal findings can include pancreatitis, gastrointestinal perforation, or hemorrhage.

Diagnostic Criteria

- The 1990 ACR criteria for CSS included the following six elements: **asthma, eosinophilia >10%, mononeuropathy or polyneuropathy, migratory or transient pulmonary opacities on CXR, paranasal sinus abnormality, and biopsy featuring eosinophils in extravascular areas** (Table 20-3). The presence of four or more of these six criteria yields a sensitivity of 85% and a specificity of >99%.[23]
- The Chapel Hill Consensus Conference described CSS, as noted above, as an eosinophil-rich and granulomatous process affecting the respiratory tract and necrotizing vasculitis involving small and medium vessels, with associated asthma and eosinophilia.[1]

TABLE 20-3 AMERICAN COLLEGE OF RHEUMATOLOGY 1990 CRITERIA FOR CHURG–STRAUSS SYNDROME

The presence of at least 4 of the following 6 are required:

- Asthma
- Eosinophilia >10%
- Mononeuropathy or polyneuropathy attributable to a systemic vasculitis
- Migratory or transient infiltrates on chest radiography
- Paranasal sinus abnormality (acute or chronic paranasal pain or radiographic opacification of paranasal sinuses)
- Extravascular eosinophils on biopsy

Adapted from Masi AT, Hunder GC, Lie JT. The American College of Rheumatology 1990 criteria for the classification of Churg–Strauss syndrome (allergic granulomatosis and angiitis). *Arthritis Rheum.* 1990;33:1094–100.

Differential Diagnosis

In the absence of proven vasculitis, the prodromal phase may be confused with typical asthma, and the eosinophilic phase may be confused with eosinophilic pneumonia, Löffler syndrome, or eosinophilic gastroenteritis.

Diagnostic Testing

Laboratories

- **Peripheral eosinophilia** is characteristic of CSS and may be present in any phase of the illness.
- ESR and CRP may be elevated in CSS, especially during active vasculitis.
- Other nonspecific laboratory abnormalities may include a normocytic anemia, leukocytosis, elevated IgE, and a positive but low-titer rheumatoid factor.
- While MPO-ANCA may be positive in approximately one-half of patients with CSS, **the utility of ANCA testing is not as well defined for CSS as for GPA or MPA.**

Imaging

- CXR findings are variable and nonspecific but can include **transient and patchy pulmonary infiltrates**, peripheral parenchymal infiltrates, pulmonary nodules (with cavitation far less frequent than in GPA), or pleural effusions.
- High-resolution CT scanning may reveal bilateral scattered ground-glass opacities and/or bronchial wall thickening.
- Cardiac MRI may have utility in assessing myocardial involvement in CSS patients.

Diagnostic Procedures

- **Bronchoalveolar lavage** is often performed and can show a **high percentage of eosinophils** in the setting of active pneumonitis.
- **Tissue biopsy** is crucial to establishing the diagnosis of CSS, and should be performed prior to initiating potentially toxic therapy. As transbronchial lung biopsy is often nondiagnostic, surgical lung biopsy may be required. The typical lung biopsy in CSS reveals **asthmatic bronchitis, eosinophilic infiltration, extravascular granulomas, and/or necrotizing vasculitis.**
- Biopsy of skin disease or peripheral neuropathy showing necrotizing, eosinophilic, and/or granulomatous vasculitis may aid in diagnosis.

TREATMENT

- The **five-factors score** (FFS) includes cardiac involvement, gastrointestinal disease, renal insufficiency (serum creatinine ≥1.58 mg/dL), proteinuria ≥1 g/d, and central nervous system involvement. The FFS, while designed for prognosis, can be used to guide initial management in CSS.[25]
- The cornerstone of therapy for CSS is **glucocorticoids**, which are used alone for an FFS score of 0. Before the use of steroids, patients with CSS faced a mortality rate of 50% within 3 months of diagnosis.
- Although the role of **cyclophosphamide** and other cytotoxic agents are less well defined for CSS than for GPA or MPA, they have been used in combination with corticosteroids for remission induction in cases with higher FFS values or in relapsed cases.[26]
- **Azathioprine and methotrexate** have been used for remission maintenance, but concurrent steroid treatment may often be required.[27,28]
- Plasma exchange, IV immunoglobulin, interferon-α, TNF-α inhibitors, and rituximab have been used in refractory cases.[17,29,30]
- At 80–90%, the remission rate for CSS is comparable to GPA and MPA but the relapse rate somewhat lower and 5-year survival slightly higher.

REFERENCES

1. Jennette JC, Falk RJ, Andrassy K, et al. Nomenclature of systemic vasculitides: proposal of an international consensus conference. *Arthritis Rheum.* 1994;37:187–92.
2. Watts RA, Carruthers DM, Scott DG. Epidemiology of systemic vasculitis: changing incidence or definition? *Sem Arthritis Rheum.* 1995;25:28–34.
3. Schwarz MI, Brown KK. Small vessel vasculitis of the lung. *Thorax.* 2000;55:502–10.
4. Hunder GG, Bloch DA, Michel BA, et al. The American College of Rheumatology 1990 criteria for the classification of giant cell arteritis. *Arthritis Rheum.* 1990;33:1122–8.
5. Dejaco C, Singh YP, Perel P, et al. 2015 Recommendations for the management of polymyalgia rheumatica: a European League Against Rheumatism/American College of Rheumatology Collaborative Initiative. *Arthritis Rheumatol.* 2015;67:2569–80.
6. Arend WP, Michel BA, Bloch DA, et al. The American College of Rheumatology 1990 criteria for the classification of Takayasu arteritis. *Arthritis Rheum.* 1990;33:1129–34.
7. Naniwa T, Maeda T, Shimuzi S, et al. Hepatitis B virus-related polyarteritis nodosa presenting with multiple lung nodules and cavitary lesions. *Chest.* 2010;138:195–7.
8. International Study Group for Behçet's Disease. Criteria for diagnosis of Behçet's disease. *Lancet.* 1990;335:1078–80.
9. International Team for the Revision of the International Criteria for Behçet's Disease (ITR-ICBD). The International Criteria for Behçet's Disease (ICBD): a collaborative study of 27 countries on the sensitivity and specificity of the new criteria. *J Eur Acad Dematol Venereol.* 2014;28:338–47.
10. Ceylan N, Bayraktaroglu S, Erturk SM, et al. Pulmonary and vascular manifestations of Behcet disease: imaging findings. *Am J Roentgenol.* 2010;194:158–64.
11. Falk RJ, Gross WL, Guillevin L, et al. Granulomatosis with polyangiitis (Wegener's): an alternative name for Wegener's granulomatosis. *Ann Rheum Dis.* 2011;70:704.
12. Knight JM, Hayduk MJ, Summerlin DJ, et al. "Strawberry" gingival hyperplasia: a pathognomonic mucocutaneous finding in Wegener granulomatosis. *Arch Dermatol.* 2000;136:171–3.
13. Leavitt RY, Fauci AS, Bloch DA, et al. The American College of Rheumatology 1990 criteria for the classification of Wegener's granulomatosis. *Arthritis Rheum.* 1990;33:1101–7.
14. Finkielman JD, Merkel PA, Schroeder D, et al. Antiproteinase 3 antineutrophil cytoplasmic antibodies and disease activity in Wegener granulomatosis. *Ann Intern Med.* 2007;147:611–9.
15. Ananthakrishnan L, Sharma N, Kanne JP. Wegener's granulomatosis in the chest: high-resolution CT findings. *Am J Roentgenol.* 2009;192:676–82.
16. Gallagher H, Kwan JT, Jayne DR. Pulmonary renal syndrome: a 4-year, single-center experience. *Am J Kidney Dis.* 2002;39:42–7.
17. Klemmer PJ, Chalermskulrat W, Reif MS, et al. Plasmapheresis therapy for diffuse alveolar hemorrhage in patients with small-vessel vasculitis. *Am J Kidney Dis.* 2003;42:1149–53.
18. Jayne DR, Gaskin G, Rasmussen N, et al. Randomized trial of plasma exchange or high-dosage methylprednisolone as adjunctive therapy for severe renal vasculitis. *J Am Soc Nephrol.* 2007;18:2180–8.
19. Walsh M, Catapano F, Szpirt W, et al. Plasma exchange for renal vasculitis and idiopathic rapidly progressive glomerulonephritis: a meta-analysis. *Am J Kidney Dis.* 2011;57:566–74.
20. Stone JH, Merkel PA, Spiera R, et al. Rituximab versus cyclophosphamide for ANCA-associated vasculitis. *N Engl J Med.* 2010;363:221–32.
21. De Groot K, Rasmussen N, Bacon PA, et al. Randomized trial of cyclophosphamide versus methotrexate for induction of remission in early systemic antineutrophil cytoplasmic antibody-associated vasculitis. *Arthritis Rheum.* 2005;52:2461–9.
22. Jayne D, Rasmussen N, Andrassy K, et al. A randomized trial of maintenance therapy for vasculitis associated with antineutrophil cytoplasmic autoantibodies. *N Engl J Med.* 2003;349:36–44.
23. Masi AT, Hunder GG, Lie JT, et al. The American College of Rheumatology 1990 criteria for the classification of Churg–Strauss syndrome (allergic granulomatosis and angiitis). *Arthritis Rheum.* 1990;33:1094–100.
24. Baldini C, Talarico R, Della Rossa A, et al. Clinical manifestations and treatment of Churg–Strauss syndrome. *Rheum Dis Clin North Am.* 2010;36:527–43.
25. Guillevin L, Lhote F, Gayraud M, et al. Prognostic factors in polyarteritis nodosa and Churg–Strauss syndrome. A Prospective study in 342 patients. *Medicine (Baltimore).* 1996;75:17–28.
26. Gayraud M, Guillevin L, le Toumelin P, et al. Long-term followup of polyarteritis nodosa, microscopic polyangiitis, and Churg–Strauss syndrome: analysis of four prospective trials including 278 patients. *Arthritis Rheum.* 2001;44:666–75.

27. Ribi C, Cohen P, Pagnoux C, et al. Treatment of Churg–Strauss syndrome without poor-prognosis factors: a multicenter, prospective, randomized, open-label study of seventy-two patients. *Arthritis Rheum.* 2008;58:586–94.
28. Metzler C, Hellmich B, Gause A, et al. Churg–Strauss syndrome—successful induction of remission with methotrexate and unexpected high cardiac and pulmonary relapse ratio during maintenance treatment. *Clin Exp Rheumatol.* 2004;22:S52–61.
29. Metzler C, Schnabel A, Gross WL, et al. A phase II study of interferon-alpha for the treatment of refractory Churg–Strauss syndrome. *Clin Exp Rheumatol.* 2008;26:S35–40.
30. Mohammad AJ, Hot A, Arndt F, et al. Rituximab for the treatment of eosinophilic granulomatosis with polyangiitis (Churg–Strauss). *Ann Rheum Dis.* 2014. doi: 10.1136/annrheumdis-2014-206095.

Pulmonary Embolism and Deep Venous Thrombosis

21

Hannah Otepka Mannem
and Roger D. Yusen

GENERAL PRINCIPLES

- Acute pulmonary embolism (PE) is a commonly diagnosed condition with a morbidity and mortality rate that varies by age, clinical presentation, and the presence of comorbid disease.
- Despite advances in diagnosis and management, PE remains an underdiagnosed condition.
- Untreated PE has a high mortality rate. In some cases, PE can be safely treated at home, while in others immediate admission to an intensive care unit may be required to prevent death.
- Accurate risk stratification remains a critical component of the initial evaluation of the patient with acute PE.
- Effective approaches for the evaluation of patients with suspected PE and the treatment of those diagnosed with PE exist.

Definition

- Thromboses or blood clots occur in veins, arteries, or chambers of the heart.
- Venous thromboembolism (VTE) refers to the presence of deep vein thrombosis (DVT) or PE.
- Thrombus, air, fat, tumor, and foreign bodies may embolize to the lung.
- PE consists of embolized thrombus in the pulmonary arterial system.

Classification

- PE classification schema uses the terms acute versus chronic.
- Acute PE classification may use terms massive, submassive, and other.
- Massive PE, associated with acute right heart failure, leads to hypotension (e.g., systolic blood pressure <90 mm Hg or a drop >40 mm Hg from baseline for at least 15 minutes) despite volume resuscitation and vasopressor therapy. Hypotension may also occur from arrhythmias and decreased cardiac output.
- Submassive PE encompasses patients with PE who have hemodynamic stability in the setting of right ventricular (RV) dysfunction.

Epidemiology

- The overall annual incidence of PE has been reported ~23–69 cases per 100,000. VTE incidence increases sharply after about 50 years of age and is consistently higher in males. Rates are also higher in Caucasians and African Americans than Hispanics and Asian-Pacific Islanders.[1–3]
- The introduction of contrast-enhanced multidetector helical chest CT scan (PE protocol CT) has been associated with a doubling of the incidence of PE.[4,5]
- Without treatment, half of patients with proximal lower extremity DVT develop PE.
- Autopsy studies suggest that many PEs remain undiagnosed.[2]

Etiology

- DVTs in the proximal lower extremities and pelvis produce most PEs.
- Only about one-half to three-quarters of the patients diagnosed with PE will have DVT found on venous compression ultrasound of the lower extremities.
- DVTs that occur in upper extremities, often secondary to an indwelling catheter, may also cause PE.

Pathophysiology

- Vascular obstruction may lead to increased pulmonary vascular resistance, which if severe enough can lead to acute right heart failure and shock.
  - This occurs commonly in cases with emboli at main pulmonary arteries or bifurcations.
  - The amount of clot burden also plays a role in the severity of hemodynamic compromise.
- Inflammatory mediators also play a role in vasoconstriction of the pulmonary vasculature, decreased perfusion, and increased vascular resistance.
- Pulmonary arterial obstruction may produce hypoxemia via impaired alveolar gas exchange and increased lung dead space ventilation.

Risk Factors

- A method of classifying VTE risk factors uses the categories of inherited, acquired, or unknown (idiopathic).
- The most common inherited risk factors for VTE include two gene polymorphisms (factor V Leiden and prothrombin gene G20210A), deficiencies of the natural anticoagulants protein C, protein S, and antithrombin, dysfibrinogenemia, and hyperhomocysteinemia.
- Spontaneous (idiopathic) thrombosis, despite the absence of an inherited thrombophilia and detectable autoantibodies, predisposes patients to future thromboses.
- Acquired hypercoagulable states may arise secondary to malignancy, immobilization, infection, trauma, surgery, collagen vascular diseases, nephrotic syndrome, heparin-induced thrombocytopenia (HIT), disseminated intravascular coagulation (DIC), medications (e.g., estrogen), and pregnancy.

DIAGNOSIS

Clinical Presentation

- PE may produce shortness of breath, chest pain (pleuritic), hypoxemia, hemoptysis, pleural rub, new right-sided heart failure, and tachycardia, but these signs and symptoms are neither sensitive nor specific.
- **Validated clinical risk factors** for a PE in outpatients who present to an emergency department include signs and symptoms of DVT, high suspicion of PE by the clinician, tachycardia, immobility in the past 4 weeks, history of VTE, malignancy, and hemoptysis (see Table 21-1).[6]
- Clinical suspicion of DVT or PE should lead to objective testing.
- Patient symptoms are usually broad, nonspecific, and not sensitive.
- **Dyspnea** commonly occurs with PE. Other symptoms include pleuritic chest pain, cough, hemoptysis, lightheadedness, syncope, and diaphoresis.
- Vital signs are the most important physical examination findings in PE. Patients with PE often have **tachycardia or tachypnea. Hypotension** suggests possible massive PE and prompt diagnostic workup is essential.
- Other physical examination findings are very nonspecific, including rales, prominent S2 and P2 on cardiac auscultation, and elevated jugular venous pressure.

TABLE 21-1 MODIFIED WELLS CRITERIA FOR PULMONARY EMBOLISM

Criterion	Point Value
Symptoms of DVT (leg edema, tenderness)	3.0
Other diagnoses less likely than PE	3.0
Heart rate >100	1.5
Immobilization or surgery within the past 4 weeks	1.5
Prior history of DVT or PE	1.5
Hemoptysis	1.0
Malignancy	1.0
Score	**Rate** (95% CI)
≤4, PE unlikely	2.3–9.4%
>4, PE likely	27.6–51.6%

DVT, deep venous thrombosis; PE, pulmonary embolism; CI, confidence interval.

Adapted from Wells PS, Anderson DR, Rodger, et al. Derivation of a simple clinical model to categorize patients probability of pulmonary embolism: increasing the models utility with the SimpliRED D-dimer. *Thromb Haemost.* 2000;83:416–20.

Differential Diagnosis

- Clinicians under diagnose PE because it mimics many other diseases and vice versa.
- The differential is broad and includes pneumonia, acute coronary syndrome, acute lung injury, pleuritis, pericarditis, and congestive heart failure.
- In a hypotensive patient, the differential broadens to include sepsis, hypovolemia, cardiac tamponade, and acute myocardial infarction.

Diagnostic Testing

- Pretest probability plays a key role in the workup of patients with suspected PE.
- The incorporation of pretest probability, using scores such as Wells score or Geneva score, with diagnostic tests improves the accuracy of diagnosis (Table 21-1).[6–9]
- CXR, ECG, and arterial blood gas all provide nonspecific information but they can assist in determining pretest probability and clinical severity, and evaluating for other disorders.

Laboratories

- d-Dimer and cross-linked fibrin degradation products may increase during PE but they are nonspecific and have a low positive predictive value (PPV) and specificity; patients with a positive test require further evaluation.
- A negative d-dimer in combination with low pretest probability can exclude almost all PEs.[10]
- In the setting of a moderate to high clinical pretest probability (e.g., patients with cancer), a negative d-dimer does not have sufficient negative predictive value (NPV) for excluding the presence of PE.
- Arterial blood gas may or may not show hypoxemia or an increased alveolar–arterial oxygen gradient.
- Cardiac biomarkers such as troponin and brain natriuretic peptide (BNP) are useful for assisting with prognosis but they have low diagnostic accuracy.[11,12]

Electrocardiography

- Sinus tachycardia occurs in most patients with PE.
- The classic findings on ECG of S1Q3T3 (S in V1, Q wave in V3, and T-wave inversion in V3) and right bundle branch block are uncommon and not diagnostic.
- Signs of RV strain that include right axis deviation and RV hypertrophy may suggest the presence of massive PE.

Imaging

- **CXR** usually shows no specific findings, but may help assess for other diagnoses in the most timely manner. Classic findings such as Westermark Sign and Hampton Hump rarely occur.
- The most common and important diagnostic modalities for assessing patients with suspected PE include multidetector helical chest CT and ventilation/perfusion scintigraphy (V/Q scan).
- The stability of the patient plays an important role in which diagnostic test to perform (see Fig. 21-1).[13]
- Contrast-enhanced multidetector **helical chest CT** scan (PE protocol CT) has become the gold standard test for evaluating patients for PE, and it may assist with the detection of alternative or concomitant diagnoses.[14]
    - The sensitivity of CT for VTE improves by combining the CT pulmonary angiography results with objective grading of clinical suspicion.
    - The accuracy of CT for diagnosis of PE decreases with poorer scan quality and for smaller and more peripheral clots.
    - Contraindications to CT include contrast allergy, severe renal dysfunction, or inability to safely travel. Patients with a contraindication to CT or inadequate CT results should undergo other testing.
    - Negative d-dimer and multidetector chest CT tests exclude most PE.
    - Advantages of CT scan over V/Q scan include more diagnostic results (positive or negative), fewer indeterminate or inadequate studies, and the detection of alternative or concomitant diagnoses, such as dissecting aortic aneurysm, pneumonia, and malignancy.
- **V/Q scan** is useful for diagnosis in correlation with pretest probability and can be used in patients with contraindications or indeterminate readings from a PE protocol CT.[15]
    - V/Q scanning remains **most useful in a patient with a normal CXR**, because nondiagnostic V/Q scans commonly occur in the setting of an abnormal CXR.
    - V/Q scans may be classified as normal, nondiagnostic (i.e., very low probability, low probability, intermediate probability), or high probability for PE.
    - Use of clinical suspicion improves the accuracy of V/Q scanning. A normal or low probability V/Q scan in the setting of a low clinical suspicion adequately rules out PE. A high probability V/Q scan in the setting of a high clinical suspicion adequately confirms PE and no further testing is warranted.
    - In the setting of an indeterminate result, further testing should be done.
- **Venous compression ultrasonography** (CUS) is an easily accessible diagnostic modality that can act as a surrogate test for PE if it detects lower extremity proximal DVT and the clinical scenario is highly suggestive of PE.
    - Lower extremity venous CUS is not a first-line modality unless the above testing is not available or indeterminate.
    - If CUS does not detect DVT and clinical suspicion for PE is high, further diagnostic testing should be performed.
- **Echocardiography** may assess cardiopulmonary reserve and evidence of end-organ damage (RV dysfunction) in patients with PE and has a role in decision-making regarding the use of thrombolytic therapy.[16–18]

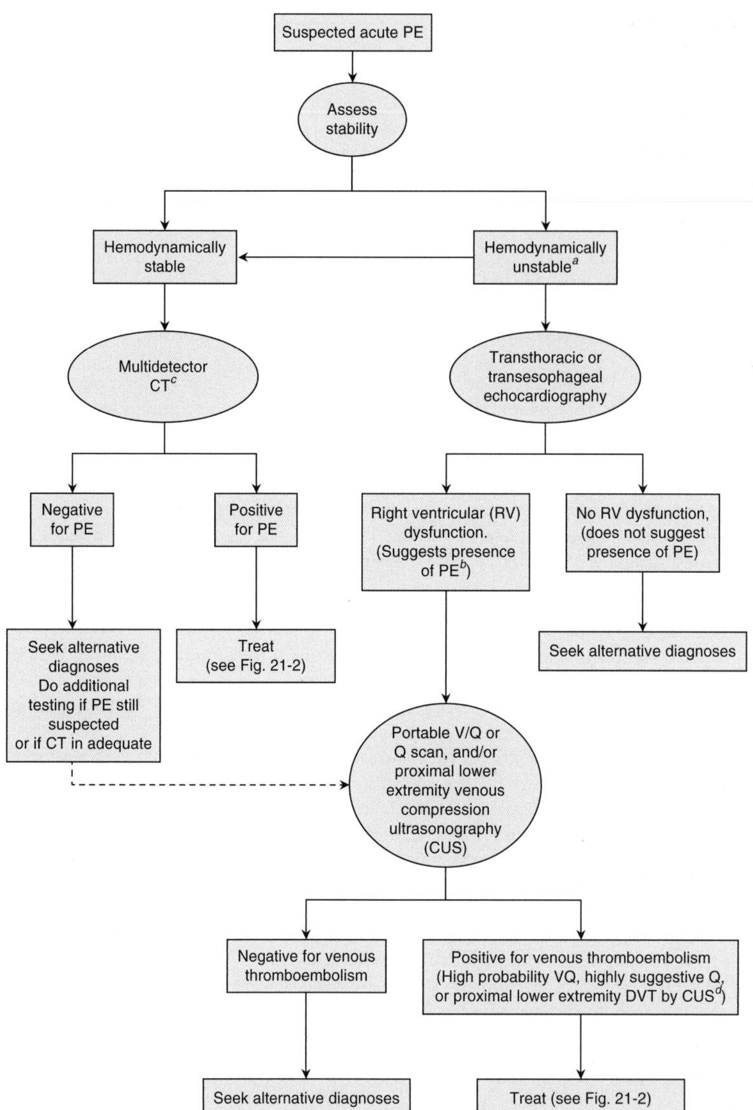

FIGURE 21-1 Diagnostic evaluation for suspected acute pulmonary embolism (PE). (From Otepka HC, Yusen RD. Pulmonary embolism. In: Kollef M, Isakow W, eds. *The Washington Manual of Critical Care*. 2nd ed. Philadelphia, PA: Lippincott Williams and Wilkins; 2013:97–104.)

- Echocardiography may detect a right heart thrombus or visualize an embolism in transit.
- Findings that suggest PE include RV dilation and hypokinesis; increase in RV/left ventricular (LV) diameter ratio; pulmonary artery dilation; tricuspid regurgitation; paradoxical septal motion; interventricular septal shift toward the LV; and McConnell sign, defined by hypokinesis of the free wall of the RV with normal motion of the apex.

TREATMENT

- Clinicians should make their treatment decisions for PE based on confidence in the diagnosis of PE, hemodynamic status, degree of RV dysfunction/injury, bleeding risk, prognosis, patient preferences, and patient-specific factors that could affect anticoagulant pharmacodynamics and pharmacokinetics. A treatment algorithm is presented in Figure 21-2.[13]
- Patients should undergo prompt initiation of empiric anticoagulation upon high clinical suspicion of PE prior to completion of diagnostic tests if the test cannot be completed in an urgent manner.
- Patients should achieve therapeutic anticoagulant levels soon after PE is diagnosed.
- Hemodynamically unstable patients should undergo prompt resuscitation in the emergency department or intensive care unit and consideration of thrombolytic therapy.[16–18]
- If diagnostic testing adequately rules out PE, then anticoagulation therapy should be discontinued and prophylaxis for VTE should be initiated.

Medications

- **Anticoagulation therapy is the mainstay of treatment** for acute PE, acting to prevent new clot formation, extension and embolism of existing clot, and recurrence.
- All patients should undergo bleeding risk assessment and evaluation for contraindications to anticoagulant therapy before their initiation.
- Anticoagulants that have efficacy for the treatment of PE demonstrated in clinical trials and approval by the FDA for this indication include unfractionated heparin (UFH), low–molecular-weight heparin (LMWH), and fondaparinux. All of these agents can be used as a bridge to warfarin for long-term therapy.
- Newer oral anticoagulants approved for other indications and currently not approved by the FDA for use in treatment of PE include the direct thrombin inhibitor dabigatran, and the direct anti-Xa inhibitors rivaroxaban and apixaban.[19]
- IV UFH was previously the mainstay of anticoagulation for stable patients with PE and it remains the primary anticoagulant for unstable patients.[20]
- **LMWHs** have become the primary short-term anticoagulant for patients with VTE.[17,20]
  - SC injection dosed once or twice daily based on body weight.
  - Caution should be used in patients with renal disease because, unlike UFH, LMWH has significant renal clearance.
- **Warfarin** inhibits vitamin K-dependent clotting factors and should be started after initiation of heparin/LMWH/fondaparinux.[17,21]
  - INR levels should be followed closely in patients on warfarin for PE with a target INR of 2.5 (goal range of 2.0–3.0).
  - Treatment of PE, with or without DVT, with warfarin requires overlap therapy with a parenteral anticoagulant (UFH, LMWH, or pentasaccharide) for at least 4–5 days and until the INR reaches at least 2.
  - It is important to counsel patients on maintaining stable diets while on warfarin and to be cautious of drug–drug interactions that may lead to rapid INR changes.
- Duration of anticoagulation for a first time VTE event is 3–6 months.

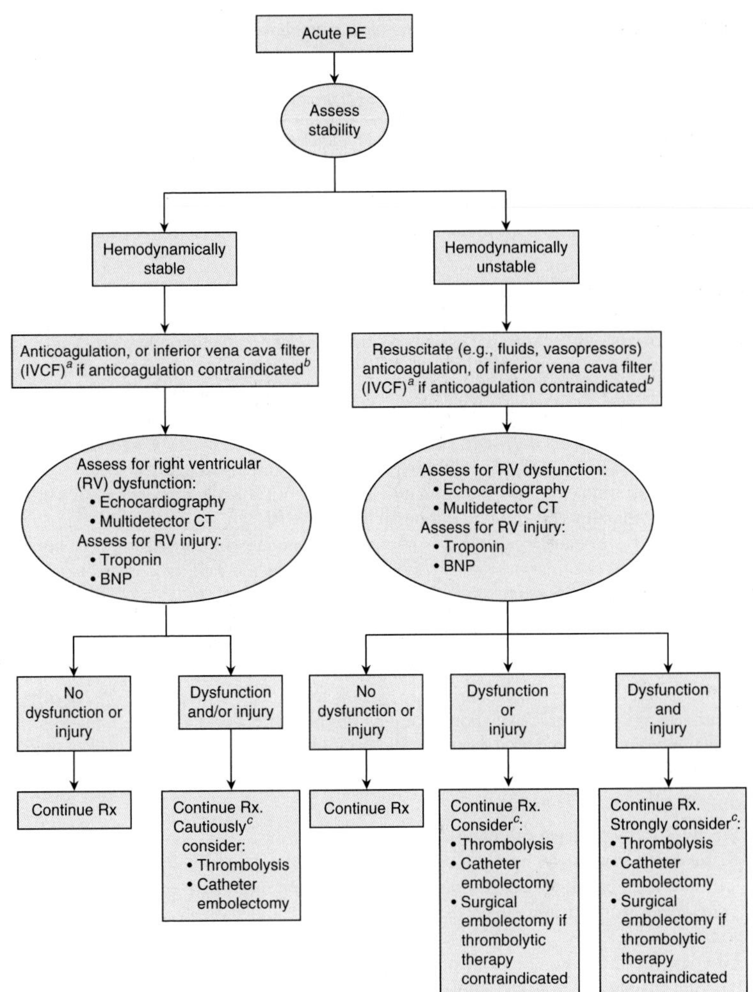

[a]Temporary or permanent IVCF.
[b]Anticoagulate after IVCF placement once contraindication to anticoagulation resolves.
[c]If contraindication do not exist.

FIGURE 21-2 Treatment of confirmed acute pulmonary embolism (PE). (From Otepka HC, Yusen RD. Pulmonary embolism. In: Kollef M, Isakow W, eds. *The Washington Manual of Critical Care*. 2nd ed. Philadelphia, PA: Lippincott Williams and Wilkins; 2013:97–104.)

- Longer-term anticoagulation is recommended in patients with a second event, a hypercoagulable state or malignancy, and possibly in patients with massive PE.
- **Thrombolytic agents** such as alteplase and reteplase have not shown a mortality benefit in clinical trials but their use should be considered in hemodynamically unstable patients with acute PE.[16–18]
    - Thrombolytics convert plasminogen to plasmin and lead to clot lysis. They are reserved for patients with massive PE, and less commonly for those with signs of right heart dysfunction on diagnostic testing.
    - Before using thrombolytic therapy, it is crucial to ensure that no contraindications exist.

Other Nonpharmacologic Therapies

- In patients who have contraindications to anticoagulation therapy a few other options are available.
- **Inferior vena cava (IVC) filters** are net devices placed into the IVC in order to help prevent embolism of pelvic or lower extremity DVT.[22–25]
    - Studies have shown a decreased risk of PE, an increased risk of DVT, and no effect on overall mortality in patients treated with IVC filters and anticoagulation.
    - Other indications for IVC filters include recurrent VTE while on therapeutic anticoagulation therapy, chronic PE, and possibly massive PE.
    - In patients who had IVC filters placed due to temporary contraindications to anticoagulation, anticoagulation therapy should be added when safe, to reduce the risk of filter-related thromboses.
    - Several types of removable IVC filters exist and can provide a temporary physical barrier against emboli from the lower extremities but they increase the risk of DVT recurrence. Filter removal requires a second procedure.
- Catheter and surgical **embolectomies** are options for patients with massive PE who have contraindications to anticoagulation, including thrombolytic agents. Catheter embolectomy lacks strong supporting data at this time, and surgical embolectomy carries a high mortality.

Complications of Therapy

- **Bleeding** is the primary risk of anticoagulation therapy.
    - The use of antiplatelet agents increases the risk of bleeding.
    - If significant bleeding occurs while on anticoagulation therapy, the anticoagulant agent should be stopped immediately, and the patient should possibly undergo IVC filter treatment.
- HIT leads to increased risk of thrombosis.
    - Clinicians should consider the possibility that HIT has occurred in patients who develop VTE in the setting of absolute or relative thrombocytopenia.
    - Patients receiving UFH or LMWH should undergo monitoring for HIT. Patients with PE and suspected or confirmed HIT **should not receive UFH, LMWH, or warfarin until the HIT has resolved.** Such patients should undergo treatment with a parenteral direct thrombin inhibitor such as **argatroban or lepirudin.**

PROGNOSIS

- The short-term mortality rate for untreated PE may be as high as 30% but treatment with anticoagulation can decrease mortality to 2–8%.[26,27]
- While treated PE in normotensive patients who do not have evidence of RV dysfunction has a short-term mortality rate of ~2%, the mortality rate increases up to 30% in patients with shock, and up to 65% in patients who present with cardiac arrest.

- Indicators of poor prognosis include hemodynamic instability, signs of RV failure, elevated troponin/BNP, coexisting DVT, RV thrombus, and hyponatremia. Hemodynamic stability is the most important factor in prognosis.
- Several prognostic scoring systems (e.g., the pulmonary embolism severity index [PESI], and the simplified PESI [sPESI], Geneva risk score, shock index) exist.[28–32]

MONITORING AND FOLLOW-UP

- All patients who are diagnosed with acute PE should have close follow-up by a physician, especially if continuing with duration of anticoagulation.
- Patients on warfarin for chronic anticoagulation should have close monitoring of INRs.

REFERENCES

1. Anderson FA Jr, Wheeler HB, Goldberg RJ, et al. A population-based perspective of the hospital incidence and case-fatality rates of deep vein thrombosis and pulmonary embolism. the Worcester DVT Study. *Arch Intern Med.* 1991;151:933–8.
2. Silverstein MD, Heit JA, Mohr DN, et al. Trends in the incidence of deep vein thrombosis and pulmonary embolism: a 25-year population-based study. *Arch Intern Med.* 1998;158:585–93.
3. White RH. The epidemiology of venous thromboembolism. *Circulation.* 2003;107:14–8.
4. Wiener RS, Schwartz LM, Woloshin S. Time trends in pulmonary embolism in the United States: evidence of overdiagnosis. *Arch Intern Med.* 2011;171:831–7.
5. Huang W, Goldberg RJ, Anderson FA, et al. Secular trends in occurrence of acute venous thromboembolism: the Worcester VTE study (1985–2009). *Am J Med.* 2014;127:829–39.
6. Wells PS, Anderson DR, Rodger, et al. Derivation of a simple clinical model to categorize patients probability of pulmonary embolism: increasing the models utility with the SimpliRED D-dimer. *Thromb Haemost.* 2000;83:416–20.
7. van Belle A, Büller HR, Huisman MV, et al. Effectiveness of managing suspected pulmonary embolism using an algorithm combining clinical probability, D-dimer testing, and computed tomography. *JAMA.* 2006;295:172–9.
8. Le Gal G, Righini M, Roy PM, et al. Prediction of pulmonary embolism in the emergency department: the revised Geneva score. *Ann Intern Med.* 2006;144:165–71.
9. Hendriksen JM, Geersing GJ, Lucassen WA, et al. Diagnostic prediction models for suspected pulmonary embolism: systematic review and independent external validation in primary care. *BMJ.* 2015;351:h4438.
10. Kearon C, Ginsberg JS, Douketis J, et al. Canadian Pulmonary Embolism Diagnosis Study (CANPEDS) Group. An evaluation of D-dimer in the diagnosis of pulmonary embolism: a randomized trial. *Ann Intern Med.* 2006;144:812–21.
11. Konstantinides S, Geibel A, Olschewski M, et al. Importance of cardiac troponins I and T in risk stratification of patients with acute pulmonary embolism. *Circulation.* 2002;106:1263–8.
12. Binder L, Pieske B, Olschewski M, et al. N-terminal pro-brain natriuretic peptide or troponin testing followed by echocardiography for risk stratification of acute pulmonary embolism. *Circulation.* 2005;112:1573–9.
13. Otepka HC, Yusen RD. Pulmonary embolism. In: Kollef M, Isakow W, eds. *The Washington Manual of Critical Care.* 2nd ed. Philadelphia, PA: Lippincott Williams and Wilkins; 2013:97–104.
14. Stein PD, Fowler SE, Goodman LR, et al.; PIOPED II Investigators. Multidetector computed tomography for acute pulmonary embolism (PIOPED II). *N Eng J Med.* 2006;354:2317–27.
15. PIOPED Investigators. Value of ventilation/perfusion scan in acute pulmonary embolism: results of the prospective investigation of the pulmonary embolism diagnosis (PIOPED). *JAMA.* 1990;263:2753–9.
16. Todd JL, Tapson VF. Thrombolytic therapy for acute pulmonary embolism: a critical appraisal. *Chest.* 2009;135:1321–9.
17. Kearon C, Akl EA, Comerota AJ, et al. Antithrombotic therapy for VTE disease: antithrombotic therapy and prevention of thrombosis, 9th ed: American College of Chest Physicians Evidence-Based Clinical Practice Guidelines. *Chest.* 2012;141:e419S–94S.

18. Konstantinides S, Geibel A, Heusel G, et al.; Management Strategies and Prognosis of Pulmonary Embolism-3 Trial Investigators. Heparin plus alteplase compared with heparin alone in patients with submassive pulmonary embolism. *N Engl J Med.* 2002;347:1143–50.
19. Weitz JI, Eikelboom JW, Samama MM. New antithrombotic drugs: antithrombotic therapy and prevention of thrombosis, 9th ed: American College of Chest Physicians Evidence-Based Clinical Practice Guidelines. *Chest.* 2012;141:e120S–51S.
20. Garcia DA, Baglin TP, Weitz JI, et al. Parenteral anticoagulants: antithrombotic therapy and prevention of thrombosis, 9th ed: American College of Chest Physicians Evidence-Based Clinical Practice Guidelines. Chest. 2012;141:e24S–43S.
21. Ageno W, Gallus AS, Wittkowsky A, et al. Oral anticoagulant therapy: antithrombotic therapy and prevention of thrombosis, 9th ed: American College of Chest Physicians Evidence-Based Clinical Practice Guidelines. *Chest.* 2012;141:e44S–88S.
22. Decousus H, Leizorovicz A, Parent F, et al. A clinical trial of vena caval filters in the prevention of pulmonary embolism in patients with proximal deep-vein thrombosis. Prévention du Risque d'Embolie Pulmonaire par Interruption Cave Study Group. *N Engl J Med.* 1998;338:409–15.
23. PREPIC Study Group. Eight-year follow-up of patients with permanent vena cava filters in the prevention of pulmonary embolism: the PREPIC (Prevention du Risque d'Embolie Pulmonaire par Interruption Cave) randomized study. *Circulation.* 2005;112:416–22.
24. Muriel A, Jiménez D, Aujesky, et al.; RIETE Investigators. Survival effects of inferior vena cava filter in patients with acute symptomatic venous thromboembolism and a significant bleeding risk. *J Am coll Cardiol.* 2014;63:1675–83.
25. Mismetti P, Laporte S, Pellerin O, et al.; PREPIC2 study Group. Effect of a retrievable inferior vena cava filter plus anticoagulation vs anticoagulation alone on risk of recurrent pulmonary embolism: a randomized clinical trial. *JAMA.* 2015;313:1627–35.
26. Horlander KT, Mannino DM, Leeper KV. Pulmonary embolism mortality in the United States, 1979–1998: an analysis using multiple-cause mortality data. *Arch Intern Med.* 2003;163:1711–7.
27. Nijkeuter M, Sohne M, Tick LW, et al.; Christopher Study Investigators. The natural course of hemodynamically stable pulmonary embolism: clinical outcome and risk factors in a large prospective cohort study. *Chest.* 2007;131:517–23.
28. Aujesky D, Obrosky DS, Stone RA, et al. Derivation and validation of a prognostic model for pulmonary embolism. *Am J Respir Crit Care Med.* 2005;172:1041–6.
29. Aujesky D, Roy PM, Le Manach CP, et al. Validation of a model to predict adverse outcomes in patients with pulmonary embolism. *Eur Heart J.* 2006;27:476–81.
30. Jiménez D, Aujesky D, Moores L, et al.; RIETE Investigators. Simplification of the pulmonary embolism severity index for prognostication in patients with acute symptomatic pulmonary embolism. *Arch Intern Med.* 2010;170:1383–9.
31. Bertoletti L, Le Gal G, Aujesky D, et al. Prognostic value of the Geneva prediction rule in patients with pulmonary embolism. *Thromb Res.* 2013;132:32–6.
32. Otero R, Trujillo-Santos J, Cayuela A, et al.; Registro Informatizado de la Enfermedad Tromboembólica (RIETE) Investigators. Haemodynamically unstable pulmonary embolism in the RIETE registry: systolic blood pressure or shock index? *Eur Respir J.* 2007;30:1111–6.

Pulmonary Hypertension

22

Murali M. Chakinala and Adam Anderson

GENERAL PRINCIPLES

Definition

- Pulmonary hypertension (PH) is defined by a **mean pulmonary artery pressure (PAP) >25 mm Hg.**[1]
- Discrimination of the type of PH (i.e., precapillary vs. postcapillary) requires additional information about the left heart's filling pressures and the pulmonary vascular resistance (PVR).

Classification

- PH is classified into five groups (Table 22-1).[2,3]
- Individuals can have more than one underlying condition leading to a so-called mixed form of PH.
- Pulmonary arterial hypertension (PAH, group 1) patients are stratified by World Health Organization (WHO) functional classes I–IV that guide therapies and provide a tool to monitor clinical response (Table 22-2).[4]

Epidemiology

- The most common type of PH in the developed world is group 2, followed by group 3.
- Group 3 PH tends to correlate with degree of severity of underlying lung disease and/or hypoxemia but exceptions include concomitant conditions having an additive effect, and a discordant degree of PH with the underlying lung disease as measured by spirometry (e.g., obstructive sleep apnea [OSA] and chronic obstructive pulmonary disease [COPD]).
- Prevalence of PAH is estimated to be **15–25 cases per million** with female/male ratio between 2:1 and 3:1. Prevalence of idiopathic pulmonary arterial hypertension (IPAH) is estimated at 6 per million.[1]
- Survival rates for PAH at 1, 3, and 5 years are 84%, 67%, and 58%, respectively with a **median survival of 3.6 years.**[5] However, survival can be substantially affected by etiology.
- Estimated cumulative incidence of PH after acute pulmonary embolism (PE) is 1.0% at 6 months, 3.1% at 1 year, and 3.8% at 2 years with cumulative burden of emboli being a risk factor.[6]

Pathophysiology

- The common finding in all forms of PH is **elevated pressures within precapillary pulmonary vessels** as blood flows across the pulmonary circuit.
- **Group 1 PH** (PAH) involves complex mechanisms that progressively narrow and stiffen the pulmonary arterioles.
  - Pathogenesis in PAH may vary with the different etiologies but converges upon **endothelial and smooth muscle cell proliferation and dysfunction** that result in the complex interplay of the following factors:
    - **Vasoconstriction** caused by overproduction of vasoconstrictor compounds such as endothelin and insufficient production of vasodilators such as prostacyclin and nitric oxide.

TABLE 22-1 2008 DANA POINT CLINICAL CLASSIFICATION OF PULMONARY HYPERTENSION (PH)

Group 1: pulmonary arterial hypertension (PAH)
- Idiopathic (IPAH)
- Heritable
  - *BMPR2*
  - ALK-1, endoglin (with or without hereditary hemorrhagic telangiectasia)
  - Unknown
- Drugs and toxins induced
- Associated with (APAH)
  - Connective tissue diseases
  - HIV infection
  - Portal hypertension
  - Congenital heart disease
  - Schistosomiasis
  - Chronic hemolytic anemia
- Persistent pulmonary hypertension of the newborn

Group 1': pulmonary veno-occlusive disease and/or pulmonary capillary hemangiomatosis

Group 2: pulmonary hypertension due to left heart disease
- Systolic dysfunction
- Diastolic dysfunction
- Valvular disease

Group 3: pulmonary hypertension due to lung disease and/or hypoxia
- Chronic obstructive lung disease
- Interstitial lung disease
- Other pulmonary diseases with mixed restrictive and obstructive pattern
- Sleep-disordered breathing
- Alveolar hypoventilation disorders
- Chronic exposure to high altitude
- Developmental abnormalities

Group 4: chronic thromboembolic pulmonary hypertension (CTEPH)

Group 5: PH with unclear and/or multifactorial mechanisms
- Hematologic disorders: myeloproliferative disorders, splenectomy
- Systemic disorders: sarcoidosis, PLCH, LAM, neurofibromatosis, vasculitis
- Metabolic disorders: glycogen storage disease, Gaucher disease, thyroid disorders
- Others: tumoral obstruction, fibrosing mediastinitis, chronic renal failure on dialysis

---

BMPR2, bone morphogenic protein receptor, type 2; ALK-1, activin receptor-like kinase 1 gene; PLCH, pulmonary Langerhans cell histiocytosis; LAM, lymphangioleiomyomatosis.

Modified from Galiè N, Hoeper MM, Humbert M, et al. Guidelines for the diagnosis and treatment of pulmonary hypertension: the Task Force for the Diagnosis and Treatment of Pulmonary Hypertension of the European Society of Cardiology (ESC) and the European Respiratory Society (ERS), endorsed by the International Society of Heart and Lung Transplantation (ISHLT). *Eur Heart J.* 2009;30:2493–537.

TABLE 22-2 WHO FUNCTIONAL CLASSIFICATION

Class I	No limitation of physical activity; ordinary physical activity does not cause undue dyspnea, fatigue, chest pain, or near syncope
Class II	Slight limitation of physical activity; comfortable at rest; ordinary activity causes undue dyspnea, fatigue, chest pain, or near syncope
Class III	Marked limitation of physical activity; comfortable at rest; less than ordinary activity causes undue dyspnea, fatigue, chest pain, or near syncope
Class IV	Unable to carry out any physical activity without symptoms; dyspnea and/or fatigue may be at rest; discomfort is increased by any physical activity

Data from Rich S. Executive summary from the World Symposium on primary pulmonary hypertension. Geneva: World Health Organization; 1998.

    - **Endothelial and smooth muscle proliferation** due to mitogenic properties of endothelin and thromboxane A2 in the setting of low levels of inhibitory molecules, such as prostacyclin and nitric oxide.
    - **In situ thrombosis** of small- and medium-sized pulmonary arteries resulting from platelet activation and aggregation.
  - The physiologic consequences of this proliferative vasculopathy are an **increase in PVR and right ventricle** (RV) **afterload.**
  - Complex origins of PAH include infectious/environmental insults in the setting of predisposing comorbidities and/or underlying genetic predisposition, for example, gene mutation of bone morphogenetic protein receptor II (BMPR II) or activin receptor-like kinase 1 (ALK1).[1,7,8]
  - *BMPR2* gene mutations are found in 75% of familial PAH and 25% of IPAH, while *ALK1* gene mutations, causative of hereditary hemorrhagic telangiectasia, rarely present with PAH.[1,9]
- Elevated pressures in **groups 2–5** result from:
  - Elevated downstream pressures on the left side of the heart (group 2),
  - Hypoxemic vasoconstriction (group 3),
  - Occlusion of the vasculature by material foreign to the lung (group 4),
  - High flow that exceeds capacitance of the pulmonary circuit (group 5), or
  - Blood vessel narrowing and destruction from processes external to the vasculature (group 3, group 5).

DIAGNOSIS

Clinical Presentation

An algorithm for evaluating PH is outlined in Figure 22-1.

History

- **Dyspnea with exertion** is the most often reported symptom for patients with PH. Orthopnea and paroxysmal nocturnal dyspnea are important clues of left heart disease and group 2 PH. Symptoms that reflect more advanced disease and secondary RV dysfunction include **fatigue, syncope, peripheral edema, and angina.**
- Hoarseness can also be encountered because of left recurrent laryngeal nerve compression by the enlarging pulmonary artery (i.e., Ortner syndrome).

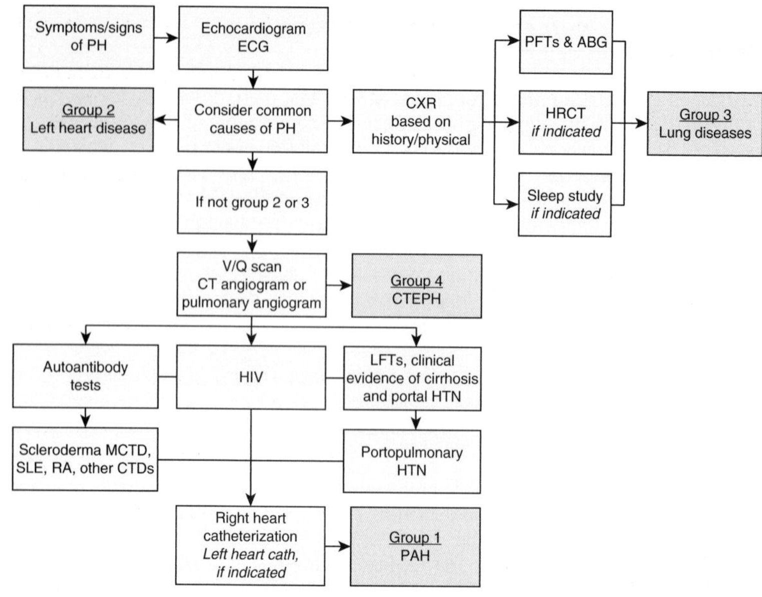

FIGURE 22-1. Diagnostic approach to pulmonary arterial hypertension. PH, pulmonary hypertension; PFT, pulmonary function tests; ABG, arterial blood gases; HRCT, high-resolution CT; V/Q scan, ventilation/perfusion scan; CTEPH, chronic thromboembolic pulmonary hypertension; LFT, liver function test; HTN, hypertension; MCTD, mixed connective tissue disease; SLE, systemic lupus erythematosus; RA, rheumatoid arthritis; CTD, connective tissue disease; PAH, pulmonary arterial hypertension.

- **Past medical history** relevant to several organ systems, including the respiratory, cardiovascular, hepatic, rheumatologic, and hematologic systems must be explored.
- Particular emphasis should be placed on prior **cardiac conditions**, including myocardial infarction, heart failure (HF), arrhythmias, rheumatic heart disease, other valvular heart disease, and congenital heart disease.
- **Social history** should focus on prior or current tobacco and alcohol use, as well as illicit or recreational drug use, particularly methamphetamines or cocaine.
- **Family history** should also be explored to exclude a genetic predisposition.
- Risk factors for exposure to **HIV** may disclose an unexpected etiology for PH.
- Careful **medication history** to document use of current or past drugs linked to development of PH is also necessary. This includes anorexigens (e.g., fenfluramine, dexfenfluramine, diethylpropion) and chemotherapeutic agents (e.g., mitomycin).[1]

Physical Examination

- A thorough physical examination to corroborate or refute suspicions of underlying medical problems should be performed; attention should be directed toward the cardiopulmonary examination.
- Auscultatory examination of the heart may reveal an accentuated S2 sound with a **prominent P2** component, systolic ejection murmur at left lower sternal border due to **tricuspid regurgitation**, and diastolic decrescendo murmur (Graham Steell murmur) along the left sternal border due to pulmonary insufficiency. Additional cardiac finding,

including continuous murmurs or rumbles and fixed-split S2, may suggest an underlying **congenital cardiac defect.**

- As PH worsens and right HF ensues, resting tachycardia, S3 gallop, elevated jugular venous pulsation of the neck, hepatomegaly, ascites, peripheral edema, diminished peripheral pulses, and cyanosis occur. Presence of these findings, in the absence of clues of left heart disease, should raise suspicion for right HF due to PH.
- **Digital clubbing** indicates underlying conditions such as interstitial lung disease (ILD), bronchiectasis, or congenital heart disease.

Diagnostic Criteria

- PH is defined as **mean PAP >25 mm Hg.**[1]
  - PAH requires **normal left ventricular** (LV) **filling pressures** (i.e., pulmonary capillary wedge pressure (PCWP), left atrial pressure, or left ventricular end-diastolic pressure (LVEDP) ≤15 mm Hg).
  - Some centers also require an elevated PVR (≥3 Wood units) to establish PAH.
- **Diagnosis of PAH requires a right heart catheterization (RHC).**
- Pulmonary artery systolic pressure (PASP) can be estimated noninvasively by transthoracic echocardiography (TTE), whereby a **PASP >40 mm Hg is considered abnormal and suggestive of PH but is not diagnostic.**

Diagnostic Testing

Laboratories

- Essential laboratory studies to evaluate unexplained PH mirror the studies of a general medical evaluation: **complete blood count** (CBC), **comprehensive metabolic panel** (CMP), **and coagulation studies** may offer diagnostic clues and direct further exploration. A prerenal pattern of blood urea nitrogen (BUN) and creatinine elevations in conjunction with passive congestion of the liver is a sign of advanced right HF and low cardiac output.
- Screening for **collagen vascular disease** with antinuclear antibody (ANA), anticentromere antibody, rheumatoid factor (RF), anti-scl-70 antibody, and antiribonucleoprotein antibody should be completed, as the associated underlying conditions are linked to PAH.
- Thyroid studies, hemoglobin electrophoresis for sickle cell disease, HIV serology, hepatitis serologies, antiphospholipid antibody, or anticardiolipin antibody should also be performed if clinical suspicions exist.
- **Arterial blood gas** can provide invaluable information. Significant resting hypoxemia should raise suspicion for right-to-left shunt, severely reduced cardiac output, or underlying pulmonary disease. **Significant hypercarbia supports a group 3 diagnosis.**

Electrocardiography

- **RV enlargement** is suspected by the presence of an R wave in V1 or an S wave in lead V6 while **RV strain** appears as a triad of S wave in lead I, Q wave in lead III, and inverted T wave in lead III. Other potential findings in cases of PH include right atrial enlargement and right bundle branch block.
- LV hypertrophy, left atrial enlargement, left axis deviation, atrial fibrillation, or evidence of prior myocardial infarction provide clues of significant left heart disease that could lead to group 2 PH.

Imaging

- **CXR**
  - Features indicative of PH are **enlarged central pulmonary arteries** on frontal views and **RV enlargement** on lateral examination. When PAPs reach systemic levels, pulmonary artery calcifications can be seen.
  - Obliteration of the distal pulmonary arteries leads to tapering of vessels in the peripheral third of the lung parenchyma, referred to as **pruning**, is classically seen in IPAH.

- In contrast, prominent pulmonary arteries extending to the periphery of the lung suggest systemic-to-pulmonary shunts and a hypercirculatory state (e.g., atrial or ventricular septal defects).
- CXR should also be reviewed for **underlying cardiopulmonary diseases**, including ILD, emphysema, or HF.

- **Ventilation/perfusion scan**
  - Provides an easy and sensitive screen for the detection of **chronic thromboembolic** disease.
  - While PH due to nonembolic processes, such as IPAH, can display a heterogeneous or mottled perfusion pattern, anatomic perfusion defects of the segmental or lobar level are more concerning for thromboembolic disease.
  - Differential diagnosis for an abnormal perfusion scan also includes pulmonary veno-occlusive disease (widespread obstruction of the pulmonary veins due to fibrous tissue), mediastinal fibrosis, or pulmonary vasculitis.
- **Chest CT**
  - While CT angiography can display features of chronic thromboembolic disease, it is less sensitive and less predictive of surgical response than the ventilation/perfusion scan.
  - Chest CT may be necessary to exclude mediastinal disease, (e.g., mediastinal fibrosis or compressive lymphadenopathy).
  - High-resolution chest CT (HRCT) can exclude ILD, if suspicion exists.
- **TTE**
  - TTE with Doppler and agitated saline injection serves as an initial test to identify PH.
  - If tricuspid regurgitation is present, Doppler interrogation allows for estimation of **PASP**.
  - TTE also identifies potential left-sided cardiac causes of PH and provides estimate of LV systolic and diastolic function.
  - The agitated saline, so-called bubble study may discover an intracardiac shunt; a patent foramen ovale allows for right-to-left shunting that could explain exertional hypoxemia in PH patients, but is not considered causative of PH.
  - Finally, presence of a pericardial effusion is a predictor of mortality in PAH.[1]

Diagnostic Procedures

- Pulmonary function testing (PFT)
  - PFTs should be inspected for obstructive lung disease while measurement of lung volumes may provide a clue for ILD.
  - DLCO values, if normal or elevated, argue against PH.
  - Classically, patients with IPAH exhibit normal spirometry, minimally reduced total lung capacity (~75%), significant reduction of DLCO, normal resting PaO_2, and exercise-induced hypoxemia.
- RHC[1]
  - **RHC is the gold standard for diagnosing PAH.**
  - Pressure measurements include PA pressures, RV end-diastolic pressure, right atrial pressure, and the PCWP; in particular, the right atrial pressure is an important predictor of survival.
  - Cardiac output is determined by either the thermodilution or Fick method. Either can be used but both have drawbacks. Thermodilution is affected by significant tricuspid regurgitation. For Fick, direct oxygen consumption (VO_2) is rarely measured and only an assumed Fick calculation is typically done.
  - Once the other aforementioned measures are made, PVR can be calculated as (mean PAP – PCWP)/cardiac output, or the ratio of pressure decline across the pulmonary circuit and the cardiac output.
  - An **acute vasodilator challenge** can also be performed to guide the choice of therapeutic agent in group 1 (PAH) patients. A short-acting vasodilator such as **inhaled nitric oxide**, IV adenosine, or IV epoprostenol is administered. A **10 mm Hg drop in the**

mean PAP and a concluding mean PAP <40 mm Hg without systemic hypotension or a decrease in cardiac output signifies a significant acute hemodynamic response.

- **Left heart catheterization** (LHC) should be performed to rule out coronary artery disease and/or directly measure the LVEDP when left heart disease is strongly suspected or the PCWP is felt to be unreliable.
- **Polysomnography** should be obtained if there is a concern for OSA or obesity hypoventilation syndrome as a contributing component to PH.

TREATMENT

- Management of PH depends on the specific category determined after a comprehensive evaluation.
- A treatment algorithm for PAH (i.e., group 1) is presented in Figure 22-2.[1]

Treatment of Groups 2–4

- **Group 2**
  - PH owing to left heart disease (group 2) should receive **appropriate therapy for underlying causative left heart conditions** with a hemodynamic goal of lowering the PCWP (and LVEDP) as much as possible.

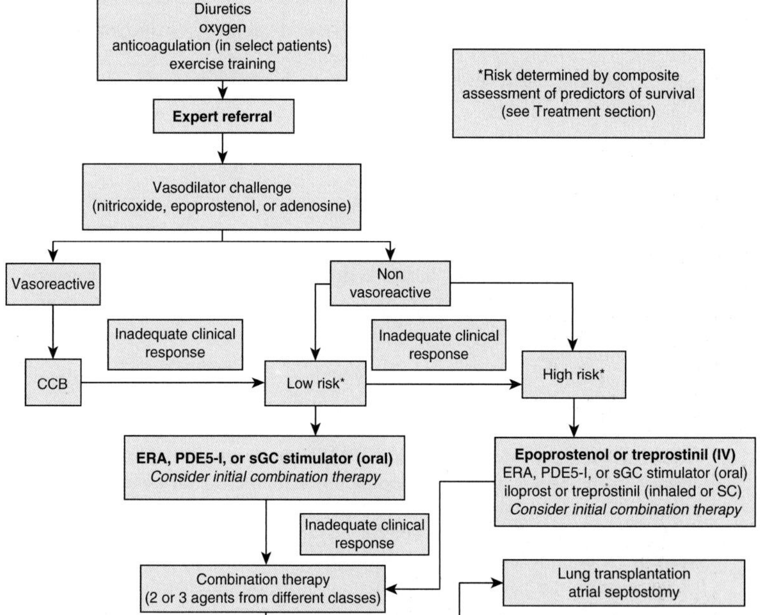

FIGURE 22-2. Pulmonary arterial hypertension treatment algorithm. Only patients with an acute vasodilator response (see text) should receive CCB treatment. Typical first-line treatment is listed first. Risk determined by variables listed in text. CCB, calcium channel blocker; ERA, endothelin receptor antagonist; PDE-5I, phosphodiesterase-5 inhibitor; sGC, soluble guanylate cyclase. (Modified from McLaughlin V, Archer S, Badesch D, et al. ACCF/AHA 2009 expert consensus document on pulmonary hypertension. J Am Coll Cardiol. 2009;53:1573–619.)

- Patients with HF with preserved ejection fraction often develop secondary PH and exertional dyspnea and require afterload-reducing agents (to minimize LV afterload), diuretics (to avoid excess volume), and negative chronotropes (to avoid tachycardic states).
- Chronic use of NSAIDs can aggravate HF and should be avoided.
- Subset of patients of LV systolic HF and associated PH appear to benefit from sildenafil (a phosphodiesterase-5 inhibitor, PDE-5I), in terms of exertional capacity, hemodynamics during exercise, and quality of life.[10,11] Sildenafil should only be used if PH is persistent after optimization of LV filling pressures (i.e., near-normal PCWP or LVEDP) and optimization of LV systolic function. Careful hemodynamic assessment should be used to demonstrate an elevated PVR.

- **Group 3**
  - PH caused by parenchymal lung diseases (group 3) should be treated with **appropriate therapies for the underlying pulmonary condition:** bronchodilators, pulmonary rehabilitation (obstructive lung disease), immunomodulators (ILDs), and noninvasive ventilation (OSA and/or hypoventilation syndrome).
  - Adequate oxygen saturation (SpO_2 ≥90%) is critical to avoid hypoxic vasoconstriction and cor pulmonale.
- **Group 4**
  - Group 4 PH (CTEPH) can be cured by **pulmonary thromboendarterectomy** at specialized centers and requires careful screening to determine candidacy and expected hemodynamic response.[1,12]
  - When the disease is considered nonsurgical due to distal predominance of the culprit lesions, medical therapy (as in PAH) can be attempted.
  - Regardless, **lifelong therapeutic anticoagulation** with warfarin should be prescribed with a goal INR of 2.0–3.0.[1]

Pharmacologic Therapy for Group 1

- **Vasodilator therapy**
  - Vasomodulator/vasodilator therapies are **only approved for treatment of group 1 conditions.**
  - Approved PAH therapies have generally been shown to improve short-term exercise capacity, functional classification, hospitalization rate, and time to clinical worsening.
  - Long-term outcomes of prolonging survival are being inferred based on observational data and large-scale contemporary registries.
  - **Calcium channel blockers** (CCBs)[13,14]
    - CCBs should only be used for treating PAH after demonstrating acute vasoresponsiveness with a short-acting vasodilator (e.g., nitric oxide) during RHC.
    - **Indiscriminate CCB use can lead to hemodynamic collapse and syncope in patients with advanced right-sided heart failure (RHF) who are not acute vasoresponders.**
    - Chronic CCB therapy, such as **amlodipine, nifedipine, or diltiazem,** can be prescribed, at an initial low dose and titrated over several weeks, while monitoring systemic pressures and guarding against aggravation of RHF.
    - **Verapamil should be avoided** due to its negative ionotropic properties.
    - Patients that do not have near normalization of PA pressures with long-term CCB usage should be considered for additional vasodilator/vasomodulator therapies.[1]
  - **Endothelin receptor antagonists** (ERAs)[1,15–19]
    - ERAs block binding of endothelin-1 to A and/or B receptors on pulmonary artery smooth muscle cells and endothelial cells.
    - Available agents include **bosentan, ambrisentan, and macitentan** which are approved for functional class II–IV patients.
    - All are teratogenic and bosentan requires monthly laboratory monitoring for hepatotoxicity.

- **PDE-5Is**[1,17,18,20,21]
  - PDE-5Is block phosphodiesterase, which degrades intracellular cyclic guanosine monophosphate (cGMP). The result is pulmonary vasodilation and, ultimately, decreased PAPs.
  - Available agents include **sildenafil and tadalafil**, which are approved for functional class II–IV patients.
  - No specific laboratory monitoring is needed but a potent drug interaction with organic nitrates must be avoided.
- **Prostanoids**[1,17,18,22–24]
  - Prostanoids are considered **the most potent, but also the most potentially toxic, class of therapies** due to their complex delivery system and wider therapeutic dosing range.
  - Prostanoids induce vasodilation, inhibit cellular growth, and inhibit platelet aggregation.
  - Commercially available prostanoids include: **epoprostenol** (IV), room temperature stable epoprostenol (IV), **treprostinil** (IV, SC, inhaled, or oral), and **iloprost** (inhaled).
  - Prostanoids are approved for functional class III–IV patients (SC treprostinil is also approved in class II).
  - The choice of therapy is variable across prescribers and dosing of parenteral agents is highly individualized to the patient and requires great expertise and impeccable nursing.
  - Prostanoids may be used as initial therapy in treatment naive patients who present in advanced RHF. However, they are most often used as add-on therapies when oral agents provide an ineffective or inadequate treatment response.
  - Several randomized controlled trials of combination therapy have confirmed the benefits of combining prostanoids with an oral agent.[1]
  - Adverse effects include drug-related side effects (e.g., jaw pain, nonpruritic rash, flushing, headache, gastrointestinal side effects, and extremity pain) and delivery system complication (e.g., bloodstream infections, catheter-related thrombosis, inadvertent interruptions of very short-acting continuous medications).
- **Soluble guanylate cyclase (sGC) stimulators**
  - The oral sGC stimulator **riociguat** increases the concentration of cGMP, and consequently vasodilation, by stimulating sGC directly and by increasing its sensitivity to nitrous oxide.
  - In the PATENT-1 and PATENT-2 trials, riociguat was shown to improve PVR, 6-minute walk test (6MWT) distance, WHO functional class, and symptoms in patients with PAH for up to 1 year.[25,26]
  - Similar results were seen in patients taking no other treatment and also in those taking prostanoids or ERAs.
  - In general, riociguat is well tolerated but syncope and rare instances of hemoptysis/pulmonary hemorrhage were reported.
  - Similar trial data suggest that riociguat is effective for CTEPH as well.[27,28]

- **Choice of vasodilator therapy**
  - Initial choice of PAH-specific therapy should be individualized based on risk factor stratification of an individual, with reliance on several clinical variables[1]:
    - Functional class, high-risk class IV (Table 22-2)
    - Clinical evidence of RHF
    - Rate of progression, rapid development high risk
    - Degree of exercise impairment (6MWT, high risk <300 m)
    - Degree of hemodynamic derangement (high-risk right atrial pressure >20 mm Hg and cardiac index <2.0 L/min/m^2)
    - Significantly elevated b-type natriuretic peptide (BNP)

- Based on these variables, individual considered high risk for significant clinical events, including hospitalization or death in the near term, should be strongly considered for a parenteral prostanoid (Fig. 22-2).[1]
- Other potentially worrisome clues are underlying PAH diagnosis (collagen vascular disease, portopulmonary hypertension, and hereditary PAH), presence of pericardial effusion, degree of BNP elevation, degree of concomitant renal dysfunction, male gender, age >60, resting systolic blood pressure (<110 mm Hg), pulse rate (92 beats/min), and diffusing capacity (<32%). The REVEAL registry has identified 19 clinical variables that may provide a simple risk calculator for any individual patient and awaits further validation.[29]
- Comorbid conditions, social support, and patient's level of sophistication are also critical in deciding a therapy, as delivery systems for PAH-specific therapies differ widely.
- If patients are declining, therapeutic classes are switched or, more likely, a second or third drug from a different therapeutic class is added.

- **Other therapies**
  - **Warfarin**
    - Warfarin to target an INR between 1.5 and 2.5 is recommended for PAH patients that have a favorable risk–benefit profile for anticoagulation, based on scant data favoring survival in IPAH patients.[1,13,30]
    - Anticoagulant therapy is not urgent and can be stopped for invasive procedures or active bleeding.
  - **Diuretic therapy**
    - Diuretics critically alleviate RHF and improve symptoms.
    - Often a combination of a loop diuretic, aldosterone antagonist, and/or a thiazide is required.
    - Overdiuresis or too rapid of a diuresis can be poorly tolerated due to preload dependency of the RV and limited ability of the cardiac output to compensate for systemic hypotension.
    - Aggravating chronic renal dysfunction, particularly in an individual with long-standing RHF or intrinsic renal disease, should be avoided.
  - **Digoxin** offers weak inotropic support and may be particularly helpful if concomitant atrial tachyarrhythmias are present.
  - **Inotropic agents** (e.g., dobutamine, dopamine, milrinone) improve right heart function and are best suited for short-term use in acutely decompensated states especially when overt organ hypoperfusion is evident.

Other Nonpharmacologic Therapies

- **Supplemental oxygen** should be used to maintain normoxemia and avoid hypoxic vasoconstriction as much as possible. Normoxemia may be impossible to achieve if significant intracardiac right-to-left shunting is occurring.
- **In-line IV filters** to prevent paradoxical air emboli in patients with significant intracardiac right-to-left shunts should be implemented.
- **Pneumococcal and influenza vaccinations** should be considered to avoid respiratory tract infections.
- Patients should **avoid high-risk behaviors** (e.g., deep **Valsalva** and **high altitudes**) that can acutely decrease RV preload and/or increase RV afterload and worsen RHF.
- Patients should **avoid pregnancy** due to marked hemodynamic alterations that can further strain a compromised RV. Contraception choice is highly variable but choosing methods that do not increase thromboembolic events is recommended.
- Systemic **sympathomimetic agents** with vasoactive properties should be avoided (e.g., over-the-counter decongestant, nicotine, and cocaine).
- Patients should **avoid NSAIDs**, which have multiple counter-productive effects in RHF.

Surgical Management

- **Transplant surgery**[1,12]
  - Lung transplantation or heart–lung transplantation is reserved for suitable PAH patients who remain in advanced functional classes (III–IV) with ominous hemodynamics despite maximal medical therapy that includes a parenteral prostanoid.
  - RV recovery after isolated lung transplantation allows for reserving heart–lung transplantation primarily for cases of irreparable complex congenital abnormalities.
  - Median survival after lung transplantation is ~6 years while survival for IPAH patients at 5 years is about 50%.
- **Atrial septostomy**[1,12]
  - Atrial septostomy percutaneously creates a right-to-left shunt across the interatrial septum and can increase systemic oxygen transport, in spite of a decrease in systemic arterial oxygen saturation, by increasing cardiac output.
  - The indications are rare but can be explored in cases of refractory RHF (e.g., recurrent syncope, severe ascites, or poor systemic end-organ perfusion).
- **Septal defect closure**
  - Septal defect closure is feasible in carefully selected cases of intracardiac defects in order to prevent or minimize progression of PAH.
  - Requirements for closure include significant net left-to-right shunting (pulmonary/systemic flow ratio ≥2.0) and low PVR (PVR <5 Wood units and pulmonary/systemic resistance ratio ≤0.3).[31]

Lifestyle/Risk Modification

- **Fluid and sodium restriction** should be employed for individuals with RHF.
- **Exercise training** and **pulmonary rehabilitation** have been shown to improve both subjective symptoms as well as WHO functional class. However, no change was seen in hemodynamic properties.[32,33] Regardless, exercise offers an economical intervention that should be recommended with caution to avoid over exertion.

REFERRAL

The field of PH is rapidly evolving with a better understanding of its pathophysiology and development of numerous pharmacologic options. Given its complex nature, most patients suspected of having PAH should be evaluated in a specialized PH center.

MONITORING/FOLLOW-UP

- PAH remains incurable and current treatments are still only palliative.
- Patients require close monitoring to detect deteriorating RV function and clinical progression.
- Patients with a favorable profile can be evaluated every 3–6 months while more unstable patients should be seen every 1–3 months.
- While no consensus exists for monitoring PAH patients, most centers utilize composite clinical variables (WHO functional class), exercise measures (e.g., 6MWT), and periodic objective RV assessments (e.g., echocardiography, catheterization, BNP, cardiac MRI).

OUTCOME/PROGNOSIS

- The prognosis of PAH is poor, with an approximate mortality of 15% within 1 year of modern therapies.[1,34]
- Predictors of a poor prognosis include[1]:

- Advanced functional class
- Poor exercise capacity as measured by 6MWT or cardiopulmonary exercise test
- Significant right ventricular dysfunction
- High right atrial pressure
- Low cardiac index
- Elevated BNP
- Underlying diagnosis of scleroderma spectrum of disease.

REFERENCES

1. McLaughlin V, Archer S, Badesch D, et al. ACCF/AHA 2009 expert consensus document on pulmonary hypertension. *J Am Coll Cardiol.* 2009;53:1573–619.
2. Galiè N, Hoeper M, Humbert M, et al. Guidelines for the diagnosis and treatment of pulmonary hypertension. *Eur Heart J.* 2009;30:2493–537.
3. Simonneau G, Robbins I, Beghetti M, et al. Updated clinical classification of pulmonary hypertension. *J Am Coll Cardiol.* 2009;54:S43–54.
4. Rich S. Executive summary from the World Symposium on primary pulmonary hypertension. Geneva: World Health Organization; 1998.
5. Benza RL, Miller DP, Barst RJ, et al. An evaluation of long-term survival from time of diagnosis in pulmonary arterial hypertension from the REVEAL Registry. *Chest.* 2012;142:448–56.
6. Pengo V, Lensing A, Prins M, et al. Incidence of chronic thromboembolic pulmonary hypertension after pulmonary embolism. *N Eng J Med.* 2004;350:2257–64.
7. Newman J, Wheeler L, Lane K, et al. Mutation in the gene for bone morphogenetic protein receptor II as a cause of primary pulmonary hypertension in a large kindred. *N Eng J Med.* 2001; 345:319–24.
8. Trembath RC, Thomson JR, Machado RE, et al. Clinical and molecular genetic features of pulmonary hypertension in patients with hereditary hemorrhagic telangiectasia. *N Engl J Med.* 2011;345:325–34.
9. Soubrier F, Cheng WK, Machado R, et al. Genetics and genomics of pulmonary arterial hypertension. *J Am Coll Cardiol.* 2013;62:D13–21.
10. Guazzi M, Samaja M, Arena R, et al. Long-term use of sildenafil in the therapeutic management of heart failure. *J Am Coll Cardiol.* 2007;50:2136–44.
11. Lewis GD, Shah R, Shahzad K, et al. Sildenafil improves exercise capacity and quality of life in patients with systolic heart failure and secondary pulmonary hypertension. *Circulation.* 2007; 166:1555–62.
12. Keogh A, Mayer E, Benza R, et al. Interventional and surgical modalities of treatment in pulmonary hypertension. *J Am Coll Cardiol.* 2009;54:S67–77.
13. Rich S, Kaufmann E, Levy PS. The effect of high doses of calcium-channel blockers on survival in primary pulmonary hypertension. *N Engl J Med.* 1992;327:76–81.
14. Sitbon O, Humbert M, Jais X, et al. Long-term response to calcium channel blockers in idiopathic pulmonary arterial hypertension. *Circulation.* 2005;111:3105–11.
15. Rubin LJ, Badesch DB, Barst RJ, et al. Bosentan therapy for pulmonary arterial hypertension. *N Engl J Med.* 2002;346:896–903.
16. Galiè N, Olschewski H, Oudiz RJ, et al. Ambrisentan for the treatment of pulmonary arterial hypertension: results of the ambrisentan in pulmonary arterial hypertension, randomized, double-blind, placebo-controlled, multicenter, efficacy (ARIES) study 1 and 2. *Circulation.* 2008;117: 3010–9.
17. Galiè N, Manes A, Negro L, et al. A meta-analysis of randomized controlled trials in pulmonary arterial hypertension. *Eur Heart J.* 2009;30:394–403.
18. He B, Zhang F, Li X, et al. Meta-analysis of randomized controlled trials on treatment of pulmonary arterial hypertension. *Circ J.* 2010;74:1458–64.
19. Pulido T, Adzerikho I, Channick RN, et al. Macitentan and morbidity and mortality in pulmonary arterial hypertension. *N Engl J Med.* 2013;369:809–18.
20. Galiè N, Ghofrani HA, Torbicki A, et al. Sildenafil citrated therapy for pulmonary arterial hypertension. *N Engl J Med.* 2005;353:2148–57.
21. Galiè N, Brundage BH, Ghofrani HA, et al. Tadalafil therapy for pulmonary hypertension. *Circulation.* 2009;119:2894–903.

22. Barst RJ, Rubin LJ, Long WA, et al. A comparison of continuous intravenous epoprostenol (prostacyclin) with conventional therapy for primary pulmonary hypertension. *N Engl J Med.* 1996;334:296–301.
23. Simonneau G, Barst RJ, Galiè N, et al. Continuous subcutaneous infusion of treprostinil, a prostacyclin analogue, in patients with pulmonary arterial hypertension: a double-blind, randomized, placebo-controlled trial. *Am J Respir Crit Care Med.* 2002;165:800–4.
24. Olschewski H, Simonneau G, Galiè N, et al. Inhaled iloprost for severe pulmonary hypertension. *N Engl J Med.* 2002;347:322–9.
25. Ghofrani HA, Galiè Nk, Grimminger F, et al. Riociguat for the treatment of pulmonary arterial hypertension. *N Engl J Med.* 2013;369:330–40.
26. Rubin LJ, Galiè N, Grimminger F, et al. Riociguat for the treatment of pulmonary arterial hypertension: a long-term extension study (PATENT-2). *Eur Respir J.* 2015;45:1303–13.
27. Ghofrani HA, D'Armini AM, Grimminger F, et al. Riociguat for the treatment of chronic thromboembolic pulmonary hypertension. *N Engl J Med.* 2013;369:319–29.
28. Simonneau G, D'Armini, Ghofrani HA, et al. Riociguat for the treatment of chronic thromboembolic pulmonary hypertension: a long-term extension study (CHEST-2). *Eur Respir J.* 2015;45:1293–302.
29. Benza R, Miller D, Gomberg-Maitland M, et al. Predicting survival in pulmonary arterial hypertension: insights from the Registry to Evaluate Early and Long-Term Pulmonary Arterial Hypertension Disease Management (REVEAL). *Circulation.* 2010;122:164–72.
30. Fuster V, Steele PM, Edwards WD, et al. Primary pulmonary hypertension: natural history and the importance of thrombosis. *Circulation.* 1984;70:580–7.
31. D'Alto M, Romeo E, Argiento P, et al. Hemodynamics of patients developing pulmonary arterial hypertension after shunt closure. *Int J Cardiol.* 2013;168:3797–801.
32. Fox BD, Kassirer M, Weiss I, et al. Ambulatory rehabilitation improves exercise capacity in patients with pulmonary hypertension. *J Card Fail.* 2011;17:196–200.
33. Weinstein AA, Chin LM, Keyser RE, et al. Effect of aerobic exercise training on fatigue and physical activity in patients with pulmonary arterial hypertension. *Respir Med.* 2013;107:778–84.
34. Thanappan T, Shah SJ, Rich S, et al. A USA-based registry for pulmonary arterial hypertension: 1982–2006. *Eur Respir J.* 2007;30:1103–10.

Pleural Diseases

23

Alexander C. Chen and Daniel J. Brown

GENERAL PRINCIPLES

- The pleural lining is a serous membrane covering the lung parenchyma, chest wall, diaphragm, and mediastinum.
- The pleural membrane covering the surface of the lung is known as the visceral pleura, the parietal pleura covers the remaining structures.
- In between the visceral and parietal pleurae of each lung is the pleural space, a potential space that contains a thin layer of fluid of ~10 mL in volume.
- **The parietal pleura secretes ~2.5 L of fluid daily**, which is reabsorbed by the visceral pleura.

Definition

- A pleural effusion is >10 mL accumulation of fluid in the pleural space.
  - A **hemothorax** refers to a pleural effusion that is comprised mainly of blood.
  - **Chylothorax** is a collection of chyle within the pleural space.
  - A **parapneumonic effusion** is any effusion caused by bacterial pneumonia and occurs in about 40% of cases of bacterial pneumonia.[1]
    - **Uncomplicated** parapneumonic effusions do not require chest tube drainage for complete resolution and are presumed to be sterile.
    - **Complicated** parapneumonic effusions are accompanied by bacterial invasion of the pleural space and typically do require thoracostomy drainage, although occasionally may improve with antibiotic therapy alone.
    - **Empyema** simply refers to a complicated parapneumonic effusion with grossly purulent pleural fluid and is presumed to be infected even though cultures may not always be positive. On occasion, empyema may not be associated with a pneumonic process.
    - Other more complicated classifications of parapneumonic effusions have also been developed.[2,3]
- A **pneumothorax** is a collection of gas in the pleural space.[4,5]
  - Primary spontaneous pneumothorax occurs when there is no obvious underlying lung disease.
  - Secondary spontaneous pneumothorax is a complication of underlying lung disease.

Epidemiology

- More than 1 million cases of pleural effusion occur annually in the United States.
- Incidence of pneumothorax varies widely by gender, country, and race.[4]

Etiology

- Pleural effusions have a variety of causes (Table 23-1).
  - **Empyema** is generally caused by extension of an infection of the lung or surrounding tissue.
    - Common microbial pathogens are *Staphylococcus aureus, Streptococcus* species, and *Haemophilus influenza.*
    - Empyemas are frequently polymicrobial in cases where aspiration is suspected.

TABLE 23-1 CAUSES OF PLEURAL EFFUSION

Exudates

- Infection (viral, bacterial, mycobacterial, fungal, protozoal)
- Neoplastic
  - Metastatic carcinoma
  - Lymphoma
  - Leukemia
  - Mesothelioma
  - Bronchogenic carcinoma
  - Chest wall tumors
- Intra-abdominal disease
  - Abdominal surgery
  - Pancreatitis
  - Meigs syndrome
  - Intrahepatic abscess
  - Incarcerated diaphragmatic hernia
  - Subdiaphragmatic abscess
  - Esophageal rupture
  - Endoscopic variceal sclerotherapy
  - Hepatitis
- Collagen vascular diseases
  - Systemic lupus erythematosus
  - Drug-induced lupus
  - Rheumatoid arthritis
  - Sjögren syndrome
  - Granulomatosis with polyangiitis
  - Churg–Strauss syndrome
- Drug induced
  - Nitrofurantoin
  - Dantrolene
  - Methysergide
  - Bromocriptine
  - Procarbazine
  - Amiodarone
- Pulmonary infarction
- Lipid laden
  - Chylous
  - Pseudochylous (chyliform, i.e., cholesterol effusion)
  - Trauma
- Miscellaneous
  - Dressler syndrome (postcardiac injury)
  - Sarcoidosis
  - Yellow nail syndrome
  - Trapped lung
  - Radiation therapy
  - Electrical burns
  - Iatrogenic injury
  - Ovarian hyperstimulation syndrome
  - Chronic atelectasis
  - Asbestos exposure
  - Familial Mediterranean fever
  - Urinoma
- Idiopathic

Transudates

- Increased hydrostatic pressure
  - Heart failure
  - Constrictive pericarditis
  - Superior vena cava obstruction
- Decreased oncotic pressure
  - Cirrhosis
  - Nephrotic syndrome
  - Hypoalbuminemia
  - Peritoneal dialysis
- Miscellaneous
  - Acute atelectasis
  - Subclavian catheter misplacement
  - Myxedema
  - Idiopathic

- The three major grouped causes of **chylothorax** are malignancy (50% of cases), trauma (25%), and idiopathic (15%). Other causes account for 10%.[6]
  - Seventy-five percent of chylous effusions related to malignancy are due to lymphomas related to obstruction of pleural lymphatics.
  - Trauma as a causative factor of chylothorax includes any cardiothoracic surgical procedure. It may take place 1–2 weeks postsurgery for the chylothorax to become apparent.
  - In a number of cases, chylothorax results from transdiaphragmatic leakage of chylous ascites. Causes of chylous ascites include nephrotic syndrome, hypothyroidism, and cirrhosis.

TABLE 23-2 CRITERIA FOR DEFINING A PLEURAL EFFUSION[9,10]

Light criteria
Pleural fluid protein to serum protein ratio of >0.5
Pleural fluid LDH to serum LDH ratio of >0.6
Pleural fluid LDH >2/3 serum upper limit of normal
Heffner criteria
Pleural fluid protein >2.9 g/dL
Pleural fluid cholesterol >45 mg/dL
Pleural fluid LDH >45% of upper limits of normal serum value

LDH, lactate dehydrogenase.

- **Hemothorax** may result from trauma or iatrogenesis, and rarely can occur spontaneously.[7]
- When the etiology for the effusion cannot be determined despite appropriate evaluation, a benign course is typical.[8]
- **Secondary pneumothorax** is often seen in chronic obstructive pulmonary disease (COPD), AIDS, cystic fibrosis, TB, sarcoidosis, pulmonary fibrosis, asthma, Marfan disease, lymphangioleiomyomatosis, pulmonary Langerhans cell histiocytosis, trauma, or any disease with pulmonary cavity formation.[4] Catamenial pneumothorax is a rare condition of spontaneous pneumothorax occurring in close proximity to menstruation and is often recurrent.[4,5] It may also cause hemopneumothorax.

Pathophysiology

- Pleural effusions can be categorized as transudates or exudates (Table 23-2).[9,10]
  - **Transudates** result primarily from passive fluid shifts that occur as a result of changes in the hydrostatic and oncotic pressures of the circulation.
  - **Exudates** imply an active pleural process such as inflammation of the pleura or underlying lung tissue.
  - There are numerous causes of both transudates and exudates (Table 23-1).
- Primary spontaneous pneumothorax is thought to result from rupture of subpleural apical blebs.[4,5]
- Secondary pneumothorax results from rupture of already pathologic lung architecture.[4]

Risk Factors

- Risk factors for pleural effusion reflect those of the underlying causative disease.
- Primary spontaneous pneumothoraces are more common in tall, thin males, and recur 50% of the time.[4]
- Smoking also increases the risk of spontaneous pneumothorax.[4,5]

DIAGNOSIS

Clinical Presentation

- Symptom onset may be chronic, subacute, or acute depending on the rapidity which the pleural pathology developed.
- If the effusion or pneumothorax is very large in nature, it may cause mass effect and even cardiac tamponade, resulting in a life-threatening condition.
- In cases of massive hemothorax requiring surgical intervention, clamping the chest tube may result in tension hemothorax and cardiovascular collapse.
- Chylothorax is nonirritating and bacteriostatic, thus secondary infection is extremely rare.[6]

History

- **Dyspnea** is the primary symptom of pleural disease, and **pain** may also be present.
  - Pain is generally pleuritic in nature.
  - Referred pain to the abdomen and ipsilateral shoulder is possible.
- Other symptoms depend on the specific etiology of the pleural disease.
  - Empyema may be associated with fevers, chills, and malaise.
  - Hemothorax may present with signs and symptoms of anemia.
  - Chylothorax contains large amounts of fat, protein, and lymphocytes, which accounts for nutritional and immunologic deficiencies observed when they are chronic in nature.

Physical Examination

- Decreased expansion on inspiration, dullness to percussion, decreased or absent breath sounds on auscultation, and absent or reduced tactile fremitus are all consistent with a pleural effusion.[11,12]
- Asymmetric chest wall, decreased breath sounds, decreased tactile fremitus, and hyperresonance to percussion are all consistent with a large pneumothorax.[4]

Differential Diagnosis

The differential diagnosis for pleural effusion or pneumothorax includes other causes of dyspnea including pulmonary edema, pneumonia, atelectasis, thromboembolic disease, or interstitial lung disease (Table 23-1).

Diagnostic Testing

Laboratories

- Categorization of pleural fluid as transudative or exudative assists with diagnosis and therapeutic management.
  - **Light criteria** compare levels of protein and lactate dehydrogenase in the effusion with those in the patient's serum to determine whether inflammation or fluid shift is responsible for the effusion. If one of the three criteria is met, the effusion is defined as an exudate (Table 23-2).[9]
  - **Heffner criteria** has similar sensitivity for identifying exudative pleural effusions when compared to Light criteria and do not require concomitant serum values for comparison (Table 23-2).[10]
- Other useful studies to differentiate the type of pleural effusion include pH, glucose, cell count, Gram stain, culture, and triglycerides. Hematocrit should be sent if hemothorax is suspected.
  - Empyema can be diagnosed by a positive Gram stain or culture. Empyema is also characterized by a low pH and glucose.[1]
  - Hemothorax is defined by a pleural hematocrit/serum hematocrit of >0.5.[7]
  - Chylothorax is diagnosed by pleural triglycerides >110 mg/dL or by the presence of chylomicrons. If chylothorax is suspected, and triglycerides are 50–100 mg/dL, a lipoprotein electrophoresis can confirm the presence of chylomicrons.[6]
  - Malignant pleural effusion is diagnosed by a positive fluid cytology and though highly specific it is not sensitive.
  - See Table 23-3 for other pleural fluid laboratory values associated with specific pleural effusions.

Imaging

- The plain CXR is generally the first imaging study obtained when a patient presents with a suspected pleural effusion or pneumothorax.
  - On a posteroanterior chest film, blunting of the costophrenic angle or blurring of the diaphragmatic margin suggests the presence of a pleural effusion. Generally 200–500 mL of fluid is needed to generate this finding.[13]

TABLE 23-3 HELPFUL FEATURES OF EXUDATIVE EFFUSIONS

Malignancy	Infection
Cytology positive for malignant cells	Gram stain and culture often reveal specific infection
TB	Empyema is accompanied by very low glucose and pH, and a markedly elevated LDH
Pleural fluid is lymphocytic	Chylothorax
Positive AFB stain is very rare	Milky fluid, triglyceride level >110 mg/dL
Pleural fluid is sanguineous	Hemothorax
Connective tissue disease	Sanguineous fluid
Pleural fluid usually lymphocytic and will often have ANA positivity	Hematocrit of pleural fluid is >50% of peripheral blood
Pancreatitis	
Increased amylase	
Drug related	
Eosinophilic fluid	

AFB, acid-fast bacillus; ANA, antinuclear antibody; LDH, lactate dehydrogenase.

- A lateral decubitus film of the affected side can reveal an effusion of ~100 mL and allows for assessment of a free-flowing versus loculated effusion.
- Uncomplicated parapneumonic effusions typically layer <10 mm on a decubitus CXR.[1,2]

- CT is more sensitive than radiography and can detect the presence of even a very small amount of fluid or air in the pleural space as well as the presence of loculations in the pleural fluid.
- Ultrasound is a modality that is increasingly being used to image the pleural space. Ultrasound can detect fluid or air and provides qualitative information regarding pleural fluid.
  - Ultrasound findings such as fluid echogenicity and the presence or absence of septations within the pleural space may change management and predict clinical outcome.
  - Ultrasound guidance is often used to direct treatments such as drainage of fluid or chest tube insertion.

Diagnostic Procedures

- **Thoracentesis** should be performed for diagnosis in cases of pleural effusion of unknown etiology.
- Thoracentesis for further characterization is often warranted with a parapneumonic effusion that layers >10 mm on decubitus CXR or >25 mm by CT.[1,2,14] Parapneumonic effusions <10 mm have a very low risk of poor outcome.[3]
- Thoracentesis may also be therapeutic and lead to symptom relief (see Treatment).
- Thoracentesis should generally be performed after ultrasound localization to decrease risk of complications.
- CXR should be performed after the procedure to rule out a complicating pneumothorax.
- The etiology of pleural effusions can often be discerned by their gross appearance during thoracentesis.
  - A serous effusion is more likely to be transudative, while an exudative effusion is more likely to have other appearances.
  - If the fluid appears bloody, a hemothorax should be suspected.
  - Grossly purulent fluid indicates an empyema.
  - Milky white and opalescent pleural fluid is indicative of a chylothorax.

TREATMENT

- Generally, treatment of a pleural effusion depends on the etiology.
  - Transudative pleural effusions are most appropriately managed by treating the underlying cause. Symptomatic treatment may involve drainage of the effusion.
  - Exudative pleural effusions should be evaluated for an underlying cause.
  - Treatment may involve drainage of the effusion or even pleurodesis to prevent reaccumulation of fluid.
- Treatment of pneumothorax generally involves draining the air from the pleural space by insertion of a chest tube.

Medications

- Pleural effusions can sometimes be treated with medications depending on the cause.
- Parapneumonic effusions and empyema are treated with **antibiotics** in conjunction with fluid drainage.[1]
- Transudative pleural effusions can sometimes be treated effectively with **diuretics**.
- Somatostatin analogs have occasionally been used to treat chylothorax.[15,16]
- There is no medical treatment for pneumothorax.

Other Nonpharmacologic Therapies

- Moderate- to large-sized pleural effusions generally require drainage by **thoracentesis** for symptomatic relief. Prior concerns about removing too much fluid (e.g., >1 L) for fear of reexpansion pulmonary edema are probably unfounded as this is a rare complication.[17]
- **Pleurodesis** involves instillation of a sclerosing agent into the pleural space to cause scarring and restriction of the space itself.[4,5] This is generally performed for recurrent malignant effusion, recurrent pneumothorax once the lung has reexpanded, and occasionally chylothorax.
- When other modalities fail, total parenteral nutrition with complete bowel rest can cause chylothoraces to resolve as oral intake results in chyle formation. Medium-chain triglyceride diets have been tried as chyle is derived from long-chain triglycerides in the diet, though this has yielded mixed results.
- If pneumothorax is small, <15% of the hemithorax volume or <3 cm apex-to-cupola distance, and the patient is clinically stable, it is safe to observe.[4,5,18] High oxygen content (e.g., 100% nonrebreather mask) administration increases the rate of pleural air reabsorption by increasing the nitrogen gradient between the air in the pneumothorax and the pleural capillaries.[4]
- In cases of persistent pneumothorax secondary to bronchopleural fistula, fiberoptic bronchoscopy with placement of endobronchial valves causing atelectasis of the distal lung can be placed in a segmental or subsegmental bronchus if the bronchopleural fistula has been localized to one location.

Surgical Management

- Pleural effusion
  - **Chest tube** insertion is often indicated for large pleural effusions.
  - Other indications for chest tube insertion include empyema, chylothorax, and hemothorax.
  - As discussed, thoracentesis can be used as a therapeutic modality.
  - Malignant pleural effusion
    - **Tunneled pleural catheter** (e.g., PleurX) is used for recurrent malignant pleural effusion and occasionally hepatic hydrothorax not amenable to dieresis.
    - The catheter can be used to drain the effusion at home once every other day with attachment of a bottle.

  - In our experience ~50% of effusions are permanently drained by way of autopleurodesis allowing for removal of the tunneled pleural catheter.
- Empyema: In cases where chest tube drainage does not effectively drain an empyema and there is continued evidence of infection, **video-assisted thoracoscopic surgery** (VATS) with decortication is often indicated.
- Hemothorax[7]
  - Requires surgical stabilization in 30% of penetrating injuries and 15% of blunt injuries.
  - Initial output of >1500 mL of blood, or continued chest tube output or >200 mL of blood over 2 hours requires surgical intervention.
  - Clotted blood in the pleural space may require VATS to prevent development of empyema or fibrothorax.
- Chylothorax[15]
  - For persistent chylothorax, surgical interventions include thoracic duct ligation via VATS in conjunction with pleurectomy or pleurodesis.
  - Pleuroperitoneal shunting is also occasionally performed, though obviously not in cases in which the pleural disease is secondary to chylous ascites.
  - Early surgical intervention for chylothorax should be considered when chest tube output is >1500 mL/d, or in a patient with malnourishment or immune compromise.
- Pneumothorax
  - Treated with chest tube insertion if they are large (>15% of the hemithorax), symptomatic, under tension, recurrent, or bilateral.[4]
  - In extreme circumstances where a large pneumothorax is causing cardiovascular collapse, immediate needle decompression is indicated by inserting a needle in the anterior chest above the nipple line in a parasternal location.
  - For recurrent pneumothorax, VATS may be indicated with endoscopic stapling and removal of the bulla or fistula, particularly if there is a bronchopleural fistula.[4,5]

REFERENCES

1. Light RW, Girard WM, Jenkinson SG, et al. Parapneumonic effusions. *Am J Med.* 1980;69:507–12.
2. Light RW. A new classification of parapneumonic effusions and empyema. *Chest.* 1995;108:299–301.
3. Colice GL, Curtis A, Deslauriers J, et al. Medical and surgical treatment of parapneumonic effusions: an evidence-based guideline. *Chest.* 2000;118:1158–71.
4. Sahn SA, Heffner JE. Spontaneous pneumothorax. *N Engl J Med.* 2000;342(12):868–74.
5. Tschopp JM, Bintcliffe O, Astoul P, et al. ERS task force statement: diagnosis and treatment of primary spontaneous pneumothorax. *Eur Respir J.* 2015;46(2):321–35.
6. Doerr CH, Miller DL, Ryu JH. Chylothorax. *Semin Respir Crit Care Med.* 2001;22:617–26.
7. Jacoby RC, Battistella FD. Hemothorax. *Semin Respir Crit Care Med.* 2001;22:627–30.
8. Ferrer JS, Muñoz XG, Orriols RM, et al. Evolution of idiopathic pleural effusion: a prospective, long-term follow-up study. *Chest.* 1996;109:1508–13.
9. Light RW, Macgregor MI, Luchsinger PC, et al. Pleural effusions: the diagnostic separation of transudates and exudates. *Ann Intern Med.* 1972;77:507–13.
10. Heffner JE, Brown LK, Barbieri CA. Diagnostic value of tests that discriminate between exudative and transudative pleural effusions. *Chest.* 1997;111:970–80.
11. Wong CL, Holroyd-Leduc J, Straus SE. Does this patient have a pleural effusion? *JAMA.* 2009; 301:309–17.
12. Kalantri S, Joshi R, Lokhande T, et al. Accuracy and reliability of physical signs in the diagnosis of pleural effusion. *Respir Med.* 2007;101:431–8.
13. Woodring JH. Recognition of pleural effusion on supine radiographs: how much fluid is required? *Am J Roentgenol.* 1984;142: 59–64.
14. Moffett BK, Panchabhai TS, Anayya E, et al. Computed tomography measurements of parapneumonic effusion indicative of thoracentesis. *Eur Respir J.* 2011;38:1406–11.

15. Bender B, Murthy V, Chamberlain RS. The changing management of chylothorax in the modern era. *Eur J Cardiothorac Surg.* 2016; 49(1):18–24.
16. Roehr CC, Lung A, Proquitté H, et al. Somatostatin or octreotide as treatment options for chylothorax in young children: a systematic review. *Intensive Care Med.* 2006;32:650–7.
17. Feller-Kopman D, Berkowitz D, Boiselle P, et al. Large volume thoracentesis and the risk of re-expansion pulmonary edema. *Ann Thorac Surg.* 2007;84:1656–62.
18. Baumann MH, Strange C, Heffner JE, et al. Management of spontaneous pneumothorax: an American College of Chest Physicians Delphi consensus statement. *Chest.* 2001;119:590–602.

Sleep-Disordered Breathing 24

Tonya D. Russell

GENERAL PRINCIPLES

Sleep-disordered breathing (SDB) is comprised of multiple different entities:

- Obstructive sleep apnea (OSA)
- Central sleep apnea (CSA)
- Sleep-related hypoventilation

Definitions

- An **apnea** is defined as ≥90% decrease in airflow as measured by thermistor, lasting at least 10 seconds in duration.
- An **hypopnea** is a ≥30% decrease in airflow as measured by pressure transducer lasting at least 10 seconds in duration and associated with a ≥4% desaturation.
- A **respiratory effort-related arousal** (RERA) is a sequence of breaths lasting at least 10 seconds with increased respiratory effort or change in airflow which is associated with an arousal.
- The **apnea–hypopnea index** (AHI) is the number of apneas and hypopneas per hour of sleep.
- The **respiratory disturbance index** (RDI) is the number of apneas, hypopneas, and RERAs per hour of sleep.
- **Sleep-related hypoventilation** is defined as an increase in $PaCO_2$ during sleep by at least ≥10 mm Hg when compared to an awake supine value.
- **Morbid obesity** is defined by a body mass index (BMI) ≥40.

Classification

- Apneas can be **obstructive, central, or mixed in nature.**[1]
  - Apneas are classified as obstructive when there is no airflow, but continued respiratory effort.
  - Central apneas have no airflow and no respiratory effort.
  - Mixed apneas have no airflow associated with a lack of respiratory effort during the first part of the event but resumption of respiratory effort during the latter part of the event.
- Severity of sleep apnea based on AHI[1]
  - An AHI <5 is normal.
  - Mild sleep apnea has an AHI of 5–15.
  - Moderate sleep apnea has an AHI of >15 and <30.
  - Severe sleep apnea has an AHI ≥30.
- Severity of sleepiness[1]
  - Mild sleepiness is when sleepiness occurs in sedentary situations such as watching TV or reading.
  - Moderate sleepiness is when sleepiness occurs in settings such as meetings or the theater.
  - Severe sleepiness is when sleepiness occurs with activities such as talking, eating, or driving.

Epidemiology

- OSA is the most common form of SDB.
  - OSA associated with daytime sleepiness (OSA-hypopnea syndrome) occurs in 2–4% of the general population.[2]
  - This percentage likely underestimates current prevalence due to the increasing prevalence of obesity in the United States and the strong association between obesity and OSA.
- Prevalence of SDB increases with age.[3,4]
  - The prevalence of OSA increases with age but CSA also becomes more prevalent.
  - The prevalence of SDB in postmenopausal women is higher than in premenopausal women.
- As BMI increases, obesity hypoventilation (OHV) is more likely to occur.[4] In patients with a BMI >50, ~50% of patients have evidence of hypoventilation.[5,6]

Etiology

- OSA occurs due to narrowing of the upper airway either due to excessive soft tissue or structural abnormalities.
- CSA can have a variety of causes
  - Stroke
  - Brain tumor
  - Congestive heart failure
  - Use of positive airway pressure devices can result in treatment-emergent central apneas.
- Sleep-related hypoventilation can be due to a variety of causes
  - Morbid obesity-OHV
  - Severe OSA
  - Neuromuscular disease with respiratory muscle weakness
  - Severe kyphoscoliosis or thoracic cage deformity
  - Diaphragmatic paralysis
  - Severe obstructive lung disease

Pathophysiology

- OSA: Narrowing of the upper airway leads to recurrent arousals.
- CSA
  - Central apneas can occur due to direct effects on the medullary respiratory centers (stroke or brain tumor).
  - In addition, central apneas may be due to increased sensitivity to small changes in carbon dioxide levels (congestive heart failure).
  - Central apneas can occur in the setting of using positive airway pressure to treat OSA.
- OHV
  - OHV may be due to frequent obstructive apneas or hypopneas that lead to a decrease in minute ventilation.[6]
  - Impairment of respiratory mechanics due to morbid obesity can also contribute to OHV.[6]
  - Leptin resistance in morbidly obese patients may impair their ability to increase their minute ventilation appropriately.[6–8]

Risk Factors

- Risk factors for OSA include the following: obesity, macroglossia, micrognathia, retrognathia, neck circumference >17 in in men and >16 in in women, enlarged tonsils, increasing age, male gender, family history, use of alcohol or sedatives, and concomitant medical conditions such as hypothyroidism.[1–4,9]
- Risk factors for CSA include the following: use of positive airway pressure, severe congestive heart failure, and stroke or brain injury.[1]

- Risk factors for sleep-related hypoventilation include the following: very severe OSA, respiratory muscle weakness, morbid obesity, severe obstructive lung disease, and thoracic cage abnormalities.[1]

Prevention

- The following factors help in the prevention of OSA:
  - Weight loss can be beneficial. However, weight loss alone may not prevent OSA if there are craniopharyngeal structural abnormalities.
  - Avoidance of alcohol and sedatives may help prevent OSA as these substances contribute to muscle relaxation and impaired arousal threshold.
  - Treatment of underlying conditions such as hypothyroidism may help prevent OSA. Hypothyroidism can result in weight gain and decreased upper airway muscle tone.
- The following factors help in the prevention of CSA:
  - Medical treatment of severe congestive heart failure may improve CSA.
  - Avoiding over titration of continuous positive airway pressure (CPAP) may help prevent CSA, as treatment-emergent CSA is more likely to occur at higher pressure settings.
- The following factors may help in the prevention of sleep-related hypoventilation: weight loss in the morbidly obese may improve underlying OSA, respiratory muscle dysfunction, and leptin resistance which can all contribute to OHV.

Associated Conditions

- Conditions associated with OSA include the following: hypertension, coronary artery disease, stroke, diabetes mellitus, metabolic syndrome, mild pulmonary hypertension, and increased risk of motor vehicle collisions due to sleepiness.[10–18]
- Conditions associated with CSA include congestive heart failure and stroke.[1,17,19]
- Conditions associated with OHV include the following: congestive heart failure, hypertension, coronary artery disease, stroke, diabetes mellitus, metabolic syndrome, pulmonary hypertension, right heart failure, and increased risk of motor vehicle collisions due to sleepiness.[1,6]

DIAGNOSIS

Clinical Presentation

History

During the history, the presence of the following symptoms should be queried[9]:

- Daytime sleepiness
- Unrefreshing sleep
- Witnessed apneas
- Awakening, snorting, or gasping
- Loud snoring (OSA and OHV)
- Morning headaches
- Nocturia
- Poorly controlled hypertension (OSA)
- Decreased concentration/memory, irritability
- Decreased libido

Physical Examination

- The physical examination to evaluate for OSA mainly focuses on the upper airway. The presence or absence of the following features should be ascertained:
  - Obesity
  - Macroglossia

  - Micrognathia
  - Retrognathia
  - Neck circumference >17 in in men and >16 in in women
  - Enlarged tonsils
  - Crowded posterior oropharynx
- Physical examination findings for CSA are examination findings that would be associated with underlying medical conditions that predispose to CSA.
  - Findings consistent with severe heart failure
  - Findings consistent with stroke or previous brain injury
- The physical examination for OHV should focus on many of the same areas as for OSA. In addition, examination findings related to complications from OHV, such as right heart failure, should be elucidated.
  - Morbid obesity, BMI >40
  - Upper airway examination findings may be similar to OSA
  - Findings consistent with right heart failure
  - Cyanosis

Diagnostic Criteria

- OSA as defined by the International Classification of Sleep Disorders[1]:
  - RDI >5 with events being associated with ongoing respiratory effort with reported complaint of daytime sleepiness, awakening gasping, loud snoring, or witnessed apneas, OR
  - RDI >15 with events being associated with ongoing respiratory effort.
- CSA as defined by the International Classification of Sleep Disorders[1]:
  - Primary CSA
    - Five or more central apneas per hour.
    - Must experience one of the following: excessive daytime sleepiness, frequent arousals or insomnia, or awakening short of breath.
  - Cheyne–Stokes respirations
    - Ten or more central apneas/hypopneas per hour with an alternating pattern of apnea/hypopnea followed by hyperpnea in a crescendo–decrescendo pattern.
    - Occurring in the setting of other serious medical conditions such as heart failure or stroke.
- Sleep-related hypoventilation/hypoxemia as defined by the International Classification of Sleep Disorders[1]:
  - Underlying disorder that can contribute to hypoventilation such as neuromuscular weakness, chest wall deformity, morbid obesity, or severe obstructive lung disease.
  - One of the following features on sleep study:
    - Oxygen saturation <90% for >5 continuous minutes while asleep with a nadir of at least 85%.
    - Oxygen saturation <90% for at least 30% of total sleep time.
    - Elevation of $PaCO_2$ that is abnormally elevated compared to waking levels.

Differential Diagnosis

- Any of the SDB entities can be in the differential diagnoses for any of the other disorders.[1]
- Consider other causes of nocturnal dyspnea: congestive heart failure and laryngospasm.
- Consider other causes of daytime sleepiness: periodic limb movement disorder, narcolepsy, and idiopathic hypersomnia.

Diagnostic Testing

Laboratories

Thyroid-stimulating hormone should be measured when hypothyroidism suspected.

Diagnostic Procedures

- **Split-night polysomnogram**
  - First 2 hours of sleep recorded to determine severity of underlying SDB.
  - Positive airway pressure initiated if AHI >40 during baseline.
- **All-night polysomnogram:** performed if SDB is mild to moderate during baseline. Allows determination of severity of SDB in different stages of sleep and sleeping positions.
- **Positive airway pressure titration:** performed if diagnosis of SDB already known.
- The use of non–sleep-laboratory (mostly at-home) portable diagnostic testing is evolving.[9]
  - Multiple different types of devices are available which record a variable number of physiologic parameters, but less than standard overnight polysomnography.
  - Sensitivity is less with these devices.
  - Treatment for a diagnosis of OSA made with just a few parameters (e.g., only arterial oxygen saturation and airflow) may not be reimbursed by insurers.
  - These portable monitors are best used in those with a high clinical pretest probability of moderate to severe OSA after a comprehensive sleep evaluation. Sensors should either be placed by an appropriately trained healthcare provider or that provider should directly educate the patient about the proper way to do so. They should not be used in patients with comorbid conditions (e.g., heart failure) or when there is suspicion of other causes of SBD. The results of such testing should be evaluated by sleep medicine specialist.

TREATMENT

Medications

- Multiple medications (e.g., certain antidepressants, theophylline, and respiratory stimulants) have been studied as primary therapy (i.e., without other forms of treatment) for OSA with largely inconclusive results. None are recommended.[9,20]
- Stimulants are approved for patients with OSA and **residual sleepiness despite adequate use of CPAP.** These include modafinil or armodafinil.[9,21]
  - First, proper adherence to and functioning of mechanical treatments should be ascertained.
  - Which patients will most benefit from the addition of pharmacotherapy is currently uncertain.
  - Both modafinil and armodafinil have been reasonably well tolerated in clinical trials. More common side effects include headache, nervousness/anxiety, dizziness, and nausea. Rare severe dermatologic and systemic hypersensitivity reactions have been reported. There are many potential drug interactions.
  - Caution is advised when used in patients with cardiovascular, hepatic, and psychiatric conditions. Lower doses should be used in the elderly.
- Nasal steroids may be useful in OSA for nasal congestion/inflammation due to allergic rhinitis.[9,22,23]
- In patients with CSA medical therapy for underlying congestive heart failure should be undertaken if present.

Other Nonpharmacologic Therapies

- OSA[9,24,25]
  - CPAP is the most effective therapy if patient is compliant, especially in severe OSA.
  - Autotitrating positive airway pressure in patients without significant comorbid conditions.
  - Positional therapy if events occur mainly in supine position—sleep belt or sleep shirt to maintain lateral position.

  - An oral appliance is less effective in severe OSA. Typically, the patient should be evaluated by a dentist specializing in sleep medicine. This is not a good choice for patients who are edentulous.
  - A nasal expiratory resistance device, which uses the patient's own breathing to produce expiratory positive airway pressure (EPAP) may be helpful but is less effective for severe OSA.[26–28]
- CSA[29]
  - Bilevel positive airway pressure (BiPAP) with a backup rate may be used for central apneas.
  - Adaptive/autoservo ventilation (ASV) may also be used in the setting of CSA. The device is equipped with an algorithm for titrating inspiratory positive airway pressure (IPAP) to help stabilize significant respiratory variations that can occur in CSA.
- OHV[6]
  - BiPAP can be used to improve hypoventilation. As patients may have concomitant OSA, the EPAP will need to be titrated to alleviate obstructive events.
  - Average volume-assured pressure support (AVAPS) allows for a targeted tidal volume. The machine allows the IPAP to be titrated to meet the goal tidal volume.
  - Nocturnal ventilation via tracheostomy may be necessary if no optimal setting can be found for noninvasive ventilation or if a patient cannot tolerate noninvasive ventilation.

Surgical Management

- OSA[30]
  - Laser-assisted uvulopalatoplasty (LAUP) is a treatment for snoring, not OSA.
  - Uvulopalatopharyngoplasty (UPPP) is less effective in severe OSA.
  - Radiofrequency ablation should only be an option for patients with mild–moderate OSA who cannot tolerate CPAP.
  - Palatal implants should only be an option for patients with mild OSA who cannot tolerate CPAP.
  - Maxillomandibular advancement is only performed at highly specialized centers.
  - Tracheostomy is essentially a cure for OSA as the site of upper airway obstruction resulting in apnea is bypassed.
  - Bariatric surgery for weight loss may be beneficial.[31]
- CSA: heart transplant in patients with severe heart failure.
- OHV[6]
  - Tracheostomy with use of nocturnal ventilator is very effective for OHV.
  - Bariatric surgery for weight loss may be beneficial.

Lifestyle/Risk Modification

The following modifications may benefit patients with OSA/OHV:

- Diet for weight loss.
- Exercise for weight loss.
- Avoidance of alcohol and other sedatives.

Special Considerations

In the elderly, the following items must be considered:

- The risk of OSA increases with age.
- Central apneas become more common.
- SDB may be associated with atypical symptoms such as nocturnal falls, enuresis, and decreased cognition.

Complications

- OSA is associated with the following medical complications:
  - Hypertension.
  - Cardiovascular disease.
  - Insulin resistance.
  - Daytime sleepiness—increased risk of motor vehicle collisions.
- CSA can also be associated with daytime sleepiness.
- OHV is associated with the following medical complications:
  - Pulmonary hypertension.
  - Right heart failure.
  - Daytime sleepiness—increased risk of motor vehicle collisions.[10,16]

Referrals

If SDB is suspected, the patient should be referred to a sleep physician for further evaluation and testing.

Patient Education

- The patient should be educated about the potential health consequences of untreated SDB and the importance of compliance with positive airway pressure.
- Counsel on weight loss if needed.
- Counsel on avoiding sedatives and alcohol.
- Counsel on driving precautions.

Follow-Up

- After initiation of positive airway pressure, the patient should be seen back within 2–3 months to assure proper use and compliance with positive airway pressure. Arrangements should be made to see the patient sooner if there is difficulty in tolerating the device.
- Newer machines have download cards so that use can be monitored.
- If the patient is stable, routine follow-up can occur every 6–12 months.

Outcome/Prognosis

Prognosis depends upon severity of underlying disorder and patient's ability to comply with therapy.[32]

REFERENCES

1. American Academy of Sleep Medicine. *International Classification of Sleep Disorders.* 3rd ed. Darien, Illinois: American Academy of Sleep Medicine; 2014.
2. Young T, Palta M, Dempsey J, et al. The occurrence of sleep-disordered breathing among middle-aged adults. *N Engl J Med.* 1993;328:1230–5.
3. Hoch C, Reynolds III C, Monk T, et al. Comparison of sleep-disordered breathing among healthy elderly in the seventh, eighth, and ninth decades. *Sleep.* 1990;13:502–11.
4. Young T, Skatrud J, Peppard PE. Risk factors for obstructive sleep apnea in adults. *JAMA.* 2004; 291:2013–6.
5. Nowbar S, Burkart K, Gonzales R, et al. Obesity-associated hypoventilation in hospitalized patients: prevalence, effects, and outcome. *Am J Med.* 2004;116:1–7.
6. Piper A, Grunstein R. Obesity hypoventilation syndrome: mechanisms and management. *Am J Respir Crit Care Med.* 2011;183:292–8.
7. Phipps PR, Starritt E, Caterson I, et al. Association of serum leptin with hypoventilation in human obesity. *Thorax.* 2002;57:75–6.
8. Shimura R, Tatsumi K, Nakamura A, et al. Fat accumulation, leptin, and hypercapnia in obstructive sleep apnea-hypopnea syndrome. *Chest.* 2005;127:543–9.

9. Epstein L, Kristo D, Strollo P, et al. Clinical guideline for the evaluation, management, and long term care of obstructive sleep apnea in adults. *J Clin Sleep Med.* 2009;5:263–76.
10. Terán-Santos J, Jiménez-Gómez A, Cordero-Guevara J, et al. The association between sleep apnea and the risk of traffic accidents. *N Engl J Med.* 1999;340:847–51.
11. Peppard PE, Young T, Palta M, et al. Prospective study of the association between sleep-disordered breathing and hypertension. *N Engl J Med.* 2000;342:1378–84.
12. Ip M, Lam B, Ng M, et al. Obstructive sleep apnea is independently associated with insulin resistance. *Am J Respir Crit Care Med.* 2002;165:670–6.
13. Punjabi NM, Shahar E, Redline S, et al. Sleep-disordered breathing, glucose intolerance, and insulin resistance: the sleep heart health study. *Am J Epidemiol.* 2004;160:521–30.
14. Yaggi HK, Concato J, Kernan WN, et al. Obstructive sleep apnea as a risk factor for stroke and death. *N Engl J Med.* 2005;353:2034–41.
15. Peker Y, Carlson J, Hedner J. Increased incidence of coronary artery disease in sleep apnoea: a long term follow up. *Eur Respir J.* 2006;28:596–602.
16. Ellen RL, Marshall SC, Palayew M. Systematic review of motor vehicle crash risk in persons with sleep apnea. *J Clin Sleep Med.* 2006;2:193–200.
17. Somers VK, White DP, Amin R, et al. Sleep apnea and cardiovascular disease: an American Heart Association/American College of Cardiology Foundation Scientific Statement from the American Heart Association Council for High Blood Pressure Research Professional Education Committee, Council on Clinical Cardiology, Stroke Council, and Council on Cardiovascular Nursing. *J Am Coll Cardiol.* 2008;52:686–717.
18. O'Connor G, Caffo B, Newman A, et al. Prospective study of sleep-disordered breathing and hypertension: the sleep heart health study. *Am J Respir Crit Care Med.* 2009;179:1159–64.
19. Constanzo MR, Khayat R, Ponikowski P, et al. Mechanisms and clinical consequences of untreated central sleep apnea in heart failure. *J Am Coll Cardiol.* 2015;65:72–84.
20. Mason M, Welsh EJ, Smith I. Drug therapy for obstructive sleep apnoea in adults. *Cochrane Database Syst Rev.* 2013;5:CD003002.
21. Sukhal S, Khalid M, Tulaimat A. Effect of wakefulness-promoting agents on sleepiness in patients with sleep apnea treated with CPAP: a meta-analysis. *J Clin Sleep Med.* 2015;11(10):1179–86.
22. Kiely JL, Nolan P, McNicholas WT. Intranasal corticosteroid therapy for obstructive sleep apnoea in patients with co-existing rhinitis. *Thorax.* 2004;59:50–5.
23. Acar M, Cingi C, Sakallioglu O, et al. The effects of mometasone furoate and desloratadine in obstructive sleep apnea syndrome patients with allergic rhinitis. *Am J Rhinol Allergy.* 2013;27: e113–6.
24. Kushida C, Littner M, Hirshkowitz M, et al. Practice parameters for the use of continuous and bilevel positive airway pressure devices to treat adults with sleep related breathing disorders. *Sleep.* 2006;29:375–80.
25. Morgenthaler T, Aurora R, Brown T, et al. Practice parameters for the use of autotitrating continuous positive airway pressure devices for titrating pressures and treating adult patients with obstructive sleep apnea syndrome: an update for 2007. *Sleep.* 2008;31:141–7.
26. Rosenthal L, Massie CA, Dolan DC, et al. A multicenter, prospective study of a novel nasal EPAP device in the treatment of obstructive sleep apnea: efficacy and 30-day adherence. *J Clin Sleep Med.* 2009;5:532–7.
27. Berry RB, Kryger MH, Massie CA. A novel nasal expiratory positive airway pressure (EPAP) device for the treatment of obstructive sleep apnea: a randomized controlled trial. *Sleep.* 2011; 34:479–85.
28. Kryger MH, Berry RB, Massie CA. Long-term use of a nasal expiratory positive airway pressure (EPAP) device as a treatment for obstructive sleep apnea (OSA). *J Clin Sleep Med.* 2011;7:449–53.
29. Aurora RN, Chowdhuri S, Ramar K, et al. The treatment of central sleep apnea syndromes in adults: practice parameters with an evidence-based literature review and meta-analyses. *Sleep.* 2012;35:17–40.
30. Aurora R, Casey K, Kristo D, et al. Practice parameters for the surgical modifications of the upper airway for obstructive sleep apnea in adults. *Sleep.* 2010;33:1408–13.
31. Sarkhosh K, Switzer NJ, El-Hadi M, et al. The impact of bariatric surgery on obstructive sleep apnea: a systematic review. *Obes Surg.* 2013;23:414–23.
32. Young T, Finn L, Peppard PE, et al. Sleep disordered breathing and mortality: eighteen-year follow-up of the Wisconsin sleep cohort. *Sleep.* 2008;31:1071–8.

Interstitial Lung Disease

25

Catherine Chen and Adrian Shifren

GENERAL PRINCIPLES

Definition

- Interstitial lung disease (ILD) describes a heterogeneous group of over 200 diseases affecting the pulmonary interstitium with varying degrees of involvement of the pleural space, airways, and pulmonary vasculature.
- ILD is also termed diffuse parenchymal lung disease (DPLD).
- These diseases account for ~15–20% of general pulmonary practice.
- Since ILDs differ greatly in presentation, clinical course, and response to therapy, establishing an accurate diagnosis is essential for determining the optimal management strategy.
- This requires effective collaboration between the pulmonologist, thoracic surgeon, radiologist, and pathologist to integrate clinical, physiologic, laboratory, radiographic, and histopathologic data.
- Accordingly, the majority of this chapter will focus on the clinical evaluation and diagnosis of ILD.

Classification

- Guidelines based on clinical, histopathologic, and radiographic findings have been proposed for subgroups of ILD including idiopathic interstitial pneumonias (IIP), hypersensitivity pneumonitis (HP), lymphangioleiomyomatosis (LAM), and others.
- However, due to the heterogeneous nature of these diseases, there is currently no universal classification system that encompasses all ILDs.
- A classification system based loosely on etiology and/or disease association is presented in Table 25-1.
- Keep in mind that this table is far from comprehensive, and the definition and classification of ILDs will continue to evolve rapidly as we learn more about the pathogenesis of these diseases.

Etiology and Pathogenesis

- Environmental and heritable factors both play a significant role in the pathogenesis of ILD, but the relative contribution and importance of these factors is quite variable between diseases and patients.
- An increasing number of occupational/environmental exposures and genetic modifiers of disease susceptibility have been elucidated through epidemiologic and genomic analyses, respectively.
- However, the complex interactions between these factors and how they affect disease development and progression remain poorly understood.
- Alveolar epithelial cell injury is a hallmark of ILD. The source of injury may be extrinsic, as in cases of HP, pneumoconiosis, or radiation pneumonitis.
- Alternatively, the injurious insult may arrive via the circulation, as suspected in collagen vascular diseases, vasculitides, or drug-induced lung diseases.
- Normally after a limited injury, the initial acute inflammatory response resolves, and tissue repair programs restore lung integrity and homeostasis.

TABLE 25-1 CLASSIFICATION OF DIFFUSE PROLIFERATIVE LUNG DISEASES

A. Known etiologies		
Collagen vascular disease:	Scleroderma Rheumatoid arthritis Polymyositis/dermatomyositis Antisynthetase syndrome Sjögren syndrome	
Drug-related:	*Antibiotics*	Cephalosporins Nitrofurantoin Sulfasalazine
	Antiarrhythmic	Amiodarone β-blockers
	Anti-inflammatory	NSAIDs Gold Penicillamine
	Neuropsychiatric	Phenytoin Carbamazepine Fluoxetine
	Chemotherapeutic	Bleomycin Methotrexate Azathioprine Busulfan Paclitaxel
Pneumoconioses:	Asbestosis Coal miner pneumoconiosis Silicosis Berylliosis Hard-metal pneumoconiosis (cobalt) Talcosis (talc) Siderosis (iron) Stannosis (tin)	
Hypersensitivity pneumonitis:	Bird fancier lung (pigeons, parakeets, others) Farmer lung (moldy hay) Humidifier lung Hot tub lung Bagassosis (sugar cane) Cheese worker lung Suberosis (cork)	
Vasculitis:	Granulomatosis with polyangiitis (GPA) Microscopic polyangiitis Goodpasture syndrome[a] Churg–Strauss syndrome Behçet disease	
B. Unkown etiologies		
Idiopathic interstitial pneumonias:	**Major IIPs** Idiopathic pulmonary fibrosis (IPF) Idiopathic nonspecific interstitial pneumonitis (NSIP)	

(*Continued*)

TABLE 25-1 CLASSIFICATION OF DIFFUSE PROLIFERATIVE LUNG DISEASES (*Continued*)

	Cryptogenic organizing pneumonia (COP)
	Acute interstitial pneumonia (AIP)
	Respiratory bronchiolitis-interstitial lung disease (RB-ILD)[a]
	Desquamative interstitial pneumonia (DIP)[a]
	Rare IIPs
	Idiopathic lymphoid interstitial pneumonia (LIP)
	Idiopathic pleuroparenchymal fibroelastosis
	Unclassifiable IIPs
Others:	Familial pulmonary fibrosis
	Sarcoidosis
	Lymphangioleiomyomatosis (LAM)
	Pulmonary Langerhans cell histiocytosis (PLCH)[a]
	Alveolar proteinosis
	Amyloidosis
	Acute eosinophilic pneumonia
	Chronic eosinophilic pneumonia
	Pulmonary alveolar microlithiasis
	Diffuse pulmonary ossification
	Combined pulmonary fibrosis and emphysema (CPFE)[a]

C. Hereditary diseases with diffuse lung involvement

Tuberous sclerosis
Neurofibromatosis
Hermansky–Pudlak syndrome
Gaucher disease
Niemann–Pick disease
Birt–Hogg–Dubé

[a]These diseases are strongly associated with tobacco smoking. In the case of Goodpasture syndrome, diffuse alveolar hemorrhage is significantly more common in smokers than nonsmokers.

Adapted from British Thoracic Society and Standards of Care Committee. The diagnosis, assessment and treatment of diffuse parenchymal lung disease in adults. *Thorax*. 1999;54(Suppl 1): S1–S28; and Schwarz M, King TE, Raghu G. Approach to the evaluation and diagnosis of interstitial lung disease. In: Schwarz M, King T Jr, eds. *Interstitial Lung Disease*. Hamilton, Ontario: BC Decker; 1998.

- However, with recurrent or persistent injury the reparative response becomes maladaptive; this leads to dysregulation of the normal injury repair response, resulting disruption of lung architecture and function.
- Indeed, lung biopsy specimens from patients with ILD frequently show varying degrees of inflammation and/or fibrosis.
- In addition to recurrent injury and aberrant repair of the airway epithelium, other factors may contribute to the pathogenesis of ILD.
- Studies have revealed an association between short telomere length and idiopathic pulmonary fibrosis (IPF); these findings are consistent with the increased prevalence of IPF in elderly patients and implicate accelerated cellular aging or stem cell exhaustion as additional mechanisms of disease in some ILDs.

DIAGNOSIS

- A suggested algorithm for the evaluation of ILD is presented in Figure 25-1.

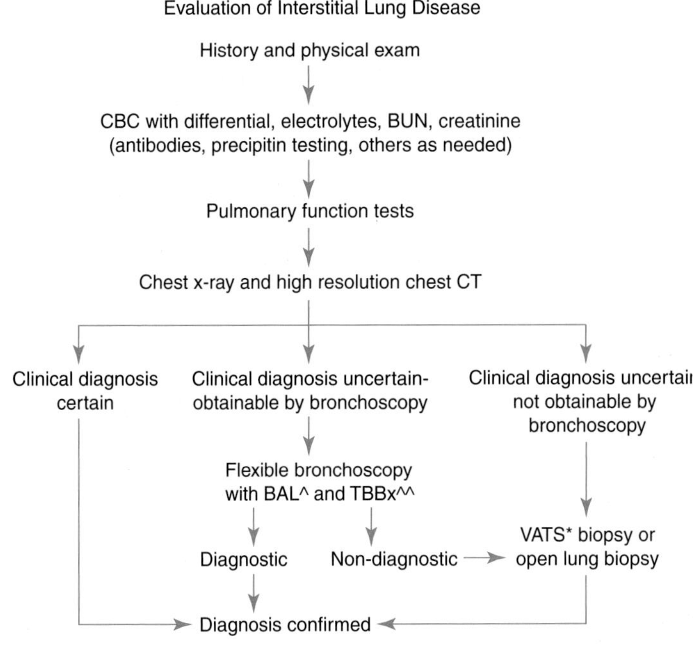

FIGURE 25-1. Evaluation of diffuse proliferative lung diseases. (Adapted from American Thoracic Society/European Respiratory Society International Multidisciplinary Consensus Classification of the Idiopathic Interstitial Pneumonias. *Am J Respir Crit Care Med.* 2002;165:277–304; and British Thoracic Society and Standards of Care Committee. The diagnosis, assessment and treatment of diffuse parenchymal lung disease in adults. *Thorax.* 1999;54(Suppl 1):S1–S28.)

Clinical Presentation

History

- A comprehensive history is a very important part of the patient evaluation.
- It can significantly narrow the differential diagnosis, guide the physical examination, and reduce the need for extensive diagnostic testing.
- **Dyspnea** is the most common presenting symptom.
  - Patients may initially present with dyspnea only with moderate or heavy exertion.
  - As the disease progresses, breathlessness with mild or minimal exertion becomes apparent.
  - Eventually patients become dyspneic at rest.
  - Depending on the specific disease, dyspnea may present insidiously over months to years as in IPF, or pursue a more aggressive course over weeks to months as in acute interstitial pneumonia or acute eosinophilic pneumonia.
  - Episodic dyspnea may occur in cases of HP where repeated exposure to an inciting environmental agent causes waxing and waning symptoms.
  - Therefore, it is important to accurately quantify the duration and severity of the patient's dyspnea.
- **Cough** is also a frequent complaint associated with ILD.
  - A nonproductive cough is common in cases of IPF, HP, and sarcoidosis.
- **Chest pain** is unusual.
  - When present it may be associated with inflammation of the pleural space (systemic lupus erythematosus, rheumatoid arthritis), pneumothorax (LAM), or an atypical cause of ILD (sarcoidosis).
  - Occult coronary artery disease is common in elderly patients with advanced lung disease and limited functional capacity. Therefore, coronary ischemia should be considered in the differential.
- **Wheezing** is less frequent in general.
  - It may be more prevalent in ILDs involving the airways such as HP, respiratory bronchiolitis-interstitial lung disease (RB-ILD), or sarcoidosis.
  - Other diseases involving the airways, such as chronic bronchitis or asthma, may occur concurrently.
- **Hemoptysis** is also infrequent. It may occur in ILDs associated with vasculitis, connective tissue diseases or diffuse alveolar hemorrhage, such as Goodpasture syndrome, microscopic polyangiitis, and granulomatosis with polyangiitis (GPA, known previously as Wegener granulomatosis).
- **Constitutional symptoms**, such as fevers, chills, weight loss, night sweats, and fatigue occur with variable frequency. Significant unintentional weight loss should also raise the possibility of a concurrent malignancy, since patients with certain ILDs such as IPF, lymphoid interstitial pneumonia (LIP), and asbestosis are known to have an increased incidence of lung malignancy.
- **Past and current medical histories** are important for diagnosing ILDs secondary to systemic conditions such as collagen vascular disease, vasculitides, and other autoimmune diseases (Table 25-1).
  - In some cases, the systemic disease is already present at the time of diagnosis.
  - However, in certain ILDs associated with systemic disease, ILD may be the initial manifestation of the disease.
  - In rare cases ILD can be the only manifestation of the disease.
  - The clinician should maintain a high index of clinical suspicion, and in the correct clinical context, such as a younger female presenting with ILD, diagnostic testing should be performed to exclude the presence of collagen vascular disease.
- **Social history** should be obtained to identify known risk factors for certain ILDs.
  - Cigarette smoking has an integral causal relationship with diseases such as RB-ILD, desquamative interstitial pneumonia (DIP), and pulmonary Langerhans cell histiocytosis (PLCH).

- In addition, diffuse alveolar hemorrhage occurs in nearly 100% of patients with Goodpasture syndrome who smoke and only around 20% of those who do not.
- Conversely, ILDs such as HP, chronic eosinophilic pneumonia, and sarcoidosis appear to be less common in cigarette smokers.
- Recreational drug abuse has also been described as a cause of ILD.

- **Occupational and environmental histories** are an essential part of any DLPD workup.
  - A large number of occupational and environmental exposures have been implicated as causative agents for ILDs.
  - The occupational history should cover the patient's entire lifetime since the time between exposure and disease onset may span many years.
  - Details of each exposure, including *duration*, *frequency*, *intensity*, and presence or absence of *respiratory protection* should be recorded.
  - The occupational history of close contacts should also be established, as exposure to an inciting agent (e.g., asbestos) may not occur only in the workplace.
  - Environmental (nonwork-related) exposures including pets, hobbies, and recreational activities should also be reviewed.
  - Finally, a detailed travel and residential history should also be obtained.
- **Family history** may be important in certain ILDs with a known heritable basis. These include diseases like familial IPF, Hermansky–Pudlak syndrome (HPS), and lysosomal storage disorders such as Gaucher disease and Niemann–Pick disease.
- **Therapeutic agents** are a common cause of ILD.
  - Therapeutic agents include not only prescription medications, but also over-the-counter medications, herbal supplements, radiation therapy for malignant diseases, and other forms of therapy the patient may have been receiving.
  - Development of disease may occur years after the initial exposure.
  - Thus it is important to obtain not only a list of current medications but also a comprehensive therapeutic agent history.

Physical Examination

- Because the pulmonary examination in patients with ILD is nonspecific, the main goal of the physical examination is to search for evidence of systemic disease that may help narrow the differential diagnosis.
- Extrathoracic manifestations of systemic diseases such as collagen vascular disease, amyloidosis, sarcoidosis, and vasculitis may be present.
- **Head and neck** examination should exclude:
  - enlarged lachrymal, parotid, and salivary glands (sarcoidosis and systemic sclerosis)
  - conjunctivitis and episcleritis (collagen vascular diseases and sarcoidosis)
  - dry mouth or eyes (primary or secondary Sjögren syndrome)
  - lymphadenopathy (sarcoidosis, lymphoma)
  - lupus pernio (sarcoidosis)
  - alopecia (systemic lupus erythematosus, sarcoidosis)
- **Pulmonary** examination is most commonly characterized by bilateral fine inspiratory crackles often described as Velcro crackles. Other findings on lung examination may include coarse crackles, and less commonly, wheezing.
- **Cardiovascular** examination should focus on detecting signs of pulmonary hypertension and right ventricular dysfunction, including:
  - elevated jugular venous pressure and peripheral pitting edema
  - pulsatile liver and hepatojugular reflux
  - right ventricular heave, accentuated second heart sound (P2), and tricuspid regurgitation
  - Left ventricular dysfunction or valvular dysfunction may also be present in systemic diseases such as amyloidosis, sarcoidosis, and Behçet disease

- **Abdominal** examination may reveal hepatomegaly and/or splenomegaly in collagen vascular diseases, amyloidosis, sarcoidosis, or lymphoma.
- **Musculoskeletal** examination may reveal digital clubbing, arthritis, effusions, joint deformities, contractures, muscle atrophy, swelling, tenderness, or weakness.
- **Skin** examination may show nonpitting edema, sclerosis, various rashes, purpura, SC nodules, telangiectasias, calcinosis, abnormal pigmentation, plaques, or ulcerations from digital ischemia.
- **Neurologic** examination may reveal a broad spectrum of central and peripheral deficits ranging from subtle cognitive defects to peripheral neuropathy and paresthesias, mononeuritis multiplex, autonomic dysfunction, or focal deficits associated with cerebral ischemia.

Diagnostic Testing

Laboratory Testing

- Laboratory testing for ILDs should be directed by history and physical examination findings.
- **General testing** should include:
  - complete blood count with differential
  - renal function panel
  - hepatic function panel
  - urinalysis (where indicated)
- **Testing for collagen vascular diseases** should be conducted in the appropriate clinical context. Where indicated, the following labs should be drawn:
  - Antinuclear antibodies (ANA) and extractable nuclear antigens (ENA)
  - Rheumatoid factor (RF) and anticyclic citrullinated peptide antibodies (anti-CCP3)
  - Creatine kinase (CK), aldolase, and anti-Jo1 antibodies
  - Scl-70 and anticentromere antibodies
  - Double-stranded DNA antibodies
  - Myositis panel
- Routine use of serum angiotensin-converting enzyme (ACE) levels in sarcoidosis is **not** recommended as ACE levels have a poor sensitivity and specificity for diagnosing the disease. Moreover, ACE levels correlate poorly with radiographic findings and physiologic impairment, and have no prognostic utility.
- **Serum precipitin testing** in HP may be used to confirm the presence of serum antibodies against a specific antigen implicated as a causative agent of disease.
  - However, the presence of specific circulating antibodies only serves as evidence of exposure, and does not confirm that the agent is responsible for the disease.
  - Furthermore, antigen panels can differ significantly between institutions and are usually directed at antigens commonly seen in each particular community. As a result, these tests often do not identify novel or rare antigens.

Physiologic Testing

- **Pulmonary function tests** (PFTs) in ILDs such as IPF are classically described as having a purely *restrictive pattern* (see Chapter 3).
  - However, the finding of restriction on PFTs is nonspecific and may be due to a number of causes including chest wall disease, obesity, neuromuscular disease, etc.
  - In reality, a significant number of ILDs show a *mixed obstructive–restrictive pattern* on pulmonary function testing.
  - A predominantly *obstructive pattern* may be seen in ILDs with small airways involvement including sarcoidosis, HP, and the smoking-related ILDs like PLCH, RB-ILD, and DIP.
  - Combined pulmonary fibrosis and emphysema (CPFE) may present with normal appearing PFTs, however, the diffusion capacity (DLCO) is universally decreased in these patients.

- **DLCO** in patients with ILDs is almost invariably reduced. This reduction may be due to a number of factors depending on the etiology of the ILD, including abnormal V/Q relationships, decreased surface area for gaseous diffusion, and in extreme cases, a thickened alveolar–capillary interface.
- The **6-minute walk test** is a useful tool in the evaluation of ILD.
  - It provides a measurement of a patient's exercise capacity, and can be used to follow a patient's disease progression and/or response to therapy.
  - Moreover, it has prognostic value in diseases like IPF.
  - A decrease of ≥5% points (e.g., from 95% to 90%) with exertion is generally considered to be a significant physiologic drop in oxygen saturation.
- **Oxygen assessments** are based on 6-minute walking tests. They allow for assessment of a patient's supplemental oxygen requirements at rest and with exertion.

Imaging

Plain Film CXR

- Despite the advent of high-resolution computed tomography (HRCT), plain film CXR is still a useful modality for evaluating DLPD.
- It is not uncommon for findings on CXR to predate the clinical presentation, sometimes by 5–10 years.
- In some cases, subclinical ILD may be incidentally detected on a CXR obtained for unrelated reasons in an otherwise asymptomatic patient.
- Thus, reviewing *old studies* as part of the initial evaluation may yield useful information on the disease course and progression.
- Certain ILDs have characteristic appearance on CXR that can assist significantly in narrowing the differential diagnosis, including:
  - LAM
  - PLCH
  - silicosis
  - asbestosis
  - sarcoidosis
  - chronic eosinophilic pneumonia
- Markings commonly found in ILD include linear (reticular) markings, nodules, opacities, and honeycombing.
  - **Honeycombing** suggests an end-stage fibrotic process, which may be the result of progression of any number of diseases (IPF, HP, sarcoidosis, and scleroderma).
  - **Ground-glass opacity**, an increased attenuation of lung parenchyma that does not obscure pulmonary vessels, can be found in both interstitial (nonspecific interstitial pneumonitis [NSIP], DIP, sarcoidosis) and alveolar diseases.
  - **Linear** (or reticular) markings (sarcoidosis, pneumoconiosis, NSIP, IPF) are almost always associated with interstitial processes.
  - **Nodular** markings (pneumoconiosis, sarcoidosis, PLCH, GPA) also have a strong association with interstitial processes.
- The presence of pleural disease on CXR may also be helpful since pleural involvement in ILD is generally uncommon.
- **Diseases that affect the pleura** include:
  - collagen vascular diseases (pleural effusion, pleural thickening)
  - asbestosis (pleural plaques, pleural calcifications, mesothelioma)
  - LAM (pneumothorax and chylous effusions)
  - PLCH (pneumothorax)
- The distribution of interstitial markings on CXR can be useful because certain diseases have a predilection for affecting particular areas of the lung.

- In general, diseases can be grouped into those affecting predominantly the upper lobes and those affecting predominantly the lower.
  - Diseases affecting the **upper lobes** include CF, ankylosing spondylitis, sarcoidosis, silicosis, eosinophilic granuloma (PLCH), TB, *Pneumocystis jiroveci* pneumonia, Crohn disease-associated ILD, ulcerative colitis-associated ILD, and ILD secondary to bischloroethylnitrosourea (BCNU) chemotherapy.
  - These can be remembered with the mnemonic **CASSET-P-CUB.**
  - Diseases affecting the **lower lobes** include bronchiectasis, asbestosis, lymphangitic carcinomatosis, DIP/usual interstitial pneumonia (UIP)/NSIP, aspiration, sarcoidosis (note, also included under upper lobe diseases), and scleroderma-associated ILD.
  - These can be remembered with the mnemonic **BALDASS.**
- Despite the aforementioned advantages of CXR in evaluating ILD, it is also important to remember that almost 10% of patients with biopsy-proven diffuse lung disease may have a normal CXR.
- Also, the clinical severity of ILDs may be difficult to predict from radiographic findings.
- In IPF, for example, the clinical severity of disease is often greater than would be predicted by the CXR.
- The converse is often true in the case of nodular diseases such as sarcoidosis, LCH, and pneumoconiosis, in which patients can be asymptomatic despite radiographic abnormalities.

High-Resolution Computed Tomography

- HRCT has revolutionized the evaluation of ILDs, as it offers far greater spatial resolution than CXR.
- The diagnostic power of HRCT scanning has increased substantially as a result of clinical, histopathologic, and radiographic experience accumulated over the last 20 years and advances in scanner technology.
- As such, characteristic HRCT findings have become diagnostic in certain ILDs, enabling clinicians to make a diagnosis with a high degree of confidence without the need for surgical lung biopsy (SLB).
- One such disease is **IPF.**
  - IPF is a lethal fibrosing interstitial pneumonia of unknown etiology characterized by progressive pulmonary fibrosis associated with histopathologic pattern of UIP.
  - Histopathologic UIP pattern is defined as patchy involvement of the lung parenchyma by fibrosis with architectural distortion, honeycombing in a predominantly subpleural/paraseptal distribution, presence of fibroblastic foci, and absence of features suggesting an alternative diagnosis such as granulomas, organizing pneumonia, or hyaline membranes.
  - HRCT has been shown in several clinical studies to be highly accurate for the presence of UIP pattern on SLB, with a positive predictive value as high as 90–100%.
  - HRCT has become an essential tool in the diagnosis of IIP. Joint International Society guidelines for diagnosing IPF recommend against SLB if UIP pattern is present on HRCT, and alternative causes of ILDs have been excluded.
  - In order for an HRCT to be consistent with the diagnosis of IPF, it has to demonstrate:
    1. reticular infiltrates in a predominantly basilar and subpleural distribution
    2. honeycombing with/without traction bronchiectasis
    3. an absence of features inconsistent with the diagnosis of UIP (e.g., ground glass, upper lung predominance, cysts, mosaic attenuation, and micronodules).
  - For full details on the noninvasive diagnosis of IPF the reader is referred to the Official ATS/ERS/JRS/ALAT Statement on the diagnosis and treatment of IPF published in 2011.

- There is good circumstantial evidence that HRCT diagnosis is similarly accurate in other ILDs. In one study of patients with ILD in which the majority had a pre-existing histologic diagnosis, the correct first choice HRCT diagnosis was made in 87% of cases, with a remarkable level of agreement between the radiologic observers.
- HRCT appearance is highly suggestive of, or sometimes pathognomonic for:
  - LAM
  - LCH
  - Pulmonary alveolar proteinosis (PAP)
  - HP
- It is very important to note, however, that many studies of HRCT in ILD utilized experienced academic radiologists in making the diagnoses. The level of accuracy is often less in community settings. In these cases, or where the radiographic findings are equivocal, it may be necessary to move to a tissue diagnosis (see following sections).
- One of the great advantages of HRCT is the ability to detect coexisting pathology at the time of scanning.
- Once all coexisting conditions are diagnosed, management of patients with ILD can be optimized.
  - One example is the coexistence of lung cancers and COPD in smokers with ILD.
  - For example, PLCH, RB-ILD, and DIP occur almost exclusively in smokers. Therefore, all these patients are at higher risk of developing COPD and lung cancers, which can be detected at the time of scanning.
- Finally, although some clinicians believe serial CT evaluation is a valuable adjunct for monitoring disease progression in selected cases of ILD, the clinical utility of HRCT scanning in this capacity is overwhelmingly anecdotal and is in need of formal evaluation.
- As such, no firm recommendations regarding the monitoring of disease progression can be made at the present time.

Lung Sampling

Bronchoalveolar Lavage

- Bronchoalveolar lavage (BAL) is a method for sampling bronchial and alveolar epithelial secretions by instilling sterile saline into the distal lung units and retrieving the fluid for microscopic analysis.
- BAL is performed during fiberoptic bronchoscopy (FOB) and the target site is usually guided by HRCT.
- In general the procedure is well tolerated, but may carry an increased risk of complications in patients with severe hypoxemia or bleeding diathesis.
- The returned fluid carries a mixture of cellular and acellular components, pathogens, proteins, and insoluble particles that can be used for culture, cytology, and histologic analysis.
- The composition of BAL fluid may be diagnostic or suggestive of certain ILDs including:
  - PAP (milky white fluid with positive periodic acid–Schiff staining)
  - acute or chronic eosinophilic pneumonia (>25% eosinophils in the cell differential)
  - diffuse alveolar hemorrhage (increasingly bloody aliquots of aspirated fluid)
  - malignancy (positive cytology)
  - infection (positive bacterial, fungal, or viral cultures)
  - pneumoconiosis (fluid contains asbestos bodies or silica)
  - drug-induced pneumonitis or HP (>50% lymphocytes)

Transbronchial Lung Biopsy

- There is some controversy about the ideal lung biopsy technique for patients with ILD.
- Essentially, two forms of biopsy exist: transbronchial biopsy (TBBx) performed via FOB, and SLB.

- When deciding on a biopsy, a number of factors need to be taken into consideration.
- These factors include:
  - the clinical condition of the patient
  - the skill of the surgeons or bronchoscopists
  - the facilities available at the medical center concerned
  - the disease process itself (this is very important)
- The overall yield for TBBx in *all* forms of ILD is ~50%.
- However, certain diseases are very amenable to diagnosis by TBBx.
- These diseases are predominantly bronchiolocentric (centered around the bronchioles) because the biopsy forceps must bite through the small peripheral bronchi to obtain lung tissue.
- Diseases with a **high diagnostic yield on TBBx** include:
  - sarcoidosis (>95% in experienced hands)
  - berylliosis
  - HP (subacute form)
  - PAP
  - lymphangitic carcinomatosis
  - bronchoalveolar carcinoma
- Conversely, TBBx cannot be used to diagnose some diseases owing to the small size of the tissue specimens.
- In these cases, TBBx may lead to an incorrect diagnosis being made.
- Examples include IPF and COP (also known as bronchiolitis obliterans organizing pneumonia).
  - IPF has a diffuse and heterogeneous pathology with numerous pathologic features being required to confirm the diagnosis. Therefore, the findings of isolated parenchymal fibrosis on a TBBx are nonspecific and inadequate for the diagnosis of IPF.
  - COP is characterized by the plugging of bronchioles by growths of myxoid connective tissue, which occur diffusely throughout the lower zones of the lungs. However, localized injury (e.g., pneumonia) can result in the formation of identical lesions as part of a reparative response.
- In addition to errors resulting from biopsy size, TBBx can yield poor results from sampling error (biopsying unaffected areas of lung), and crush artifact (crushing of the tissue by the biopsy forceps).
  - To overcome these sampling errors and increase the TBBx yield, the lung is sampled multiple (10–20) times in different lobes.
  - Yields are further increased by the use of HRCT to localize affected areas that are then targeted for biopsy.

Surgical Lung Biopsy

- Indications for SLB include diseases such as vasculitis, NSIP, COP, DIP, and cases of suspected IPF in which HRCT findings are equivocal.
- SLB may be performed using two different techniques:
  - video-assisted thoracoscopic surgery (VATS)
  - open thoracotomy
- **VATS biopsy** is less invasive than open lung biopsy obtained through an open thoracotomy.
- It results in similar diagnostic yields with less morbidity and shorter hospital stays.
- It is, however, unavailable in some centers and quite dependent on the skill of the surgeon.
- Similar to BAL and TBBx, SLB should be guided by HRCT to target areas of lung with abnormal findings.
- In general, obtaining biopsy samples from more than one lobe in a targeted fashion improves the diagnostic yield and accuracy.
- As with all biopsies, histopathologic data from SLBs should be correlated with a detailed clinical history, physical examination, and radiographic data to establish a diagnosis.

TREATMENT

General Treatment

- A comprehensive review of specific treatments for the various ILDs is well beyond the scope of this discussion.
- In general, if a causative agent is identified, withdrawal and avoidance of the offending agent (e.g., drugs, occupational exposures, and cigarette smoke) should be implemented immediately.
- Nonpharmacologic interventions such as pulmonary rehabilitation and supplemental oxygen should be initiated based on physiologic testing results to maintain functional status.
- Other comorbidities such as coronary artery disease, pulmonary hypertension, gastroesophageal reflux disease, and thromboembolic disease should be addressed as indicated.
- Treatment may involve both pharmacologic and nonpharmacologic therapies such as lung transplantation.
- For patients with progressive disease and severe physiologic impairment, who are ineligible for therapy or lung transplantation, end-of-life care issues should be addressed in the inpatient and outpatient setting.

Pharmacologic Treatment

- Pharmacologic treatment depends on the specific etiology of the ILD.
- In general **collagen vascular, hypersensitivity, and autoimmune diseases** are treated with glucocorticoids and/or immunosuppressive agents with varying degrees of success.
- Targeted therapies, such as granulocyte macrophage colony–stimulating factor (GM-CSF) for **PAP** may be considered.
- There have been promising advances in the field of **LAM**, which is now treated with sirolimus in selected cases. Other drugs for the treatment of LAM are currently in clinical trials.
- In 2014, two new drugs were approved by the FDA for treatment of IPF: pirfenidone and nintedanib. Both drugs were shown to slow the progression of disease, but did not reverse fibrosis. No significant mortality benefit has been demonstrated for either agent.
  - **Pirfenidone** is an antifibrotic agent that reduces fibroblast proliferation, inhibits collagen production, and reduces production of fibrogenic mediators. Primary side effects include photosensitivity and GI upset.
  - **Nintedanib** is a tyrosine–kinase inhibitor that targets vascular endothelial growth factor receptor (VEGFR), fibroblast growth factor receptor (FGFR), and platelet-derived growth factor receptor (PDGFR). Primary side effects include diarrhea, nausea, and other GI effects.

Lung Transplantation

- For selected patients without multiple comorbidities, lung transplantation may be an option.
- More detail on lung transplantation can be found in Chapter 29.

CONCLUSION

- ILD comprises a wide spectrum of diseases accounting for a considerable portion of everyday pulmonary practice.
- The pathogenesis of many of these diseases remains poorly understood and requires further investigation to facilitate development of novel therapies.
- Management of patients with ILD requires the clinician to integrate radiographic, physiologic, and histopathologic information with a detailed history and physical examination to make an accurate diagnosis and determine the optimal course of treatment.
- Many of these patients should be referred to clinical centers experienced in their treatment, or that offer clinical trials or lung transplant programs to appropriately facilitate their management.

REFERENCES

1. Deconinck B, Verschakelen J, Coolen J, et al. Diagnostic workup for diffuse parenchymal lung disease: schematic flowchart, literature review and pitfalls. *Lung.* 2012;191(1):19–25.
2. Meyer KC, Raghu G, Baughman RP, et al. An official American Thoracic Society clinical practice guideline: the clinical utility of bronchoalveolar lavage cellular analysis in interstitial lung disease. *Am J Respir Crit Care Med.* 2012;185(9):1004–14.
3. Raghu G, Collard HR, Egan JJ, et al. An official ATS/ERS/JRS/ALAT statement: idiopathic pulmonary fibrosis: evidence-based guidelines for diagnosis and management. *Am J Respir Crit Care Med.* 2011;183(6):788–824.
4. Wuyts WA, Agostini C, Antoniou K, et al. The pathogenesis of pulmonary fibrosis: a moving target. *Eur Respir J.* 2012;41(5):1207–18.
5. Ferguson EC, Berkowitz EA. Lung CT: Part 2, the interstitial pneumonias—clinical, histologic, and CT manifestations. *AJR Am J Roentgenol.* 2012;199(4):W464–76.
6. Swensen SJ, Aughenbaugh GL, Myers JL. Diffuse lung disease: diagnostic accuracy of CT in patients undergoing surgical biopsy of the lung. *Radiology.* 1997;205:229–34.
7. Garcia CK. Idiopathic pulmonary fibrosis. Update on genetic discoveries. *Proc Am Thorac Soc.* 2011; 8(2):158–62.
8. Kligerman SJ, Groshong S, Brown KK, et al. Nonspecific interstitial pneumonia: radiologic, clinical, and pathologic considerations. *Radiographics.* 2009;29(1):73–87.
9. Doyle TJ, Hunninghake GM, Rosas IO. Subclinical interstitial lung disease: why you should care. *Am J Respir Crit Care Med.* 2012;185(11):1147–53.
10. Jankowich MD, Rounds SI. Combined pulmonary fibrosis and emphysema syndrome: a review. *Chest.* 2012;141(1):222–31.
11. Fischer A, du Bois R. Interstitial lung disease in connective tissue disorders. *Lancet.* 2012;380(9842):689–98.
12. Capobianco J, Gimberg A, Thompson BM, et al. Thoracic manifestations of collagen vascular diseases. *Radiographics.* 2012;32(1):33–50.
13. Selman M, Pardo A, King TE. Hypersensitivity Pneumonitis. Insights in diagnosis and pathobiology. *Am J Respir Crit Care Med.* 2012;186(4):314–24.
14. Hirschmann JV, Pipavath SN, Godwin JD. Hypersensitivity pneumonitis: a historical, clinical and radiologic review. *Radiographics.* 2009;29(7):1921–38.
15. Chong S, Lee KS, Chung MJ, et al. Pneumoconiosis: comparison of imaging and pathologic findings. *Radiographics.* 2006;26(1):59–77.
16. Frankel SK, Cosgrove GP, Fischer A, et al. Update in the diagnosis and management of pulmonary vasculitis. *Chest.* 2006;129(2):452–65.
17. Statement on sarcoidosis. Joint Statement of the American Thoracic Society (ATS), the European Respiratory Society (ERS) and the World Association of Sarcoidosis and Other Granulomatous Disorders (WASOG) adopted by the ATS Board of Directors and by the ERS Executive Committee, February 1999. *Am J Respir Crit Care Med.* 1999;160(2): 736–55.
18. Criado E, Sanchez M, Ramirez J, et al. Pulmonary sarcoidosis: typical and atypical manifestations at high-resolution CT with pathologic correlation. *Radiographics.* 2010;30(6):1567–86.
19. Johnson SR, Cordier JF, Lazor R, et al. European Respiratory Society guidelines for the diagnosis and management of lymphangioleiomyomatosis. *Eur Respir J.* 2010;35(1):14–26.
20. Caminati A, Cavazza A, Sverzellati N, et al. An integrated approach in the diagnosis of smoking-related interstitial lung diseases. *Eur Respir Rev.* 2012;21(125):207–17.
21. Ghafoori P, Marks LB, Vujaskovic Z, et al. Radiation-induced lung injury. Assessment, management, and prevention. *Oncology (Williston Park).* 2008;22(1):37–47.
22. Borie R, Danel C, Debray MP, et al. Pulmonary alveolar proteinosis. *Eur Respir Rev.* 2011; 20(120):98–107.
23. Raghu G, Brown KK. Interstitial lung disease: clinical evaluation and keys to an accurate diagnosis. *Clin Chest Med.* 2004;25(3):409–19.
24. Travis WD, Costabel U, Hansell DM, et al. An Official American Thoracic Society/European Respiratory Society Statement: update of the International Multidisciplinary Classification of the Idiopathic Interstitial Pneumonias. *Am J Respir Crit Care Med.* 2013;188(6):733–48.

Occupational Lung Disease 26

Peter G. Tuteur and Barbara Lutey

INTRODUCTION

- The workplace contains a wide range of materials and conditions that can potentially aggravate pre-existing conditions or cause pulmonary disease in susceptible hosts. Table 26-1 lists a number of some relatively common potentially hazardous agents.
- Diagnosis of workplace-related pulmonary disease requires a high index of suspicion because there may be no clear temporal relationship between an exposure and the subsequent development of signs and symptoms, which may be nonspecific and fleeting.
- Obtaining a detailed occupational history from a patient with a possible workplace-related pulmonary disease is an essential part of the diagnostic evaluation.[1]
  - The occupational history is a comprehensive list of the activities and environments of all remunerative or volunteer work the patient has ever performed, including short-term/temporary/military jobs and hobbies, which is compiled to identify all exposures (Table 26-2).
  - Assessment of the home environment, especially during childhood, emphasizing biomass fuel exhaust, radon, and mineral dust exposures may also be important.
- General management principles
  - The patient should **avoid further exposure** to the offending agent. This intervention may involve a change in job responsibilities and patients should be made aware of the fact.
  - Supportive care measures which will depend upon individual patient requirements:
    - Supplemental oxygen
    - Pulmonary rehabilitation
    - Tobacco cessation
    - Bronchodilators
    - Influenza/pneumonia vaccinations
  - Because disease can progress even after exposure has ended, serial imaging and pulmonary function tests (PFTs) are recommended in the first years after retirement.
- Issues of impairment, disability, and workers' compensation frequently arise with a diagnosis of workplace-related pulmonary disease.
  - Impairment means objectively determined abnormality of functional assessment.
  - Disability implies inability to perform certain tasks owing to impairment.
  - The disability certification process often involves multiple agencies and procedures that vary from state to state.
  - For assistance with definitions and criteria, the American Medical Association Guides to the Evaluation of Permanent Impairment is a valuable resource.[2]

ASBESTOS-ASSOCIATED LUNG DISEASE

General Principles

- Asbestos is composed of hydrated silicates with varying combinations of other elements such as sodium, magnesium, and iron.
- Asbestos can be classified according to the shape of its fibers: amphibolites which are linear fibers or serpentines which are curly fibers.

TABLE 26-1 POTENTIALLY HAZARDOUS AGENTS IN THE WORKPLACE

Gases/vapors
- Carbon monoxide
- Formaldehyde
- Hydrochloric acid
- Sulfuric acid
- Sodium hydroxide
- Bleach
- Hydrogen sulfide
- Ethylene oxide
- Nitrogen dioxide
- Ozone
- Phosgene
- Smoke
- Sulfur dioxide
- Fumes from welding and metal processing
- Acids/alkalis
- Ammonia
- Chlorine

Biologic agents
- Bacteria
- Fungi
- Molds
- Rickettsia
- Spores

Inorganic dusts
- Asbestos
- Silica
- Coal mine dust
- Nickel
- Talc
- Beryllium

Organic dusts
- Cotton dust
- Wood dust

Solvents
- Benzene
- Carbon tetrachloride
- Methanol
- Chloroform
- Trichloroethylene
- Xylene

Metals
- Aluminum
- Arsenic
- Cadmium
- Cobalt
- Iron
- Lead
- Mercury
- Chromium

Other
- Plastics
  - Vinyl chloride
  - Acrylonitrile
  - Styrene
- Dyes
- Petrochemicals
  - Creosote
  - Asphalt and tar
- Poisons
  - Insecticides
  - Herbicides
- Products of combustion
  - Biomass fuel
  - Diesel exhaust

- Asbestos fibers can damage lung parenchyma and pleura, causing both benign and malignant disease by complex processes that are incompletely understood.[3,4]
  - Fibers can be suspended in air and inhaled.
  - Inhaled fibers penetrate deeply into the lungs and cellular structures.
  - Fibers are incompletely cleared.
- All asbestos-containing materials, whether made from amosite, crocidolite, tremolite, or chrysotile, can cause fibrosis, lung cancer, and diffuse malignant mesothelioma.
- Clinical and radiographic manifestations of disease may be delayed for decades.
- Asbestos was widely used in construction and manufactured products until 1975. Routes for exposure include:
  - The manufacture of asbestos-containing products.

TABLE 26-2 SAMPLE OCCUPATIONAL HISTORY

1. **List all jobs you have ever held and the dates of employment beginning with the very first one.**
2. **For each job identify:**
   a. Chemicals/dusts or other substances you may have been exposed to? Nature of exposure risk: contact/inhalation/ingestion?
   b. Protective equipment:
      1) Was equipment available? Did you use it? Describe
      2) Was the equipment fit tested?
      3) Did you use the equipment as instructed? When? What percentage of the time? Under what circumstances did you not use it?
   c. Air quality:
      1) What kind of active ventilation was provided? What was the maintenance schedule?
      2) Were there strong odors/taste in the air?
      3) Could you see haze/dust in the air?
      4) Did your eyes burn/water?
   d. Facilities for washing/showering present?
   e. Were uniforms provided? Did you wear them? Were they washed at home? By whom?
   f. Did you eat, drink, or smoke in the workplace?
   g. Procedures for accidental exposure?
   h. Your symptoms:
      1) Date of onset?
      2) Relationship to exposure: Worse at beginning/end of shift/week? Better after weekend off/vacation?
      3) Do you blow dust from your nose or cough it up?
   i. Coworkers with similar symptoms? Other problems?
   j. Were there animals/insects in the workplace?
   k. Is the workplace damp? Is there standing water?
   l. Any usual event such as spills, excessive exposure, or fires?
3. **Other exposures:**
   a. Smoking history?
   b. Alcohol history?
   c. Chemicals used at home in housekeeping/hobbies/lawn care/automobile maintenance?
   d. Animals at home: pets, livestock, birds?

   - Removal of floor tiles, insulated pipes, roofing materials, brake linings, and other asbestos-containing materials currently in place.
   - Employment in the construction, maintenance, textile, or roofing industries.

Diagnosis

- The exposure history may be essential to making the diagnosis. The patient should have a history of exposure to asbestos fibers and a suitable latency period before development of symptoms or radiographic findings.
   - Pleural effusions >1 year
   - Pleural plaques >10 years
   - Asbestosis, lung cancer, diffuse malignant mesothelioma (DMM) >20 years
- The presentation, examination, PFTs, and radiologic findings can be nonspecific.[3]

- Patients may complain of cough, persistent progressive dyspnea, and sometimes chest discomfort.
- Late inspiratory crackles may be heard on auscultation and clubbing may be seen in some cases.
- PFTs show decreased lung volumes, especially total lung capacity (TLC) and decreased forced vital capacity (FVC), along with decreased diffusing capacity of the lung for carbon monoxide (DLCO).
- Impairment of gas exchange is most sensitively determined by arterial blood gas (ABG) analysis conducted at rest and during exercise.
- CT is more sensitive than CXR for detecting subtle findings as well as for characterizing pleural processes.[5–7]
- Special studies such as bronchoalveolar lavage, tissue biopsy, and sputum evaluations may be necessary to find asbestos fibers if exposure requires documentation.

- **Asbestosis**
  - The presence of asbestos fibers may result in a persistent inflammatory process culminating in diffuse interstitial fibrosis, with distortion of the lung parenchyma. Diffuse interstitial fibrosis usually develops no sooner than 20 years after the first and heavy exposure.
  - CT scan shows multiple abnormalities: curving subpleural lines, parenchymal banding, short peripheral lines, and honeycombing in advanced disease.
  - Both bilateral pleural plaques and parenchymal processes must be present to make the diagnosis.
- **Pleural disease**[5–7]
  - Pleural disease may result from translocation of fibers into the pleural space to stimulate an inflammatory and fibrotic response.
  - Pleural thickening
    - Fibrosis of the visceral pleural with adhesions to the parietal pleura occurs, obliterating the pleural space and extending into lung parenchyma.
    - CXR shows widely distributed plaques that do not spare the apices or the costophrenic angles.
    - Plaques are invariably asymptomatic.
  - Rounded atelectasis
    - Pleural thickening may entrap a section of lung, causing atelectasis and associated volume loss.
    - CXR shows thickened pleura surrounding a section of atelectatic lung with a so-called comet tail extending in the direction of the hilum.
  - Pleural effusion
    - This is the earliest clinical phenomenon, occurring as early as 1 year, but more typically, longer than 10 years after exposure.
    - Patients may complain of chest pain and breathlessness.
    - CXR usually shows a unilateral effusion but it may be bilateral, either synchronous or metachronous.
    - Thoracentesis yields an exudative, sometimes bloody effusion. Fibers are not often found in pleural fluid.
- **DMM**
  - DMM is a malignant process of the parietal surface of the thoracic and/or abdominal cavities that invades heart and lung by direct extension.
  - Almost all DMM in the United States is due to asbestos exposure. Exposure may have been apparently minimal, indirect, and not occupational. For example, helping a parent to clean work clothes as a child or being present during a ship refitting.
  - Exposure almost always occurred >20 years before clinical manifestations.
  - Radiographic findings include lobulated growth over the parietal pleural surface.[5]

- The diagnosis is usually established by the surgeon's description and confirmed by tumor biopsy.
- There is no curative treatment. The prognosis for this malignancy is very grim but new combined surgical and chemotherapeutic regimens show some therapeutic promise.

- There is an association of asbestos-related lung disease and **lung cancer**.[3,4,6–9]
  - Asbestos has been classified by the International Agency for Research on Cancer (IARC) as **group 1, carcinogenic to humans**.[10] Exposure to asbestos, both in amphibole or serpentine forms, clearly is associated with increased lung cancer risk.
  - **Tobacco smoking additively, and possibly synergistically, increases lung cancer risk** in persons who have even short-term exposure to asbestos. Therefore, tobacco cessation is imperative.
  - Because asbestos exposure has been associated with a substantial increased risk for lung cancer and early diagnosis may improve outcome, CT surveillance may be employed with expected outcome benefit.

COAL DUST–ASSOCIATED PULMONARY DISEASE

General Principles

- Coal is ranked according to its carbon content, which is determined by the geologic setting in which it was formed.
- Coal dust is primarily carbon but silica, kaolin, mica, metal dusts, and other potentially harmful contaminants may also be present.
- The amount and nature of exposure during coal mining depends upon the rank of coal, quality of dust control measures, and the individual's work responsibilities.
  - Exposure is greatest working underground at the coal face.
  - Above-ground workers who operate drills or transport coal may also have sufficient exposure to produce disease in a susceptible host.
- The National Institute for Occupational Safety and Health (NIOSH) estimated that 4% of coal workers develop a coal dust-associated pulmonary disease for the period 1995–1999. However, the prevalence increased to 9% during 2005–2006.[11]

Diagnosis

- The spectrum of clinical manifestations is wide. Patients may be asymptomatic with mild radiographic abnormalities or severely disabled with obvious and advanced radiographic abnormalities.
- **Coal workers' pneumoconiosis**
  - The hallmark symptom is shortness of breath.
  - Persistent late inspiratory crackles are heard on examination.
  - PFTs may show a restrictive ventilatory defect, with impaired O_2 exchange seen first during exercise. Obstructive ventilatory defects are rarely due to coal mine dust and difficult to distinguish from the more common tobacco-associated disease in smoking miners.
  - CXR shows small nodular opacities in the upper lobes in the early stages, which become more numerous and confluent as disease progresses.
- **Progressive massive fibrosis**
  - Patients complain of shortness of breath and cough.
  - PFTs may show both obstructive and restrictive ventilatory defects.
  - CXR shows coalescence of nodules >12 mm in size.
- **Chronic obstructive pulmonary disease** (COPD) **phenotype**[12,13]
  - Rarely, never-smoking miners present with cough, expectoration, and/or wheezing with manifestations of airflow obstruction on physical examination and confirmed by PFTs.
  - CXR is free of interstitial changes.

- If no other cause for this clinical presentation is found (e.g., bronchiectasis, asthma, chronic exposure to biomass fuel combustion smoke, cystic fibrosis, α1-antitrypsin deficiency) it should be attributed to coal dust.

- **Industrial bronchitis:** This diagnosis is associated with a clinical picture of cough during times of exposure that resolves with cessation of coal mine dust exposure. No other associated impairment is seen.
- There is no specific association between coal mining and lung cancer, though there is some possible uncertainty in this regard.[14] As with the general population, when miners are exposed to multiple carcinogens, including radon gas and cigarette smoke, they are at increased risk for lung cancer.

SILICA-ASSOCIATED LUNG DISEASE

General Principles

- Silica (SiO_2), in its amorphous form, is noncrystalline and relatively nontoxic if inhaled. In its crystalline form, most commonly occurring as quartz, it clearly can cause pulmonary toxicity if inhaled.[15–17]
- A detailed occupational history may be necessary to determine all possible routes of silica exposure.
  - Found in soil and rock, it is a hazard for tunnelers, sandblasters, millers, and foundry workers.
  - It is also found in manufactured materials as diverse as plaster and toothpaste.
- Workers who believe they worked under safe conditions may still have significant potential risk of developing disease regardless of the chronology of exposure.

Diagnosis

- **Acute silicosis**
  - Acute silicosis may develop within weeks to months after exposure to very high concentrations of silica in small particles of airborne dust, such as may occur when sandblasting, rock drilling, tunneling, or quartz milling in an unprotected manner.
  - Patients develop dyspnea, hypoxemia, and possible respiratory failure, which may be lethal.
  - PFTs show restrictive and/or obstructive ventilatory defects, usually with impaired oxygen gas exchange.
  - Radiographic findings include abundant ground-glass infiltrates seen on both CXR and CT.
  - A subset of acute silicosis patients develop silicoproteinosis, which mimics pulmonary alveolar proteinosis radiographically and pathologically.
- **Accelerated silicosis**
  - Accelerated silicosis develops 2–10 years after heavy exposure.
  - Patients complain of progressive exertional dyspnea and cough.
  - Patients may have restrictive and/or obstructive ventilatory defects.
  - CXR and CT show multiple small nodules in the upper and midzone regions of the lungs.
- **Chronic silicosis**
  - Chronic silicosis develops after ≥10 years of exposure to relatively low concentrations of silica.
  - Patients report progressive exertional dyspnea and cough.
  - Patients may have restrictive and/or obstructive ventilator defects.
  - CXR and CT demonstrate multiple small nodules in the upper and midzone regions of the lungs, becoming larger and more diffusely distributed with disease progression. Characteristic egg shell calcification may outline enlarged hilar and mediastinal lymph nodes.

  - Progressive massive fibrosis results from enlargement and confluence of nodules.
  - Progression may occur after cessation of exposure.
- Patients with silicosis are **prone to infection with both TB and nontuberculous mycobacteria**. Patients who are tuberculin skin test positive should be given lifelong TB prophylaxis.
- The IARC has classified silica as **group 1, carcinogenic to humans**.[18]
  - This classification has been somewhat controversial decision because not all studies have shown a clear relationship between exposure to silica and the development of cancer. In many studies, smoking history and other confounding factors must be taken into account. Some studies used unvalidated and unreliable death certificates.
  - It should be stated, however, that silica exposure, especially with silicosis, **might cause a slight increase in the risk for malignancy**.[19–21]
  - An official statement of the American Thoracic Society published in 1997 noted that, "the balance of evidence indicates that silicotic patients have increased risk for lung cancer. It is less clear whether silica exposure in the absence of silicosis carries increased risk for lung cancer."[22]
  - Until the relationship among silica exposure, silicosis, and the development of lung cancer can be clarified, it seems prudent to recommend that abnormalities seen on CXR should be followed closely, and any findings concerning for malignancy should be evaluated with chest CT and tissue diagnosis as appropriate.

WORKPLACE- AND ENVIRONMENT-ASSOCIATED BRONCHIAL REACTIVITY

General Principles

- Occupational asthma is characterized by variable airflow limitation and/or airway hyperresponsiveness attributable to the workplace environment, although the syndrome can develop outside the workplace as well.
- IgE-mediated immunologic mechanisms are not necessarily responsible.
- Individual variability in genetic susceptibility to disease, symptom presentation, and response to therapy, in addition to the differences in apparently similar workplaces produce a very diverse clinical picture.
- The clinician may be required to opine if such a worker has occupational asthma or a pre-existing asthma phenotype aggravated by the workplace.
- In almost all settings, there is **substantial individual variation of the dose–response and the type of symptoms that result**.
  - Several workers may experience apparently similar exposures in an industrial spill but not all are adversely affected.
  - Workers with either retrospectively identified or extremely quiescent atopy may have a greater susceptibility to develop latency-associated occupational asthma of any sort (immunologic and nonimmunologic), especially with repeated exposures.[23]
- **Nonantigenic chemicals** such as hydrochloric acid, sulfuric acid, diacetyl sodium hydroxide, chlorine, other inorganic acids, alkalis, and low–molecular-weight irritants can induce this syndrome either immediately after a single massive exposure, or, more slowly, after multiple, less intense exposures. Chronic exposure to formaldehyde, pesticides, insecticides, solvents, isocyanates (toluene diisocyanate, methylene diphenylisocyante, hexamethylene diisocyanate), and cleaners can produce similar clinical responses.[24]
- Consideration should also be given to **immunologic agents** such as cotton, textile dust exposures, animal, insect, or shellfish allergies; western red cedar dust in the lumber industry; wheat or rye dusts in the baking industry; or other food industry exposures to garlic dust, cinnamon, and mushrooms.
- Flour and isocyanates are the most common culprits in the developed world.[25]

Diagnosis

- The patient complains of some combination of breathlessness, cough, expectoration, wheezing, and chest tightness.
- Persistent bronchial reactivity is manifested over time by different symptom patterns triggered by irritants differing from the initial etiologic agent.
- In general, irritant triggers include extremes of temperature and humidity, ambient tobacco smoke, perfumes, colognes, hairspray, cooking fumes, products of combustion, and cleaning materials.
- The physical examination may be normal; intermittently, wheezing may be heard on auscultation.
- PFTs are often normal at baseline but may demonstrate airflow obstruction with or without improvement after bronchodilator administration.
  - Methacholine challenge test is generally considered diagnostic for the presence of bronchial reactivity.[26,27]
  - Specific inhalation challenge is sometimes necessary.[27]
  - In some cases, airflow limitation may be demonstrated years after exposure.[28]
  - If only small airways dominant disease is present, such as occurred among first responders to the World Trade Center disaster, conventional methacholine test may be normal. In such cases, the only measurable abnormality identifiable may be through the use of impedance oscillometry (IOS).[29,30]
- CXR is typically normal.

Treatment

- Environmental
  - Environmental control is foremost; patients should not return to the workplace without proper respiratory protection, which can be difficult to achieve.[27]
  - Persons must be fastidious in their avoidance of other non–workplace-associated triggers, both allergic and irritant.
- Pharmacologic
  - Treatment with β2 agonists and inhaled corticosteroids should be the first-order approach to blunt the effect of inadvertent breaches in environmental control.
  - Anticholinergics and systemic steroids seem less successful.
- Reports to patients and third parties
  - Because of the nature of reversible or partially reversible airflow obstruction, and because appropriate treatment may preclude an individual's return to the workplace, the physician may be faced with difficulty in explaining the apparent inconsistency between no measurable impairment on PFTs and the presence of disability owing to dysfunction that develops when returning to the workplace.
  - Although this situation is well understood by the worker, others may be less accepting.
- Family and social problems
  - Because regularly occurring irritants in the household initiate bronchial narrowing, not only may a former wage earner be unable to return to work, but s/he may also be limited in ability to perform household chores (cooking, cleaning, transport, and shopping).
  - This limitation may result in unsuccessful role reversal and substantial family stress for which appropriate counseling may be helpful.
- Special cases
  - **World Trade Center disaster**[29–31]
  - Many first responders exposed to the mixed dusts and fumes at the site developed persistent and chronic respiratory symptoms.
    - Symptoms were triggered by a wide variety of exposures.
    - Most had poor response to traditional bronchodilator and anti-inflammatory treatment.

    - Spirometry was normal and small airway abnormalities were only found through the use of frequency dependence of compliance and IOS.
  - **Popcorn lung**[32]
    - In 2002, workers in popcorn factories developed pulmonary symptoms that were sometimes disabling.
    - CT images suggested bronchiolitis obliterans.
    - Those who mixed butter flavoring were most frequently affected.
    - Flavoring compounds (diacetyl) appeared to have more severe disease developing after months of exposure.
  - **Biomass fuel combustion fumes**
    - Biomass products such as wood, coal, charcoal, or agricultural residue are often used to fuel cook stoves in many parts of the world, including North America.[33]
    - Never-smoking homemakers and children were most frequently exposed.
    - The clinical picture resembled COPD.
    - When studying COPD epidemiology, biomass fume exposure must be considered as well as genetic propensity, α1-antitrypsin deficiency, and workplace exposures.

HYPERSENSITIVITY PNEUMONITIS

General Principles

- Hypersensitivity pneumonitis (also known as extrinsic allergic alveolitis) develops when susceptible hosts become sensitized and are then repeatedly exposed to any of an enormous number of offending antigens (Table 26-3) that can be found in virtually any environment.
- Although many persons may be exposed to a particular antigen, few develop disease.[34,35]
- Multiple exposures may be necessary to become sensitized.
- Smokers may be less prone to developing the disease.[35,36]
- Some attempts have been made to formalize the diagnostic process with major and minor diagnostic criteria but these criteria have not been universally accepted.

Diagnosis

Clinical Presentation

- A high level of clinical suspicion is necessary for diagnosis.
- Patient presentation and radiographic studies can vary according to the stage of the disease.[35,37]
- Findings are not pathognomonic. Hypersensitivity pneumonitis should be considered when symptoms improve with avoidance of the suspected agent, and recur or worsen with reexposure.[34]
- **Acute phase**
  - The acute phase resembles an infectious process usually develops between 4 and 12 hours after antigen exposure.
  - The patient complains of cough, dyspnea, fever, chills, arthralgia, and malaise.
  - The physical examination findings are fever, tachypnea, significant hypoxemia, and respiratory crackles.
- **Subacute phase**
  - This phase develops after continued, prolonged, low-level exposure.
  - Patients report progressive dyspnea, cough, fatigue, anorexia, and weight loss.
  - The examination may be normal or may reveal findings such as crackles.
- **Chronic phase**
  - These patients often lack a history of acute episodes.
  - Patients have an insidious onset of cough, progressive dyspnea, fatigue, and weight loss.
  - The examination frequently reveals basilar crackles.
  - Up to 50% of patients demonstrate clubbing.

TABLE 26-3	HYPERSENSITIVITY PNEUMONITIS—CAUSATIVE AGENTS

Organisms
- Bacteria
  - Thermophilic actinomycetes
    - Moldy hay, grain, compost
    - Air conditioners, humidifiers
  - *Mycobacterium avium* complex-contaminated water
  - Mixed bacteria/fungi-contaminated metal-working fluids
- Fungi
  - *Aspergillus* species—moldy malt dust
  - *Alternaria* species—moldy wood dust
  - *Cryptostroma corticale*—wet maple bark
  - *Pullularia* species—moldy redwood dust
  - *Trichosporon cutaneum*—Japanese house mold
- Amoebae
  - *Naegleria gruberi*-contaminated ventilation system
  - *Acanthamoeba castellanii*-contaminated ventilation system

Animal proteins
- Bovine/porcine protein
- Rat urinary protein—rat urine
- Oyster/mollusk shell protein—shell dust
- Animal fur protein
- Fish meal dust
- Birds (pigeons, doves, domestic pet birds)

Plants
- Soybean hulls
- Coffee bean dust
- *Lycoperdon* species (puffball mushrooms)

Chemicals and manufactured products
- Amiodarone
- Procarbazine
- Toluene diisocyanate—paints, plastics
- Diphenylmethane diisocyanate—paints, plastics
- Phthalic anhydride—plastics
- Trimellitic anhydride—plastics
- Nylon flock

- **Farmer's lung**
  - Disease results from exposure to the fungi *Saccharopolyspora rectivirgula* (previously known as *Micropolyspora faeni*) and *Thermoactinomyces vulgaris*, which are found in moldy hay.[36,38]
  - Spores become airborne and are inhaled by susceptible persons.
  - The risk of disease is increased by weather conditions conducive to mold growth, frequent and heavy exposures to hay, and poor-quality ventilation in the workplace.
- Some very unusual routes of exposure have been reported including a saxophone contaminated with *Ulocladium botrytis* and *Phomo* spp.[39]

Diagnostic Testing

- Laboratory evaluation is not helpful because elevations in erythrocyte sedimentation rate (ESR), C-reactive protein (CRP), and immune globulin levels are nondiagnostic.[37]

- In the **acute phase**, PFTs show decreased TLC, decreased DLCO, and oxygen desaturation with exercise. CXR and CT show diffuse ground-glass opacification, but a nodular or reticulonodular pattern may be seen.[35,37]
- In the **subacute phase**, CXR and CT show nodular or reticular opacities that are most prominent in mid or lower lung zones.[35,37]
- In the **chronic phase**, CXR and CT scans show irregular linear opacities, traction bronchiectasis, lobar volume loss, honeycombing, and traction emphysema.[35,37] PFTs may demonstrate any combination of restrictive and obstructive ventilatory defects. Desaturation with exercise is commonly seen.
- **Bronchoalveolar lavage** may show increased cellularity, usually lymphocyte predominant, with variable proportions of CD8 and CD4 cells.
- Precipitin tests are of limited usefulness.[37]
  - Specific tests do not exist for all potential antigens and both test reagents and testing procedures vary widely in quality.
  - A positive result shows only that the patient has had sufficient exposure to develop an immunologic response, but is not proof the particular antigen is responsible for the disease.
- Inhalation challenge, in which the expected offending agent is inhaled in a similar fashion to that used in a methacholine challenge, is not necessary for diagnosis. Such testing is usually most useful if symptoms appear promptly after exposure and improve after removal from offending agents.[37]

Treatment

- Acute hypersensitivity pneumonitis usually resolves within 1–3 days without specific intervention once the antigen exposure is removed.
- Removal/avoidance of antigen exposure is essential to prevent progression to fibrosis, reactive airway disease, and obstruction.
  - Protective equipment includes masks and filters.
  - Workplace exposure to the antigen should be decreased or eliminated.
- Corticosteroids (initially 1 mg/kg maximum, 60 mg) PO daily until clinical improvements are noted, then tapered off over 3–6 months while monitoring symptoms may help to resolve the acute/subacute phases.
- Supportive measures include smoking cessation, bronchodilators if PFTs show a reactive airway component to the disease, supplemental oxygen if needed, and pulmonary rehabilitation.
- Acute disease has a good prognosis if further exposure is avoided. Subacute and chronic diseases are unpredictable, and some patients progress despite antigen avoidance.

TOXIC LUNG INJURY

Silo Filler's Disease

- Workers who upload silage without appropriate ventilation and protective gear can develop pulmonary injury from **exposure to nitrogen oxides**.
- Patients may present with moderate breathlessness and cough, or full-blown respiratory failure with pulmonary edema.
- Death occurs in 20–30% of those seriously exposed.
- Survivors of the toxin-induced process may have permanent lung injury characterized by airway obstruction and/or an interstitial process causing impairment of oxygen gas exchange and a restrictive abnormality.

Chronic Beryllium Disease

- Chronic beryllium disease (CBD) is a granulomatous pulmonary process also known as **berylliosis**.

- Workers may be exposed to beryllium aerosols in the manufacture of nuclear weapons, viscose rayon, electronics, and when employed by dental laboratories.
- Not all persons with beryllium sensitization develop CBD.
- Previous studies have shown a disconnect between disease severity and intensity of exposure, beryllium sensitization, and the development of disease.
- Recent studies have shown that the odds of developing beryllium sensitization and CBD are differentially distributed by genotype.[40]
  - The risk for beryllium sensitization and CBD increases among persons with a glutamic acid at position 69 of the HLA-DPB1 gene (HLA-DPB1 E69).
  - Non-*02 E69 carriers and E69 homozygotes are at higher risk of developing sensitization and disease compared to those with *02 genotypes.

REFERENCES

1. Goldman RH, Peters JM. The occupational and environmental health history. *JAMA.* 1981; 246:2831–36.
2. American Medical Association. *Guides for the Evaluation of Permanent Impairment.* 6th ed. Chicago: American Medical Association; 2007.
3. Levin SM, Kann PE, Lax MB. Medical examination for asbestos-related disease. *Am J Ind Med.* 2000;37:6–22.
4. Kamp DW. Asbestos-induced lung diseases: an update. *Transl Res.* 2009;153:143–52.
5. Roach HD, Davies GJ, Attanoos R, et al. Asbestos: when the dust settles—an imaging review of asbestos-related disease. *Radiographics.* 2002;22:S167–82.
6. Chapman SJ, Cookson WOC, Musk AW, et al. Benign asbestos pleural diseases. *Curr Opin Pulm Med.* 2003;9:266–71.
7. Ross RM. The clinical diagnosis of asbestosis in this century requires more than a chest radiograph. *Chest.* 2003;124:1120–8.
8. Hillerdal G, Henderson DW. Asbestos, asbestosis, pleural plaques and lung cancer. *Scand J Work Environ Health.* 1997;23:93–103.
9. Weiss W. Asbestosis: a marker for the increased risk of lung cancer among workers exposed to asbestos. *Chest.* 1999;115:536–49.
10. International Agency for Research on Cancer Working Group on the Evaluation of Carcinogenic Risks to Humans. Arsenic, metals, fibres, and dusts. Volume 100C. World Health Organization; 2009. Available at http://monographs.iarc.fr/ENG/Monographs/vol100C/index.php. Accessed 6/4/2015.
11. Centers for Disease Control and Prevention, National Institute of Occupational Safety and Health. Respiratory diseases. Available at http://www.cdc.gov/niosh/programs/resp/risks.html. Accessed 6/4/2015.
12. Lapp NL, Morgan WKC, Zaldivar G. Airways obstruction, coal mining, and disability. *Occup Environ Med.* 1994;51:234–8.
13. Kuempel ED, Wheeler MW, Smith RJ, et al. Contributions of dust exposure and cigarette smoking to emphysema severity in coal miners in the United States. *Am J Respir Crit Care Med.* 2009;180:257–64.
14. Graber JM, Stayner LT, Cohen RA, et al. Respiratory disease mortality among US coal miners; results after 37 years of follow-up. *Occup Environ Med.* 2014;71:30–9.
15. Mossman BT, Churg A. Mechanisms in the pathogenesis of asbestosis and silicosis. *Am J Respir Crit Care Med.* 1998;157:1666–80.
16. Castranova V, Vallyathan V. Silicosis and coal workers' pneumoconiosis. *Environ Health Perspect.* 2000;108:675–84.
17. Greaves IA. Not-so-simple silicosis: a case for public health action. *Am J Ind Med.* 2000;37:245–51.
18. National Institute for Occupational Safety and Health. *NIOSH Hazard Review—Health Effects of Occupational Exposure to Respirable Crystalline Silica.* DHHS (NIOSH) Publication No. 2002-129. Cincinnati, OH: U.S. Department of Health and Human Services, Centers for Disease Control and Prevention, National Institute for Occupational Safety and Health; 2002.
19. Checkoway H, Franzblau A. Is silicosis required for silica-associated lung cancer? *Am J Ind Med.* 2000;37:252–9.
20. Finkelstein MM. Silica, silicosis, and lung cancer: a risk assessment. *Am J Ind Med.* 2000;38:8–18.

21. Steenland K, Mannetje A, Boffetta P, et al. Pooled exposure-response analyses and risk assessment for lung cancer in 10 cohorts of silica-exposed workers: an IARC multicentre study. *Cancer Causes Control.* 2001;12:773–84.
22. Adverse effects of crystalline silica exposure. American Thoracic Society Committee of the Scientific Assembly on Environmental and Occupational Health. *Am J Respir Crit Care Med.* 1997;155:761–8.
23. Brooks SM, Hammad Y, Richards I, et al. The spectrum of irritant-induced asthma: sudden and not-so-sudden onset and the role of allergy. *Chest.* 1998;113:42–9.
24. Pronk A, Preller L, Raulf-Heimsoth M, et al. Respiratory symptoms, sensitization, and exposure response relationships in spray painters exposed to isocyanates. *Am J Respir Crit Care Med.* 2007; 176:1090–7.
25. Nicholson PJ, Cullinan P, Taylor AJ, et al. Evidence based guidelines for the prevention, identification, and management of occupational asthma. *Occup Environ Med.* 2005;62:290–9.
26. Brooks S, Weiss MA, Bernstein IL. Reactive airways dysfunction syndrome: persistent asthma syndrome after high-level irritant exposure. *Chest.* 1985;88:376–84.
27. Tarlo SM, Balmes J, Balkissoon R, et al. Diagnosis and management of work-related asthma: American College of Chest Physicians Consensus Statement. *Chest.* 2008;134:1S–41S.
28. Malo JL, L'archevêque J, Castellanos L, et al. Long-term outcomes of acute irritant-induced asthma. *Am J Respir Crit Care Med.* 2009;179:923–8.
29. Rom WN, Reibman J, Rogers L, et al. Emerging exposures and respiratory health: World Trade Center dust. *Proc Am Thorac Soc.* 2010;7:142–5.
30. Friedman SM, Maslow CB, Reibman J, et al. Case-control study of lung function in World Trade Center Health Registry area residents and workers. *Am J Respir Crit Care Med.* 2011;184:582–9.
31. Banauch GI, Alleyne D, Sanchez R, et al. Persistent hyperreactivity and reactive airway dysfunction in firefighters at the World Trade Center. *Am J Respir Crit Care Med.* 2003;168:54–62.
32. vanRooy FG, Rooyackers JM, Prokop M, et al. Bronchiolitis obliterans syndrome in chemical workers producing diacetyl for food flavorings. *Am J Respir Crit Care Med.* 2007;176:498–504.
33. Boman C, Forsberg B, Sandström T. Shedding new light on wood smoke: a risk factor for respiratory health. *Eur Respir J.* 2006;27:446–7.
34. Merrill W. Hypersensitivity pneumonitis: just think of it! *Chest.* 2001;120:1055–7.
35. Patel A, Ryu JH, Reed CE. Hypersensitivity pneumonitis: current concepts and future questions. *J Allergy Clin Immunol.* 2001;108:661–72.
36. McSharry C, Anderson K, Bourke SJ, et al. Takes your breath away—the immunology of allergic alveolitis. *Clin Exp Immunol.* 2002;128:3–9.
37. Glazer CS, Rose CS, Lynch DA. Clinical and radiologic manifestations of hypersensitivity pneumonitis. *J Thorac Imaging.* 2002;17:261–72.
38. Schuyler M, Cormier Y. The diagnosis of hypersensitivity pneumonitis [editorial]. *Chest.* 1997; 111:534–6.
39. Metzger F, Haccuria A, Reboux G, et al. Hypersensitivity pneumonitis due to molds in a saxophone player. *Chest.* 2010;138:724–6.
40. Van Dyke MV, Martyny JW, Mroz MM, et al. Risk of chronic beryllium disease by HLA-DPB1 E69 genotype and beryllium exposure in nuclear workers. *Am J Respir Crit Care Med.* 2011;183: 1680–8.

Solitary Pulmonary Nodule 27

Michael D. Monaco

GENERAL PRINCIPLES

- The solitary pulmonary nodule (SPN) is a common incidental finding on CXR or CT scan.
- The primary goal of working up an SPN is to determine whether the nodule is malignant or benign. Early removal of malignant nodules can significantly increase survival rate.
- After an SPN is detected, all prior CXR and CT scans should be reviewed. If the nodule is unchanged over 2 years, no further evaluation is necessary.
- For nodules with low malignancy likelihood, serial imaging is recommended.
- Intermediate malignancy likelihood requires additional diagnostic studies.
- Nodules with high likelihood of malignancy should be removed and further treatment is indicated.
- The SPN is defined as **a single opacity <3 cm within and surrounded by aerated lung parenchyma without evidence of atelectasis or hilar enlargement**. These were previously referred to as coin lesions.
- **Lesions >3 cm are referred to as a mass**, and have a higher likelihood of being malignant.
- **Prevalence of malignant SPN varies widely** depending on population and reason for imaging (i.e., in the setting of a screening study or detected incidentally).
- Over 150,000 patients per year evaluated for SPN, almost all are asymptomatic.[1]
- Of benign nodules, >80% are infection related.[2]
- **Malignant nodules are usually primary neoplasms of the lung**—about 50% are adenocarcinoma, 22% squamous cell carcinoma, 8% solitary metastasis, 7% undifferentiated non–small-cell carcinoma, and 4% small-cell carcinoma. Uncommon causes include large cell carcinoma, carcinoid, and lymphoma.[3]
- SPNs are relatively common, particularly by CT scan.

DIAGNOSIS

Clinical Presentation

History

- SPN is radiographic diagnosis, but one should obtain a complete history with an emphasis on risk factors for malignancy or granulomatous disease.
- A detailed smoking history is essential because tobacco is the leading risk factor for primary lung cancer, with relative risk 10–30-fold greater than that of nonsmokers.
- Age is also important. In patients >50 years old, an SPN has a 65% chance of being malignant, whereas in patients <50 years old the chance is 33%.[4]
- Other risk factors include
  - Exposures to asbestos, second-hand smoke, radon, arsenic, radiation, haloethers, nickel, and polycyclic aromatic hydrocarbons.
  - Environmental exposures such as living in an area with pathogenic endemic fungi.
  - Risk factors for or having resided in an area with a high prevalence of *Mycobacterium tuberculosis*.

- Details on symptoms if present:
  - Chest pain, especially pleuritic, may indicate pleural, mediastinal, or pericardial involvement.
  - New diffuse pain or bone pain may indicate metastatic disease or hypertrophic osteoarthropathy.
  - Weight loss is nonspecific but if present with malignancy is a poor prognostic factor.
  - Cough may or may not be present and is nonspecific.
  - Hemoptysis with an SPN can suggest malignancy such as a squamous cell carcinoma or proximal lesion.
  - Hoarseness may be present from compression or invasion of the left recurrent laryngeal nerve.
- Past medical history can yield risk factors for infection or malignancy.
  - Any immunosuppressed state including HIV, autoimmune disease, chronic corticosteroid or other immune-modulating medications, or post-transplantation status broadens the differential diagnosis for infection as well as malignancy.
  - History of chronic obstructive pulmonary disease (COPD) may indicate past or current smoking history.
  - History of any malignancy, but especially cancers that metastasize to the lung (e.g., lung cancer, malignant melanoma, sarcomas, and colon, breast, renal, germ cell, and bladder cancers), raises suspicion of a metastatic lung nodule.

Physical Examination

- A thorough examination can yield clues to complications of direct involvement of the SPN, metastatic disease, paraneoplastic disease, or evidence of infection.
- Focal wheezing may suggest intraluminal tumor.
- Signs to look for include clubbing and long bone swelling (hypertrophic osteoarthropathy), hepatomegaly, bone tenderness (metastases), plethoric face, engorged neck, and superficial veins (superior vena cava syndrome), wasting, lymphadenopathy, and focal neurologic deficits.

Differential Diagnosis

- The differential diagnosis can be divided into malignant and nonmalignant causes (Table 27-1).
- Malignant causes include primary lung cancers (adenocarcinoma, squamous cell carcinoma, large-cell carcinoma, small-cell carcinoma, adenocarcinoma-in-situ [fomerly referred to as bronchoalveolar cell carcinoma]), metastatic cancers, and carcinoid tumors.
- Nonmalignant causes include benign neoplasms, vascular malformations, developmental abnormalities, inflammatory nodules, and infections (granulomatous and nongranulomatous).

Diagnostic Testing

Laboratories

- Laboratory evaluation should include a complete blood count, electrolyte panel, creatinine, and hepatic function panel.
- Hypercalcemia may be due to bony metastases or release of parathyroid hormone (PTH)-related peptide from a squamous cell carcinoma.
- Hyponatremia may be due to the syndrome of inappropriate antidiuretic hormone secretion (SIADH), which can be seen in small-cell carcinoma or significant pulmonary or neurologic disease.
- Liver abnormalities may suggest liver metastases.
- If the history includes risk factors for endemic fungi or TB, additional focused laboratory testing should be obtained.

TABLE 27-1 DIFFERENTIAL DIAGNOSIS OF THE SOLITARY PULMONARY NODULE

Malignant
- Primary lung cancer (adenocarcinoma, squamous cell carcinoma, large cell carcinoma, small cell carcinoma, adenocarcinoma-in-situ)
- Lymphoma
- Carcinoid
- Metastasis (breast, kidney, thyroid, lung, melanoma, sarcoma, bladder, colon, kidney, testicle)

Benign
- **Infectious granuloma**
  - Histoplasmosis
  - Coccidioidomycosis
  - TB
  - Atypical mycobacteria
  - Cryptococcosis
  - Blastomycosis
- **Other infections**
  - Bacterial abscess
  - *Dirofilaria immitis*
  - Echinococcal cyst
  - Ascariasis
  - *Pneumocystis carinii*
  - Aspergilloma
- **Benign neoplasms**
  - Hamartoma
  - Lipoma
  - Fibroma
- **Vascular**
  - Arteriovenous malformation
  - Pulmonary varix
- **Developmental**
  - Bronchogenic cyst
- **Inflammatory**
  - Amyloidoma
  - Antineutrophil cytoplasmic antibody (ANCA)-positive vasculitis
  - Foreign body
  - Posttransplant lymphoproliferative disorder
  - Rheumatoid nodule
  - Rounded atelectasis
  - Sarcoidosis

Imaging

- Multiple characteristics on CXR or CT scans of SPN can help in risk stratification.
  - Size is the most important characteristic.
    - SPN >2 cm in size should be considered malignant unless proven otherwise.[2]
    - SPN <2 cm, 50% are malignant.
  - Calcification patterns can suggest a benign or malignant process.[2]
    - Central calcifications suggest infectious granuloma.

- Popcorn calcifications can occur in hamartomas.
- Stippled or eccentric calcifications are indeterminate and can occur in benign or malignant disease.
- All other patterns of calcification are suggestive of malignancy.

◦ Doubling time refers to volume of nodule rather than two-dimensional size.
- One doubling time corresponds to 26% increase in diameter on CXR.[5]
- Doubling times vary widely for both malignant and benign lesions.
- The doubling time of malignant tumors ranges from 30 to 400 days, while benign lesions may be shorter or longer in their doubling time.[5]

◦ Appearance of SPN edge and shape may suggest etiology.
- Smooth or lobulated edge suggests benign process.
- Scalloped, speculated, and corona radiata appearance suggests a malignant SPN.
- Rounded atelectasis is thought to be due to inflammatory process, often after exposure to asbestos.
- Halo sign can indicate fungal infection.

◦ Cavitation of a nodule on CT is indicative of malignancy but can be present in benign nodules. Refer to Chapter 28.
- Cavity wall thickness <5 mm is most likely benign.
- Cavity wall thickness >15 mm are malignant 95% of the time.[1]

◦ CT can detect multiple nodules, mediastinal lymphadenopathy, or pleural involvement, all suspicious for malignancy and can be used for staging once pathology is obtained.
◦ CT density can assist in identification. SPN with fat density suggests hamartoma.
◦ Contrast can identify feeding artery and draining vein such as arteriovenous fistulas.
◦ Parenchymal findings such as pulmonary fibrosis suggest systemic inflammatory disease.
◦ Pleural retraction or dilated bronchus near an SPN suggests malignancy.

- MRI is generally not additionally helpful or indicated.
- Positron emission tomography (PET) with 18-fluorodeoxyglucose (FDG) identifies metabolically active lesions.
  - PET can discriminate between malignant and nonmalignant nodules with sensitivity of 95% and specificity of 82%.[6]
  - Specificity will vary depending on area and likelihood of granulomatous disease.[7]
  - False positives can occur with infectious or inflammatory lesions.
  - False negatives may occur with slow-growing tumors such as carcinoid or adenocarcinoma-in-situ.
  - This modality is of limited use in very small nodules due to lower resolution.
  - Can provide benefit in management of nodules with intermediate risk of malignancy.
  - PET scanning is not indicated for low-risk or high-risk lesions.

Approach to Evaluation of the SPN

- It is important to first discuss with the patient the possible causes and determine his or her desire for further evaluation or suitability for invasive testing.
- When an SPN is detected on incidental imaging, every effort should be made to review all prior CXRs and CT scans. An opacity that is present and stable for >2 years can be considered benign; no serial imaging needed.
- All other SPN noted on CXR should be evaluated with CT scan with IV contrast if not contraindicated.
- Determine the pretest probability of malignancy by either expert clinical judgment or quantitatively by using a model. Current predictive models are as accurate as expert clinicians.[8,9]
  - Most recent American College of Chest Physicians (ACCP) guidelines evaluate SPN based on size and risk of malignancy.[10]
  - SPN grouped as low risk (<5%), low to moderate risk (5–65%), and high risk of malignancy (>65%).

- Evaluation of nodules >8 mm in diameter without prior images[10]:
  - Low-risk nodules (<5%) should be followed on serial thin-section, low-dose CT scan imaging at 3–6 months, 9–12 months, and 18–24 months.
  - Low-to-moderate-risk nodules (5–65%) need functional imaging such as PET scan to further characterize the nodule.
  - High-risk nodules (>65%), nodules with evidence of malignant growth on serial CT scans, and nodules hypermetabolic on PET scan should undergo surgical evaluation unless contraindicated.
  - For nodules with discordant test results, patients with high-risk nodules who do not desire surgery, or patients not suitable for surgery, consider nonsurgical biopsy.
- The evaluation of nodules ≤8 mm without prior imaging is based on risk for malignancy and size[10]:
  - For low-risk nodules and patients with no risk factors for malignancy:
    - Nodules <4 mm do not need any additional evaluation but patients should be notified.
    - Nodules 4–6 mm should be monitored with a single thin section, low-dose CT scan imaging at 12 months.
    - Nodules 6–8 mm should be followed with thin section, low-dose CT scan imaging at 6–12 and 18–24 months.
  - For higher-risk nodules or patients with risk factors for malignancy:
    - Nodules <4 mm should be monitored with a single thin section, low-dose CT scan imaging at 12 months.
    - Nodules 4–6 mm should be followed by thin-section, low-dose CT scan imaging at 6–12 and 18–24 months.
    - Nodules 6–8 mm should be followed by serial thin-section, low-dose CT scan imaging at 3–6, 9–12, and 24 months.
- Surgical evaluation of SPN is usually thoracotomy, open or video assisted, to obtain wedge biopsy. If frozen sectioning indicates malignancy, additional resection, often lobectomy, and lymph node sampling should be performed during the same operation.
- For low to moderate risk of malignancy nodules (5–65%) or patients with high risk of malignancy lesions who either are not surgical candidates or refuse surgery should undergo additional testing to make the diagnosis.[10]
  - For nodules >8 mm in size FDG-PET scan can help characterize the nodule.
  - Nodule sampling can be performed.
    - Transthoracic needle biopsy has a diagnostic accuracy of 93–97%.[11–14] However, the operating characteristic of this diagnostic test will vary depending on factors such as lesion size and location.
    - Bronchoscopy with or without endobronchial ultrasound can be performed to sample proximal and peripheral lesions depending on institutional expertise.

TREATMENT

- Many benign disease processes causing SPN do not require additional treatment.
- Malignant or infectious causes should be treated and managed accordingly.

REFERENCES

1. Tan BB, Flaherty KR, Kazerooni EA, et al. The solitary pulmonary nodule. *Chest.* 2003;123:89S–96S.
2. Erasmus JJ, Connolly JE, McAdams HP, et al. Solitary pulmonary nodules: part I. Morphologic evaluation for differentiation of benign and malignant lesions. *Radiographics.* 2000;20:43–58.
3. Gould MK, Fletcher J, Iannettoni MD, et al. Evaluation of patients with pulmonary nodules: when is it lung cancer?: ACCP evidence-based clinical practice guidelines (2nd edition). *Chest.* 2007;132:108S–30S.

4. Toome H, Delphendahl A, Manke HG, et al. The coin lesion of the lung. A review of 955 resected coin lesions. *Cancer.* 1983;51:534–7.
5. Erasmus JJ, McAdams HP, Connolly JE. Solitary pulmonary nodules: part II. Evaluation of the indeterminate nodule. *Radiographics.* 2000;20:59–66.
6. Cronin P, Dwamena BA, Kelly AM, et al. Solitary pulmonary nodules: meta-analytic comparison of cross-sectional imaging modalities for diagnosis of malignancy. *Radiology.* 2008;246:772–82.
7. Deppen SA, Blume JD, Kensinger CD, et al. Accuracy of FDG-PTE to diagnose lung cancer in areas with infectious lung disease: a meta-analysis. *JAMA.* 2014;312:1227–36.
8. Swensen SJ, Silverstein MD, Edell ES, et al. solitary pulmonary nodules: clinical prediction model versus physicians. *Mayo Clin Proc.* 1999;74:319–29.
9. Gould MK, Simkovich S, Mestaz PJ, et al. Predicting the probability of malignancy in patients with pulmonary nodules: comparison of clinic judgment with two validated models. *Am J Respir Crit Care Med.* 2012;185:A4425.
10. Gould MK, Donington J, Lynch WR, et al. Evaluation of individuals with pulmonary nodules: when is it lung cancer? Diagnosis and management of lung cancer, 3rd ed: American College of Chest Physicians evidence-based clinical practice guidelines. *Chest.* 2013;143:e93S–120S.
11. Hiraki T, Mimura H, Gobara H, et al. CT fluoroscopy-guided biopsy of 1,000 pulmonary lesions performed with 20-gauge coaxial cutting needles: diagnostic yield and risk factors for diagnostic failure. *Chest.* 2009;136:1612–7.
12. Choi SH, Chai EJ, Kim JE, et al. Percutaneous CT-guided aspiration and core biopsy of pulmonary nodules smaller than 1 cm: analysis of outcomes of 305 procedures from a tertiary referral center. *AJR Am J Roentgenol.* 2013;201:964–70.
13. Lee SM, Park CM, Lee KH, et al. C-arm cone-beam CT-guided percutaneous transthoracic needle biopsy of lung nodules: clinical experience in 1108 patients. *Radiology.* 2014;271:291–300.
14. Takeshita J, Masago K, Kato R, et al. CT-guided fine-needle aspiration and core needle biopsies of pulmonary lesions: a single-center experience with 750 biopsies in Japan. *AJR Am J Roentgenol.* 2015;204:29–34.

Cavitary Lung Disease

28

Desh Nandedkar

GENERAL PRINCIPLES

- Cavitary lung diseases may arise from a broad range of disease processes.
- Cavitation may represent an active, latent, or resolved condition.

Definition

- Pathologic definition: air-filled spaces within a nodule, mass, or area of consolidation produced by expulsion of the necrotic debris via the bronchiolar tree.
- Radiologic definition: lucent areas within the lung that may or may not contain an air–fluid level that is surrounded by a wall, usually of varied thickness.
- Other conditions such as cysts, bullae, and pneumatoceles may be incorrectly referred to as cavities.

Epidemiology

- The epidemiology of cavitary lung disease is related to the epidemiology of the underlying disease process.
- There is limited data on what the incidence of cavitation by itself is in the overall population.

Etiology

- The differential diagnosis of cavitary lung lesions is presented in Table 28-1.
- **Pyogenic infections**
  - **Necrotizing pneumonia** can lead to cavitation in the setting of (or after) an acute febrile illness with productive cough.
  - **Pyogenic abscesses** develop as the ongoing infection destroys the surrounding lung parenchyma. Liquefaction necrosis and communication with the airways may develop, which leads to evacuation and expectoration of the abscess fluid, thereby producing a cavity.
  - Causative organisms commonly include:
    - *Staphylococcus aureus, Klebsiella, Legionella,* and other gram-negative bacteria (*Pseudomonas, Escherichia coli, Proteus,* and *Serratia*).[1]
    - Anaerobes and mixed gram-negative organisms are more common with comorbid risk factors such as alcoholism, poor dentition, existence of otolaryngologic pathology, and aspiration pneumonia.
    - It is rare for pneumonias caused by *Mycoplasma, Chlamydia psittaci,* viruses, *Streptococcus pneumoniae,* or *Haemophilus influenzae* to produce cavitary lesions, although these bacteria may still be cultured from airway secretions.
- **Mycobacterial infections**[1,2]
  - TB: cavitation is found in most cases of reactivation TB and in ~10% of primary cases.
  - The most common non-TB mycobacterial organisms are *Mycobacterium avium-intracellulare* complex and *M. kansasii.*
- **Fungal infections**[1]
  - Coccidioidomycosis: a common fungal pathogen associated with cavitary lung diseases. Endemic to the southwestern United States, Mexico, and Central and South America. Lives in the soil, and infectious airborne spores are transmitted via inhalation.[3]

TABLE 28-1 DIFFERENTIAL DIAGNOSIS OF CAVITARY LUNG DISEASE

Infection
- Bacterial
  - *Staphylococcus aureus*
  - *Klebsiella, Legionella,* and other gram-negative bacteria (e.g., *Pseudomonas, Escherichia coli, Proteus,* and *Serratia*)
  - Anaerobes
  - *Nocardia*
  - Infective endocarditis
- Mycobacterial
  - *Mycobacterium tuberculosis*
  - Atypical mycobacteria (e.g., *M. avium* complex and *M. kansasii*)
- Fungal
  - Coccidioidomycosis, histoplasmosis, blastomycosis, aspergillosis, cryptococcosis, actinomycosis, sporotrichosis, mucormycosis, and invasive candidiasis
- Parasitic
  - *Pneumocystis jirovecii*, echinococcosis (hydatid disease), amebiasis, paragonimiasis

Neoplasm
- Primary (particularly squamous cell bronchogenic carcinoma)
- Metastatic
- Lymphoma (Hodgkin or non-Hodgkin)

Vascular
- Granulomatosis with polyangiitis
- Rheumatoid arthritis
- Thromboembolic (pulmonary emboli, infective endocarditis/septic emboli)

Congenital
- Congenital cysts
- Congenital adenomatoid malformation
- Pulmonary sequestration

Other
- Pneumoconiosis
- Pulmonary Langerhans cell histiocytosis
- Pulmonary lymphangioleiomyomatosis
- Diaphragmatic hernia
- Sarcoidosis
- Bronchiectasis
- Lucite plombage

- Histoplasmosis: found most commonly in the southeastern, mid-Atlantic, and central United States.
- Blastomycosis: seen in the Missouri and Ohio river valley states (southeastern and south central United States), the Canadian provinces bordering the Great Lakes, and the area adjacent to the St. Lawrence river in New York and Canada.
- *Aspergillus fumigatus*: a ubiquitous soil fungus.
- *Cryptococcus neoformans*: usually an indolent infection found incidentally on immunocompetent patients, cavitation is typically seen in immunocompromised patients.
- Actinomycosis, sporotrichosis, mucormycosis, and invasive candidiasis.

- **Other infections**[1,4]
  - *Pneumocystis jirovecii* (formerly *Pneumocystis carinii*): seen in HIV patients with CD4 count <200, transplant patients on immunosuppression, or cancer patients undergoing chemotherapy. The rate of cavitation tends to be higher in HIV-positive patients.
  - Parasites: hydatid cysts, amebic lung abscess, and pulmonary paragonimiasis.
  - *Nocardia*: a well-described cause of pulmonary infection, consolidation, and cavitation in those who are immunosuppressed or in those with alveolar proteinosis.
- **Malignancy**
  - Can lead to cavitation in two ways: central necrosis of the tumor itself or occludes its own blood supply, or postobstructive pneumonitis with abscess formation distal to the neoplasm.
  - Cavitation detected by CXR is seen in 7–11% of primary bronchogenic carcinomas cavitate.[1] **Squamous cell carcinoma is the most common variant**, cavitating >30% of the time.[1,5]
  - Sarcomas cavitate more frequently than do lung carcinomas but are relatively less common.
  - Both Hodgkin and non-Hodgkin lymphoma can cause pulmonary cavitation.
  - Metastatic disease is often multifocal but can present as a solitary lesion as well. Few metastatic lung lesions cavitate (about 4%).[1] In addition, the metastatic lesions that cavitate are most likely of squamous cell origin and can, therefore, create a diagnostic conundrum in differentiating primary versus metastatic malignancies.[6]
  - Keep in mind that infection can also lead to cavitary lung disease in malignant lung lesions (e.g., postobstructive pneumonia, reactivation TB from chemotherapy).[1]
- **Vascular**
  - **Granulomatosis with polyangiitis** and **rheumatoid arthritis** are the most common autoimmune conditions that cavitate. Perivascular inflammation within the granulomas and rheumatoid nodules leads to tissue necrosis and cavity formation in multiple locations.[4]
    - Cavitation occurs in up to 50% of cases of granulomatosis with polyangiitis on CT scanning, typically with a thick wall and irregular inner lining.[7]
    - Cavitary rheumatoid nodules are usually preceded by signs and symptoms of extrapulmonary rheumatoid disease. Caplan syndrome is the occurrence of pulmonary masses in coal miners with comorbid rheumatoid arthritis; a pneumoconiosis that is accelerated by the patient's pre-existing autoimmune disease.
  - **Thromboembolic disease**
    - Septic emboli: from right-sided endocarditis or infected thrombi. Lesions tend to be at the periphery of the lungs and, when cavitated, have thick walls.
    - Pulmonary emboli (PE): rare for sterile PEs to cavitate unless there is superimposed infection.
- **Congenital abnormalities**
  - Developmental abnormalities in the primitive foregut or lung bud may produce various cystic lesions that can be mistaken as lung cavities.
  - Congenital adenomatoid malformation is an entity marked by multiple circumscribed radiographic lung lucencies; it is usually discovered in childhood.
  - **Pulmonary sequestration** leads to an isolated portion of the lung possessing an independent blood supply without communication with a normal bronchus. The intralobar variant is particularly susceptible to recurrent infections and cystic or cavity formation.
- Miscellaneous
  - Pneumoconioses: Coal workers' pneumoconiosis and silicosis have been associated with cavities. They produce discrete masses secondary to progressive massive fibrosis that become centrally necrotic and cavitate. Cavitation is rare, however, and its presence should always prompt one to rule out pyogenic or mycobacterial infection.

- ◦ Pulmonary Langerhans cell histiocytosis is seen in young adults, almost always associated with a significant smoking history.[8]
- ◦ Diaphragmatic hernia may be mistaken for a cavitary lung lesion on routine CXR.
- ◦ Lucite plombage: a formerly used surgical practice of placing inert substances in the extrapleural space to induce collapse of adjacent lung for treatment of TB, produces a very characteristic appearance of multiple, tightly packed, spherical, cavitary-appearing lesions over an upper lung field.
- ◦ Other rare causes include pulmonary sarcoidosis, bronchiectasis, and amyloidosis.

DIAGNOSIS

Clinical Presentation

Patients usually present with respiratory complaints or other systemic symptoms. Cavitation is then usually initially diagnosed on imaging during evaluation of these conditions. Once cavitation is seen, the patient's history becomes important in narrowing down the differential diagnosis.

History

- Hemoptysis indicates the invasion of pulmonary vessels, which can be seen with malignancy, invasive aspergillosis, TB, pyogenic infections, and vasculitides.
- Fever, malaise, productive cough, and pleuritic chest pain are typical for infectious, granulomatous processes, and malignancies.
- Weight loss may occur.
- Sinusitis and hematuria can be associated symptoms in granulomatosis with polyangiitis.
- Advanced age.
- Tempo of disease, that is, acute versus chronic.[9]
  - ◦ A process that presents symptomatically and radiographically in a matter of days to a few weeks is more likely infectious, thromboembolic, traumatic, or perhaps immunologic.
  - ◦ Chronic processes point toward neoplastic, congenital, or chronic inflammatory conditions.
- History of malignancy.
- Immune status.
- Exposures: TB risk factors, industrial exposures.
- Travel history: recent travel or residence in regions of endemic mycoses, mycobacterial, and parasitic infections should be inquired.
  - ◦ Coccidioidomycosis: southwestern United States, Central and South America, Mexico.
  - ◦ Histoplasmosis: southeastern, mid-Atlantic, and central United States.
  - ◦ Blastomycosis: Missouri and Ohio river valley, Canadian provinces bordering the Great Lakes, and St. Lawrence river region in New York and Canada.
  - ◦ TB: particularly prevalent in China, India, the southeastern islands of Asia, and sub-Saharan Africa.
  - ◦ Amebiasis: developing countries, particularly those with conditions of poor sanitation.
  - ◦ Hydatid disease (echinococcosis): rural South and Central America, China, Russia, Middle East, sub-Saharan Africa. While most cases in the United States are seen in immigrants from endemic countries, unusual cases of local transmission have been reported.
  - ◦ Paragonimiasis: Central and South America, West Africa, Far East. A few locally acquired cases have been reported in the United States, mostly due to consuming undercooked or raw crayfish.
- Social history: alcohol, tobacco, illicit drug use, HIV risk factors.

Physical Examination

- The physical examination is not very helpful in the recognition of cavitary lung disease but may be helpful in the differential diagnosis.

- Lymphadenopathy suggests lymphoma, metastatic disease, or infection.
- Dermatologic examination can reveal signs of many infectious, immunologic, rheumatologic, and fungal infections.

Diagnostic Testing

Laboratories

- Complete blood count
- Connective tissue disease serologies
  - Antineutrophil cytoplasmic antibodies (ANCA), specifically c-ANCA or antiproteinase 3 are elevated in granulomatosis with polyangiitis.
  - Rheumatoid factor: elevation may suggest cavitated rheumatoid nodules.
- Fungal antigens in serum and urine.
- Blood cultures may reveal a causative organism in lung abscess or endocarditis.
- Sputum can be evaluated for infection (bacterial, fungal, mycobacterial), and cytology.

Imaging

- Radiologic characteristics of cavitary lesions can help guide workup but must be interpreted in the context of history, physical examination findings, and laboratory diagnostics, to identify the cause.
- CXR: appropriate first step in identifying cavitary lesions.
  - May miss small cavitary lesions, especially those near mediastinal structures, or within areas of lung opacification (consolidation, atelectasis, effusion).
  - Even if well seen on CXR, CT imaging is warranted for better characterization of the cavitation, as well as in preparation for further diagnostic testing.
  - Remember to check upright and even decubitus films to identify air–fluid levels.
- CT
  - Sensitive and specific for evaluating the characteristics of cavitary lesions.
  - High-resolution CT allows for greater detail, with thinner slices providing more accurate depictions of the cavity, the cavity wall, and the surrounding lung parenchyma.
- Magnetic resonance angiography may be required if intralobar sequestration is suspected.
- **Air–fluid levels** indicate communication with airways allowing partial drainage and the entrance of air into the space.
  - Often found in pyogenic abscesses and infection. However, any cavity of any etiology is capable of having an air–fluid level.
  - Never exclude malignancy the setting of an air–fluid level because a malignancy may become secondarily infected, potentially masking itself as a more benign process, or sterile fluid may also occupy the space created by a cavitated neoplasm.[9]
- **Cavity wall thickness**
  - The maximum thickness of a cavity wall can help to stratify the risk of a malignant process.[1,9–12]
    - Maximum thickness <1 mm: virtually always benign.
    - Maximum thickness <4 mm: 92% benign.
    - Maximum thickness 5–15 mm: 51% benign and 49% malignant.
    - Maximum thickness >15 mm: 95% malignant.
  - Most thin-walled cavities **<4 mm** are more appropriately termed **cystic masses** and, in adults, are usually blebs, bullae, or pneumatoceles.[9]
  - Coccidioidomycosis is classically described as producing thin-walled cysts, but on further study, appears to produce thick-walled cysts as well.
- **Cavity wall characteristics**
  - Eccentric cavitation with a septate, nodular inner cavity is highly suspicious for malignancy.

  - Cavitation within surrounding consolidation is consistent with necrotizing pneumonia or TB.
  - Irregular inner wall contour is often described in cavitated granulomatosis with polyangiitis or lymphomatoid granulomatosis.
  - Smooth, thin walls are seen in benign cysts (congenital cysts, pneumatoceles, blebs, bullae).
- **Focality of lesions**[9]
  - Single, isolated cavitary lung lesions are usually bronchogenic carcinomas.
  - Multifocal cavitary lesions are usually found in septic emboli, connective tissue diseases, and metastatic disease, or occasionally sarcoidosis, idiopathic pulmonary fibrosis, and bronchiectasis.
- **Location**
  - Upper lobe cavities (apical or posterior): consider mycobacterial and fungal disease.[2]
  - Lower lobes: consider pyogenic abscesses from aspiration or pulmonary sequestrations.
- Other findings
  - **Meniscus sign or air crescent sign** refers to the characteristic appearance of a mass within a cavitated lesion that may be produced commonly by a fungus ball or a hydatid cyst (which are usually mobile within the lesion) and less commonly by pulmonary gangrene, cavitating neoplasm, or abscesses.
  - **Fibrocalcific findings** are often indicative of old granulomatous disease. However, active TB should be investigated.
  - **Secondary spontaneous pneumothorax** is a potential complication of cavitary lung disease with rupture into the pleural space and potential seeding of infectious or malignant material.

Diagnostic Procedures

- Skin testing can be considered for coccidioidomycosis, aspergillosis, and histoplasmosis; however, positive tests do not distinguish between previous and current exposures.
- Mantoux test (PPD) and newer blood tests (interferon-γ release assay) for TB are helpful in the diagnosis of TB but will not differentiate active versus latent disease.
- **Bronchoscopy**
  - Minimally invasive procedure and useful to obtain microbiologic cultures, brushing, and biopsies.
  - The diagnostic success is influenced greatly by the size and positioning of the lesion. Newer modalities such as endobronchial ultrasound can improve diagnostic yield.
- Percutaneous biopsy[13]
  - Typically CT- or ultrasound-guided biopsy.
  - Similar to bronchoscopy, percutaneous biopsy can provide material for microbiologic and histologic diagnosis.
  - Increased risk of secondary spontaneous pneumothorax and spillage of infectious or malignant material into the pleural space.
- Video-assisted thoracoscopy and/or surgical open lung biopsy
  - Can be used for diagnosis and excision of lesion.
  - Typically used when other less invasive modalities have given nondiagnostic results and definitive diagnosis is required.

TREATMENT

- Treatment and prognosis depends on the etiology of the underlying process and is discussed in the appropriate chapters.
- In some cases (e.g., mycetomas, benign cavitary lesions, bulla), cavities can be followed with serial imaging examinations and no intervention is needed.

REFERENCES

1. Gadowski LB, Stout JE. Cavitary pulmonary lesions. *Clin Microbiol Rev.* 2008;21:305–13.
2. Goo JM, Im JG. CT of tuberculosis and nontuberculous mycobacterial infections. *Radiol Clin North Am.* 2002;40:73–81.
3. Stevens DA. Coccidioidomycosis. *N Engl J Med.* 1995;332:1077–82.
4. Vourtsi A, Gouliamos A, Moulopoulos L, et al. CT appearance of solitary and multiple cystic and cavitary lung lesions. *Eur Radiol.* 2001;11:612–22.
5. Chaudhuri MR. Primary pulmonary cavitating carcinomas. *Thorax.* 1973;28:354–66.
6. Chaudhuri MR. Cavitary pulmonary metastases. *Thorax.* 1970;25:375–81.
7. Dordier JF, Valeyre D, Guillevin L, et al. Pulmonary Wegener's granulomatosis. A clinical and imaging study of 77 cases. *Chest.* 1990;97:906–12.
8. Sundar KM, Gosselin MV, Chung HL, et al. Pulmonary Langerhans cell histiocytosis: emerging concepts in pathobiology, radiology, and clinical evolution of disease. *Chest.* 2003;123:1673–83.
9. Ryu JH, Swenson SJ. Cystic and cavitary lung diseases: focal and diffuse. *Mayo Clin Proc.* 2003; 78:744–52.
10. Woodring JH, Fried AM, Chuang VP. Solitary cavities of the lung: diagnostic implications of cavity wall thickness. *AJR Am J Roentgenol.* 1980;135:1269–71.
11. Woodring JH, Fried AM. Significance of wall thickness in solitary cavities of the lung: a follow-up study. *AJR Am J Roentgenol.* 1983;140:473–4.
12. Tan BB, Flaherty KR, Kazerooni EA, et al. The solitary pulmonary nodule. *Chest.* 2003;123:89S–96S.
13. Wong PW, Stefenac T, Brown K, et al. Role of fine-needle aspirates of focal lung lesions in patient with hematologic malignancies. *Chest.* 2002;121:527–32.

Lung Transplantation

29

Jennifer Alexander-Brett
and Ramsey Hachem

GENERAL PRINCIPLES

- This chapter briefly touches on the background of lung transplantation, common terminology, and candidate selection. The primary focus, however, is on postoperative management of adult lung transplant patients, including a review of immunosuppressive agents as well as common complications and their management.
- There are three general arms to the **organ transplantation system** in the United States:
  - **United network for organ sharing** (UNOS) operates the organ procurement and transplantation network (OPTN) and maintains a national registry for organ matching.
  - **Organ procurement organizations** (OPOs) are nongovernmental organizations that recover organs in their respective service areas and allocate them based on UNOS policies.
  - **Transplant centers:** as of November 2011, there were 246 transplant centers in the United States and 63 of these were performing lung transplantation.
- The most common underlying lung diseases leading to transplantation are chronic obstructive pulmonary disease (COPD)/emphysema (including α_1-antitrypsin deficiency), idiopathic pulmonary fibrosis (IPF), cystic fibrosis (CF), sarcoidosis, and idiopathic pulmonary arterial hypertension (IPAH).
- Heart–lung transplantation is generally reserved for patients with Eisenmenger syndrome and an uncorrectable congenital heart defect.
- The majority of lung transplant recipients are between 18 to 64 years of age, though the percentage of recipients >65 years has increased in recent years.[1]
- Candidates should be in relatively good health except for their lung disease. When referring a patient for transplantation, absolute and relative contraindications must be considered (Table 29-1).[2–4]

DIAGNOSIS AND CANDIDATE EVALUATION

Donor Selection

- Donor organs remain in short supply.
- Given the limitation in the organ pool, donor criteria have become increasingly liberalized. Standard criteria for acceptance are listed in Table 29-2.[5]
- Efforts to broaden the donor pool include acceptance of marginal donors, donation after cardiac death (so-called DCD donor), and development of *ex vivo* organ reconditioning protocols.
- Potential donors are screened for social and medical history, physical examination findings, cause of death, vital signs, documentation of arrest or hypotensive episodes, use of vasopressors and/or hydration, echocardiogram and ECG, and bronchoscopy.
- Donors are also tested for HIV, hepatitis B and C, human T-cell leukemia virus type 1 (HTLV-1), syphilis, and cytomegalovirus (CMV, pretransfusion preferred). Organs that are positive for HIV or HTLV-1 are excluded from transplantation.
- Malignancy usually prevents transplantation, except for localized skin cancers, cervical cancer, or neurologic tumors that rarely metastasize.

TABLE 29-1 CONTRAINDICATIONS TO LUNG TRANSPLANTATION

Absolute

Significant dysfunction of major nonpulmonary organs, especially renal dysfunction (which can worsen with immunosuppression); patients with cardiomyopathy or heart disease refractory to medical therapy or revascularization may be considered for heart–lung transplantation
HIV infection
Active malignancy (other than basal or squamous cell carcinoma of the skin); in general, previous cancer should be in continuous remission for 5 years before transplantation
Hepatitis B and C
Poor rehabilitation potential
Active extrapulmonary infection

Relative

Symptomatic osteoporosis (disease must be treated before transplantation)
Ideal body weight <70% or >130%
Substance abuse (a minimum of 6 months cessation of alcohol, tobacco, and illicit drugs is needed)
Psychosocial issues and medical noncompliance
Mechanical ventilation

Recipient Selection and Organ Allocation

- Each transplant center has its own specific evaluation requirements. Patients usually undergo a thorough battery of history, physical examination, pulmonary function and imaging tests. Cardiac, kidney, liver, and other vital organ functions are evaluated as needed based on the results of screening tests.
- Following this evaluation, the suitability for transplantation and appropriate timing for listing are decided.
- The donor and the recipient are matched for ABO blood groups, height, and the absence of circulating antidonor HLA antibodies (discussed further in the section on Rejection).
- Prior to 2005, priority for lung organ allocation was determined primarily by waiting time. In 2005, the Lung Allocation System (LAS) was developed with the goal to allocate organs based primarily on medical urgency and expected outcome (i.e., success) after transplantation.[6]

TABLE 29-2 STANDARD LUNG TRANSPLANT DONOR CRITERIA

Age <55 yrs
ABO compatibility
Clear CXR
PaO_2 ≥300 mm Hg, ventilated with a fraction of inspired oxygen = 1, and positive end-expiratory pressure = 5 cm H_2O
≤20 pack-year smoking history
Satisfactory bronchoscopic examination and gross inspection (before harvest)

Adapted from Snell GI, Westall GP. Selection and management of the lung donor. *Clin Chest Med.* 2011;32:223–32.

- This new system generally favors high-urgency candidates and transplantation in sicker patients, although the overall outcomes after transplantation have not been affected substantially based on current data.

Surgical Considerations

- Single (SLT) and bilateral lung transplantation (BLT) are possible for COPD, α_1-antitrypsin deficiency emphysema, IPF, IPAH, and in some cases of Eisenmenger syndrome.
- BLT is mandatory for diffuse bronchiectasis associated with CF or other diseases.
- Heart–lung transplantation is usually reserved for complex congenital heart diseases with pulmonary hypertension.
- BLT is the most common procedure performed currently.

TREATMENT

Immunosuppressive Therapy

- **Induction:** Some, but not all centers use induction immunosuppressive therapy immediately following transplantation. Treatment options have included interleukin (IL-2) receptor antagonists, antilymphocyte antibody preparations, or alemtuzumab (anti-CD52).[7]
- **Maintenance:** Immunosuppression strategies vary among transplant centers but most use a triple-drug maintenance regimen consisting of a corticosteroid (methylprednisolone perioperatively, followed by prednisone), an antimetabolite (azathioprine or mycophenolate mofetil [MMF]), and a calcineurin inhibitor (cyclosporine [CsA] or tacrolimus).[7]

Specific Agents

Corticosteroids

- Steroids have anti-inflammatory effects in both the innate and adaptive arms of the immune system. Dosing is variable.
- Metabolism and excretion: Hepatic metabolism, including cytochrome P450-3A4 isoform (CYP3A4), and urinary excretion.
- Interactions: Barbiturates, phenytoin, rifampin, and St. John's wort decrease corticosteroid effectiveness by inducing CYP3A4. Conversely, inhibitors of CYP3A4, such as azole antifungals and macrolides, may increase steroid levels. Steroids may also increase CsA levels and potentiate aspirin- or NSAID-induced gastritis.
- Adverse drug reactions: Complications are common with chronic steroid use and include skin thinning, impaired wound healing, fat redistribution, hypertension, hypokalemia, hyperglycemia, adrenal insufficiency, osteoporosis, and mental status changes (ranging from restlessness and poor sleep to agitation and steroid psychosis). Corticosteroids may also increase or decrease the prothrombotic effect of warfarin.

Azathioprine

- Azathioprine is a **purine analog** that inhibits DNA and RNA synthesis, ultimately blocking proliferation of activated lymphocytes.
- Initial dosing is 1–3 mg/kg PO/IV daily.
- Bioavailability: Azathioprine is well absorbed after oral administration. Azathioprine and its metabolite 6-mercaptopurine are 30% bound to plasma proteins.
- Metabolism and excretion: Hepatic metabolism and urinary excretion.
- Interactions: Allopurinol may reduce metabolism and increase levels of azathioprine. Drugs with bone marrow suppression or toxicity should be avoided, as the effects can be additive. Warfarin levels may increase via unknown mechanisms.
- Adverse drug reactions: **Bone marrow toxicity** can occur (thrombocytopenia, anemia, and leukopenia). Leukopenia is especially common in patients with mutations in

thiopurine S-methyltransferase, which can be screened with genetic testing if needed. Gastrointestinal (GI) side effects can include hepatitis, cholestatic jaundice, and pancreatitis.

Mycophenolate Mofetil

- MMF was initially developed as an antibiotic/antineoplastic/antipsoriatic agent. It is a selective, noncompetitive, and **reversible inhibitor of inosine monophosphate dehydrogenase**, blocking de novo purine synthesis. As B and T cells lack the salvage pathway of purine synthesis, they are selectively inhibited.
- Initial dosing is 1–1.5 g PO/IV bid.
- Bioavailability: MMF is given as an ester derivative owing to poor absorption. In this form it is rapidly absorbed orally. It is 97% albumin bound in plasma.
- Metabolism and excretion: MMF is rapidly hydrolyzed to an active metabolite mycophenolic acid (MPA) in the liver. Also, it is later inactivated in the liver by glucuronidation. MPA is eliminated primarily in the urine as MPA glucuronide. In renal failure, accumulated MPA glucuronide may be converted to MPA, causing toxicity.
- Interactions: Relatively few drug interactions occur. Antacids may reduce absorption. Cholestyramine and antibiotics that alter gut flora can decrease levels by reducing enterohepatic circulation. Drugs that interfere (e.g., probenecid) or compete for renal tubular secretion may increase MPA glucuronide levels. High doses of salicylates may increase free MPA levels.
- Adverse drug reactions: MMF is generally well tolerated with GI side effects being most common (abdominal pain, nausea, vomiting, dyspepsia, diarrhea); these can be overcome by splitting doses or administering the drug with small amounts of food. Bone marrow toxicity is seen as well (anemia, leukopenia, and thrombocytopenia).
- Monitoring: **Therapeutic monitoring is not routinely performed.** Concentrations may be monitored in renal failure or coadministration with CsA.

Cyclosporine

- CsA is a fat-soluble fungal polypeptide that inhibits production of IL-2 from CD4+ cells. It binds cyclophilin in lymphocytes, and the complex then **binds calcineurin, inhibiting cytokine gene transcription and lymphocyte proliferation**.
- Initial dosing is 5–10 mg/kg/d split into two doses.
- Bioavailability: Oral bioavailability is variable and dependent on the drug formulation (sandimmune 10–90%, neoral 30–45%). It is also bile dependent and can be influenced by fat intake, diarrhea, and GI motility. CsA is mostly distributed outside of the blood volume and the fraction in plasma is 90% lipoprotein bound.
- Metabolism and excretion: CsA is extensively metabolized in liver and intestine (CYP3A4). Elimination is primarily by excretion of metabolites in the bile. Only a small fraction is excreted unchanged via GI and genitourinary tracts.
- Interactions: Drug interactions are very common as a result of CYP3A4 induction or inhibition. Drugs that decrease CsA levels include rifampin, phenytoin, carbamazepine, phenytoin, St. John's wort, and hydroxymethylglutaryl (HMG) coenzyme A reductase inhibitors. Increased levels are seen with azole antifungals, macrolides, calcium channel blockers (verapamil and diltiazem; nifedipine has less effect), and grapefruit juice. Many nephrotoxic drugs have synergistic toxicity with CsA. Potassium-sparing diuretics should be avoided owing to the potential for hyperkalemia. Concomitant use of HMG coenzyme A reductase inhibitor therapy increases the risk of myopathy and rhabdomyolysis.
- Adverse drug reactions: Renal side effects are common (hyperkalemia, hypomagnesemia, hypertension). Metabolic side effects include hyperlipidemia, gout, osteoporosis, hirsutism, and hyperglycemia. Neurologic effects include tremors, peripheral neuropathy, headaches, mental status changes, and, in rare instances, reversible posterior leukoencephalopathy. Gingival hypertrophy (especially in conjunction with nifedipine), a thrombotic thrombocytopenic purpura–like syndrome, and hepatotoxicity can be seen as well.

- Monitoring: **Therapeutic monitoring is performed** due to intra- and interpatient variability of absorption, metabolism, and excretion, as well as the considerable side effect profile. Levels measured include trough, area under the curve, and C2 pseudopeak levels. Target levels vary with time interval after transplant, organ type, and rejection history.

Tacrolimus

- Tacrolimus is a fungal-derived macrolide that inhibits IL-2 production. It binds to immunophilin FKBP12, and **blocks calcineurin activity** in a fashion similar to that of CsA.
- Initial dosing range is ~0.1 mg/kg/d PO divided into two doses.
- Bioavailability: Oral bioavailability is poor (20–25%) but not bile acid dependent. It is fat soluble, and ~80% of serum drug is RBC membrane bound.
- Metabolism and excretion: Tacrolimus is metabolized in the liver and intestine (CYP3A4). Tacrolimus is excreted unchanged in bile, thus there is no need for adjustment in renal failure or hepatic disease.
- Interactions: Similar to those with CsA.
- Adverse drug reactions: Similar to those with CsA.
- Monitoring: **Trough levels are routinely used** (and correlate with area under the curve measurements).

Sirolimus

- Sirolimus is a fungal-derived macrolide, also known as rapamycin. Unlike the calcineurin inhibitors tacrolimus and CsA, the sirolimus–immunophilin complex **inhibits the mammalian target of rapamycin (mTOR)** and blocks cytokine-mediated cell cycling and B- and T-cell function.
- Initial dosing is 2 mg/d. It is diluted with water or juice (except grapefruit juice). A long half-life allows for once-daily dosing.
- Bioavailability: Sirolimus is rapidly absorbed after oral administration but has poor bioavailability (~14% with the oral solution but higher with tablets). It is 92% bound to plasma proteins.
- Metabolism and excretion: It is metabolized in the liver and intestine (CYP3A4). More than 90% is eliminated via the gut.
- Interactions: Similar to those with CsA. There is marked interaction with CsA itself, increasing the levels of CsA by >300%. CsA can be dosed 4 hours before sirolimus (but this complicates monitoring of blood levels).
- Adverse drug reactions: Side effects include hypertension, hypercholesterolemia, and hypertriglyceridemia. Bone marrow toxicity (thrombocytopenia and anemia) may occur. Other effects include interstitial pneumonitis and hepatotoxicity. Sirolimus has a **boxed warning** regarding immediate use after lung transplant, as it has been associated with bronchial anastomotic dehiscence. It can be safely used later (after anastomotic healing), but caution is warranted if other surgeries are required.
- Monitoring: **Monitoring is essential** as target levels also depend on whether CsA or tacrolimus is used.

Interleukin-2 Receptor Antagonists

- IL-2 receptor antagonists are chimeric murine–human monoclonal antibodies. They bind the IL-2 receptor on the surface of activated T lymphocytes and **inhibit proliferation and differentiation of T cells.** Basiliximab is a true chimeric antibody (25% mouse) used for induction immunosuppression. Daclizumab is a humanized antibody (10% mouse) that is no longer available.
- Basiliximab has a half-life of ~14 days. It is given as a 20-mg IV infusion once before transplant and then again on the fourth day posttransplantation.

- Adverse effects: Basiliximab is fairly well tolerated, much better than predecessors OKT3 and muromonab-CD3. Side effects are generally similar to placebo but there remains a theoretical risk for infection and posttransplant lymphoproliferative disorder (PTLD). A severe, acute hypersensitivity syndrome (including a pulmonary edema/acute respiratory distress [ARDS]-like picture) can occur with basiliximab and is a contraindication to continued use.

Antithymocyte Globulin

- Antithymocyte globulin (ATG) is a polyclonal antilymphocyte globulin used for treatment of rejection and also for induction immunosuppression in some centers. Atgam is derived from horses, whereas thymoglobulin is of rabbit origin. There is **profound B- and T-cell depletion** after administration owing to complement-mediated cytolysis of antibody-coated cells.
- Dosing: Atgam: 10–20 mg/kg IV infusion. Thymoglobulin: 1–1.5 mg/kg IV infusion. Atgam has a half-life of 6 days, whereas thymoglobulin has a half-life of 30 days. Thymoglobulin is ~10 times more potent than atgam.
- Adverse drug reactions: There are numerous reactions, including **flu-like symptoms** secondary to cytokine release syndrome (IL-1, IL-6, tumor necrosis factor-α). These symptoms can be attenuated with premedication (using a combination of prednisone, acetaminophen, diphenhydramine, and IV fluids). There is a potential risk of infection and PTLD, but the data in lung transplantation are variable. Leukopenia is the most serious complication of therapy. Thrombocytopenia may complicate therapy and anaphylaxis is documented but rare.
- Monitoring: Some centers monitor CD3+ levels to gauge adequacy of therapy.

Other Agents

- Alemtuzumab (anti-CD52) has been used by a few centers for induction immunosuppression or for treatment of rejection. However, this drug is no longer widely available and is used under a special distribution program.
- Azithromycin is a macrolide antibiotic that has demonstrated efficacy to delay the development of bronchiolitis obliterans syndrome (BOS) and chronic rejection in several studies. Dosing schedules are usually three times per week.
- Leflunomide is an antimetabolite that blocks pyrimidine synthesis and lymphocyte proliferation, similar to purine synthesis inhibitors.
- Rituximab (anti-CD20) is a chimeric monoclonal antibody that destroys B cells and commonly used for connective tissue diseases, such as lupus. It is also used in the treatment of antibody-mediated rejection (AMR) in some centers.
- Bortezomib is a proteasome inhibitor used in the treatment of multiple myeloma. Given the effect on plasma cells, some centers have used bortezomib in patients with severe AMR.

COMPLICATIONS

Hyperacute Rejection

- Immediate response due to **preformed circulating antibodies** to donor antigens (HLA, ABO, and other antigens) that bind the vascular endothelium and initiate the host immunologic response and lead to thrombus formation, inflammatory cell infiltrates, and fibrinoid necrosis of the vessels.[8]
- Clinically, this results in fulminant allograft failure, although there have been reported cases of successful management with intensive immunosuppression and plasma exchange.
- This complication has become exceedingly rare in recent years because of sensitive screening methods to avoid donors with reactivity to preformed anti-HLA antibodies in potential transplant recipients.

Antibody-Mediated Rejection

- AMR is a more indolent antibody-mediated process that develops over weeks to months and arises from **newly developed circulating antibodies** to donor antigens.[8,9]
- No formal diagnostic criteria for AMR have been developed, but the detection of new donor-specific anti-HLA antibodies with allograft dysfunction, pulmonary infiltrates, and evidence of C4d complement deposition and associated pathologic changes in transbronchial lung biopsies help to confirm the diagnosis.[9]
- Treatment may include a combination of rituximab, plasma exchange, IV immune globulin, and even bortezomib in the most severe cases.

Acute Rejection

- Despite standard three-drug immunosuppressive therapy, **many lung transplant patients still experience one or more episodes of acute rejection**, especially in the first 6 months after transplantation.[8]
- Acute rejection is **primarily a cell-mediated immune response** triggered by recognition of major histocompatibility complex antigens. Pathologic findings include perivascular and/or peribronchiolar lymphocytic infiltrate, with the extent of the inflammation into the surrounding tissue determining the grade of rejection.[9]
- Most cases of mild acute rejection are asymptomatic and discovered only with surveillance bronchoscopy during the first year following transplantation. More severe cases may present with shortness of breath, nonproductive cough, low-grade fever, and decline in exercise oximetry and spirometry (forced expiratory volume at 1 second [FEV_1] decrease by >10%).[9]
- Examinations may be notable for crackles or rhonchi, with CXR demonstrating nonspecific infiltrates, and blood tests showing leukocytosis.
- Pathologic findings in transbronchial biopsies are the gold standard. Since early stages of acute rejection may be asymptomatic, surveillance bronchoscopies can improve early detection are used by some centers during the first year after transplantation. However, surveillance biopsies still remain controversial, as it does not necessarily improve survival nor decrease the incidence of chronic rejection.[9]
- The International Society for Heart and Lung Transplantation (ISHLT) criteria for acute rejection are listed in Table 29-3 and are based on severity and location.[10] Most centers treat acute rejection grades A2 and higher, but practices vary for grade A1 depending on clinical parameters such as lung function or history of prior episodes of acute rejection.
- **Initial treatment** includes high-dose IV corticosteroids (methylprednisolone, 0.5–1 g IV daily for 3 days). An oral prednisone taper starting at 0.5–1 mg/kg/d over a few weeks may also be used.[8,9]
- Refractory cases of acute cellular rejection may be retreated with steroids, by alteration of maintenance immunosuppression, with antilymphocyte antibody therapy, or, very rarely, total lymphoid irradiation.[8]

Chronic Rejection

- Two forms of chronic rejection may be observed: **Chronic airway rejection** is the most common and is characterized histologically by bronchiolitis obliterans (BO). **Chronic vascular rejection** manifests by atherosclerosis within the pulmonary vasculature.
- **BO** is the end result of multifactorial insults to the transplanted tissue. Table 29-4 lists the risk factors linked to chronic rejection.[11–19] BO is a fibroproliferative process that begins with lymphocytic infiltration of the submucosa. As the infiltrate migrates into the epithelium, destruction and loss of bronchiolar mucosa follow. Fibroblasts and myofibroblasts are stimulated by this reaction, and subsequently lay down intraluminal granulation tissue. Some airways may remain patent, whereas others are obliterated.

TABLE 29-3 CLASSIFICATION AND GRADING OF LUNG ALLOGRAFT REJECTION

A. Acute vascular rejection (vascular rejection of any grade may occur with or without acute airway rejection)
   A0: none
   A1: minimal
   A2: mild
   A3: moderate
   A4: severe
B. Lymphocytic bronchiolitis
   B0: none
   B1R: mild
   B2R: severe
C. Chronic airway rejection
   C1: bronchiolitis obliterans
D. Chronic vascular rejection
   Accelerated graft vascular sclerosis

Adapted from Stewart S, Fishbein MC, Snell GI, et al. Revision of the 1996 working formulation for the standardization of nomenclature in the diagnosis of lung rejection. *J Heart Lung Transplant.* 2007;26:1229–42

TABLE 29-4 MECHANISMS OF CHRONIC AIRWAY REJECTION

Immune mechanisms

Acute rejection: The risk of BO has been correlated with higher grades of histologic rejection, persistent rejection, or recurrent rejection after treatment; patients with more than three episodes of acute rejection were also noted to be at increased risk of developing subsequent BO; there is some suggestion that in certain cases, severe acute rejection may lead directly to airway fibrosis

HLA mismatching: Lung transplants are not HLA matched with recipients; however, although the significance of HLA mismatch remains controversial, the development of donor-specific HLA antibodies after transplantation is strongly linked to BO

Nonimmune mechanisms

Primary graft dysfunction (PGD): PGD has been identified as an independent risk factor for BO

CMV infection: CMV pneumonitis is a risk factor for developing BO; prophylaxis may attenuate this risk

Hemodynamic factors: Donor cold ischemic time at the time of transplantation (between procurement and surgery) increases the risk of BO; reperfusion injury, after vascular anastomosis, may cause oxidative damage to the allograft tissue; disruption of the bronchial circulation in the transplanted lung may be a contributing factor

Community-acquired respiratory tract infection

Gastroesophageal reflux disease

BO, bronchiolitis obliterans; CMV, cytomegalovirus.

TABLE 29-5 CLASSIFICATION OF BRONCHIOLITIS OBLITERANS SYNDROME (2002)

BOS 0: FEV_1 >90% of baseline and FEF_{25-75} >75% of baseline
BOS 0p: FEV_1 81–90% of baseline and/or FEF_{25-75} ≤75% of baseline
BOS 1: FEV_1 66–80% of baseline
BOS 2: FEV_1 51–65% of baseline
BOS 3: FEV_1 ≤50% of baseline

BOS, bronchiolitis obliterans syndrome; FEF_{25-75}, midexpiratory flow rate; FEV_1, forced expiratory volume over 1 second.

Adapted from Estenne M, Hertz MI. Bronchiolitis obliterans after human lung transplantation. *Am J Respir Crit Care Med.* 2002;166:440–4.

- Chronic rejection manifests as **progressive decline in spirometric lung function.** Patients may present with worsening dyspnea, cough, wheezing, and low-grade fever. These symptoms may resemble asthmatic bronchitis, usually without improvement after bronchodilators or inhaled corticosteroids.
- Histologic confirmation of BO is difficult, as transbronchial biopsies may not offer adequate tissue for diagnosis.
- **BOS** is the *sine qua non* of chronic rejection and is diagnosed based on pulmonary function testing parameters (Table 29-5).[8,15,16,19] Since BO primarily affects the small airways, the earliest stages of BOS are detected by a decline in midexpiratory flow rates (forced expiratory flow [FEF] 25–75), followed by a decline in FEV_1 and FEV_1 to forced vital capacity (FVC) ratio.
- The prevalence of BOS approaches 50% within 3–5 years after lung transplantation.
- Several **approaches to treatment** include[8]:
  - Intensified or modified immunosuppression (e.g., switch azathioprine to MPA)
  - Initiation of azithromycin three times a week[19]
  - ATG therapy
  - Extracorporeal photopheresis (ECP)
  - Total lymphoid irradiation, rarely used and only in cases of rapidly progressive BOS
  - Repeat lung transplantation
- **Prevention of chronic rejection** with empiric three-drug immunosuppression, early and aggressive treatment of respiratory infections, management of gastroesophageal reflux disease (GERD), and regular spirometric testing are important aspects of prevention and management.

Infection in the Lung Transplant Patient

- Infections confer a risk of increased morbidity and mortality in the transplant population. The combination of immunosuppression, denervated lung, impaired lymphatic drainage, abnormal mucociliary clearance, and suboptimal cough reflex all increase the susceptibility to infection in lung transplant recipients disproportionate to other solid organ transplant recipients.
- Empiric broad-spectrum antibiotics at the time of transplantation help to prevent early postoperative pneumonia after transplantation. Vancomycin and cefepime or meropenem are reasonable choices while awaiting culture results.

Bacterial Pneumonia

- Bacterial infections account for >50% of infection-related transplant deaths.
- Most of these infections occur within the first 2 weeks after transplantation, but can also reemerge in the setting of BOS or with chronic airway colonization (e.g., CF).

- **Gram-negative pneumonia:** Gram-negative rods are consistently the most common bacterial organisms involved.[20,21]
  - Multidrug-resistant *Pseudomonas* and related species are a considerable problem in transplant recipients colonized with these organisms before transplant.
  - There is no consensus regarding management of these multidrug-resistant infections in the perioperative period, and institutions vary their prophylaxis based on individual culture data and sensitivities.
  - Lung transplant patients are more prone to *Legionella* infection, but the rates of infection are widely variable among institutions.
- **Gram-positive pneumonia:** *Staphylococcus aureus* (including methicillin-sensitive and resistant strains) is the most common gram-positive bacterial airway infection in lung transplant recipients. This often occurs in the early posttransplant or perioperative setting and can be transferred from the donor.[22]
- Atypical pneumonia: *Listeria* and *Nocardia* infections are uncommon perhaps because they are susceptible to trimethoprim-sulfamethoxazole (TMP-SMX), used as *Pneumocystis jirovecii* prophylaxis (PJP). TB is an uncommon infection in lung transplant recipients. However, antimycobacterial treatment can be problematic owing to frequent interactions between these agents and immunosuppressive medications. Patients undergoing transplantation should receive a tuberculin skin test and receive appropriate therapy before surgery.

Viral Pneumonias

- **CMV** is the second most frequent infection in lung transplant patients.
  - CMV can be acquired via the allograft from a seropositive donor, transfusion of seropositive blood products, or activation of latent disease in a seropositive recipient.
  - Pneumonitis is the most common manifestation, but patients may also present with colitis, gastroenteritis, and hepatitis. CMV pneumonia may be confused with acute rejection but usually does not develop until 7–8 weeks after transplantation.
  - Risk of reactivation is linked to the serologic status of donor and recipient[23,24]:
    - Donor CMV Ig–/recipient CMV Ig–: low risk
    - Donor CMV Ig–/recipient CMV Ig+: moderate risk
    - Donor CMV Ig+/recipient CMV Ig+: moderate risk
    - Donor CMV Ig+/recipient CMV Ig–: highest risk
  - Symptoms include low-grade fever, cough, and shortness of breath.
  - Decreased spirometric function may occur and CXRs may demonstrate perihilar infiltrates, interstitial edema, or pleural effusions.
  - Quantitative **polymerase chain reaction** (PCR) is now widely used but there is no standardized assay. Hence, threshold levels vary from assay to assay and between centers.[20,23]
  - Shell vial **cultures** of bronchoalveolar lavage (BAL) fluid (or blood or urine) can rapidly determine active infection in 24–48 hours via fluorescent antibodies to CMV antigen.
  - **Bronchoscopy** for culture of airway secretions and transbronchial lung biopsies may be done. Viral cytopathic effect on transbronchial biopsy is the gold standard for diagnosis of CMV pneumonitis. Some centers also use immunohistochemical stains to aid in diagnosis.
  - **Prevention:** The most common method of prophylaxis is antiviral therapy, that is, valganciclovir or human CMV immunoglobulin (cytogam). Centers differ on approach and duration of prophylactic therapy.[20,23] Our center uses the following approach:
    - Prophylactic strategy for high-risk patients: valganciclovir, 450–900 mg/d, for 6 months after transplantation. Some centers may extend prophylaxis to 12 months.
    - Preemptive strategy for medium- and low-risk patients: serum CMV PCR is monitored once a week for the first 3 months.
  - Treatment[20,23]:
    - Acyclovir has no role in the treatment of CMV.

- ■ **Valganciclovir PO or ganciclovir IV** for 2–3 weeks is the therapy of choice. The major side effect is leukopenia. Relapses are frequent after therapy and can be attenuated by maintenance therapy for 3–6 weeks after treatment. Ganciclovir resistance must be considered in patients who do not respond to therapy.
- ■ Other therapies may include cytogam, foscarnet, or cidofovir.

- **Other herpesviruses** Epstein–Barr virus (EBV) is implicated in development of posttransplant lymphoproliferative disease. Varicella zoster virus (VZV) manifests as chickenpox with primary exposure and as zoster with reactivation. The American Society of Transplantation recommends seronegative transplant patients be vaccinated against VZV before transplantation.[20] Immunocompromised patients with acute exposure may receive VZV immune globulin or acyclovir prophylaxis to protect against or attenuate infection.
- Community-acquired **respiratory viruses** (e.g., respiratory syncytial virus [RSV], influenza virus, parainfluenza virus, adenovirus, rhinovirus, and metapneumovirus) have been implicated in the development of BOS.
  - **Ribavirin** may be used for RSV and even parainfluenza virus, although the evidence to support these therapies is limited.[20,25]
  - **Neuraminidase inhibitors** are recommended for immunosuppressed patients infected with influenza viruses.[20,25]

Fungal Infections

- The most common fungal infections are *Candida* and *Aspergillus* following transplantation.
- **Candidal infections** of particular relevance to lung transplant recipients include candidal tracheobronchitis (fairly common but candidal pneumonitis/pneumonia is rare), thrush (especially with higher doses of steroids and/or concurrent treatment with broad-spectrum antibiotics), wound infections/cellulitis (CT scanning can help to determine the extent of disease), and disseminated disease (patients with indwelling catheters are at higher risk).
  - Candidal infections were once associated with a high mortality but now they are easier to control with newer and more effective therapies. **Treatment options include azoles, echinocandins, and liposomal amphotericin B** (minimize kidney toxicity).[26]
  - Azoles increase the levels of calcineurin inhibitors, so therapeutic monitoring and dose adjustment are necessary.
  - Resistance is also an increasing problem, especially with nonalbicans species: *C. glabrata* and *C. tropicalis* (high minimum inhibitory concentration [MIC] to fluconazole), *C. krusei* (resistant to fluconazole); *C. lusitaniae* (resistant to amphotericin B), and *C. guilliermondii* (resistant to amphotericin B and caspofungin).
- ***Aspergillus*** is contracted via inhalation of spores. Common species include: *A. fumigatus* (most common), *A. flavus, A. terreus*.
  - Disease manifestations include tracheobronchial aspergillosis (occurs within 3 months following transplantation, early colonization increases the risk of developing more invasive disease), pulmonary aspergillosis (develops after tracheobronchial aspergillosis), and disseminated aspergillosis (can be devastating, central nervous system [CNS] involvement should be identified).[20]
  - Infection can be detected clinically by screening sputum or BAL fluid for hyphae but invasive pneumonia is confirmed only by biopsy (transbronchial or surgical). Serum galactomannan may aid in diagnosis.[27]
  - **Treatment:** Bronchitis can be treated with itraconazole, voriconazole, or inhaled amphotericin B.[20,27] Disseminated disease is usually treated with liposomal amphotericin B but nephrotoxicity is a major source of morbidity, especially with calcineurin inhibitors. Voriconazole is superior to amphotericin B in invasive disease. Echinocandins may prove to be a less toxic option.
- ***Pneumocystis jirovecii* pneumonia**
  - Infection with *P. jirovecii* is uncommon as the result of widespread routine **prophylaxis with TMP-SMX.**[20,28]

- Prophylaxis is accomplished with one double-strength tablet three times a week. Alternatives include dapsone, atovaquone, and monthly inhaled pentamidine.
- Treatment for *Pneumocystis* pneumonia is TMP-SMX, 15–20 mg of the TMP component/kg/d PO/IV in 3–4 divided doses daily. IV pentamidine can also be used for treatment.

Posttransplant Lymphoproliferative Disorder

- PTLD falls in the spectrum of non-Hodgkin lymphoma and is predominantly of B-cell lineage.[29,30]
- PTLD is often, although not always, associated with EBV infection. B lymphocytes are transformed by EBV and undergo uncontrolled clonal expansion in the setting of drug-induced T-lymphocyte suppression.
- Intrathoracic PTLD, with or without involvement of the allograft, typically occurs within the first year after transplant. Intrathoracic PTLD presents as a pulmonary nodule, pulmonary infiltrate, or lymphadenopathy on routine CXR.
- Extrathoracic PTLD, especially the GI tract, is more common after the first posttransplant year. It can present as nonhealing ulcers, bowel perforations, GI bleeding, and masses.
- **Deescalation of immunosuppression** is the first step in management.
- Other approaches include a combination of rituximab, chemotherapy, and surgical excision.
- A retrospective analysis demonstrated no difference in survival based on time of PTLD diagnosis (early vs. late), but disease involving the allograft had a better prognosis than PTLD without allograft involvement (median survival postdiagnosis 2.6 vs. 0.2 years).[31]

Other Complications

- **Primary graft dysfunction** (PGD) (so-called reperfusion edema or primary graft failure) is a form of acute lung injury that occurs in the immediate postoperative period (72 hours). Up to 25% of patients develop PGD following lung transplantation. PGD severity is graded (0–3) based on PaO_2/FiO_2 ratio and radiographic infiltrates, analogous to ALI/ARDS. PGD 3 is associated with significant posttransplant morbidity and mortality, as well as increased risk for the development of BOS.
- Lung transplant recipients have a **higher risk of malignancy** than individuals in the general population. Squamous cell carcinoma of the skin is more common, as are cancers of the cervix, anogenital region, and the hepatobiliary system. Routine cancer screening and prevention are therefore essential.
- Lung transplant recipients are at a **higher risk for venous thromboembolism and hypercoagulability**. Initial treatment with low–molecular-weight heparin (LMWH) should be initially dosed at 0.8 mg/kg q12h, instead of standard 1 mg/kg q12h regimens. Monitoring of antifactor Xa levels is encouraged to avoid over-anticoagulation.
- **GI complications:** Lung transplant recipients are at an increased risk for chronic gastritis, peptic ulcer disease, and gastroparesis. GERD is a risk factor for the development of BOS and medication refractory cases are often treated with fundoplication. Secondary malnutrition can lead to a number of other systemic problems.
- **Recurrent primary disease** has been reported in sarcoidosis, bronchoalveolar carcinoma, lymphangiomyomatosis, Langerhans cell histiocytosis, pulmonary alveolar proteinosis, diffuse panbronchiolitis, and giant cell pneumonitis.

OUTCOMES

- Survival after transplant is a complicated issue.
- Based on data from the International Society of Heart and Lung Transplantation registry, the unadjusted median time to survival was 5.7 years for all adult lung transplants between

1994 and 2012.[32] Rates of long-term survival improve for those who survive to year 1. Thus, the conditional median survival for recipients who are alive at 1 year is 7.9 years.[32]

- Initial differences in 1-month survival usually reflect perioperative mortality associated with the complexity and severity of the surgery for each disease type (e.g., lung transplantation for IPAH has higher perioperative mortality than for COPD). These outcomes must be considered in light of the fact that these patients would probably have a higher mortality without transplantation when compared to a patient with COPD.
- **Retransplantation** may occur in settings of early acute graft failure, severe airway complications, and chronic rejection. Although the rate of retransplantation for BOS has increased slightly over the past few years, outcomes are worse compared to outcomes following primary lung transplantation.[32]
- A number of **risk factors have been associated with an increased risk of death** at 1 and 5 years posttransplantation.[32]
  - Severity of disease process: BOS (retransplantation) > IPAH > bronchiectasis (including CF) > IPF > COPD
  - Renal failure, requiring hemodialysis
  - Diabetes mellitus
  - Hospitalization (requiring IV inotropes, respiratory failure)
  - Pulmonary embolism
  - CMV mismatch (donor positive, recipient negative)

REFERENCES

1. Patterson GA. Indications: unilateral, bilateral, heart–lung, and lobar transplant procedures. *Clin Chest Med.* 1997;18:225–30.
2. American Thoracic Society. ATS guidelines: lung transplantation: report of the ATS workshop on lung transplantation. *Am Rev Respir Dis.* 1993;147:772–6.
3. American Thoracic Society. ATS guidelines: international guidelines for the selection of lung transplant candidates. *Am J Respir Crit Care Med.* 1998;158:335–9.
4. Orens JB, Estenne M, Arcasoy S, et al. International guidelines for the selection of lung transplant candidates: 2006 update—a consensus report from the Pulmonary Scientific Council of the International Society for Heart and Lung Transplantation. *J Heart Lung Transplant.* 2006;25:745–55.
5. Snell GI, Westfall GP. Selection and management of the lung donor. *Clin Chest Med.* 2011;32:223–32.
6. Eberlein M, Garrity ER, Orens JB. Lung allocation in the United States. *Clin Chest Med.* 2011;32:213–22.
7. Floreth T, Bhorade SM, Ahya VN. Conventional and novel approaches to immunosuppression. *Clin Chest Med.* 2011;32:265–77.
8. Hachem RH. Lung allograft rejection: diagnosis and management. *Curr Opin Organ Transplant.* 2009;14:477–82.
9. Martinu T, Pavlisko EN, Chen DF, et al. Acute allograft rejection: cellular and humoral processes. *Clin Chest Med.* 2011;32:295–310.
10. Stewart S, Fishbein MC, Snell GI, et al. Revision of the 1996 working formulation for the standardization of nomenclature in the diagnosis of lung rejection. *J Heart Lung Transplant.* 2007;26:1229–42.
11. Bando K, Paradis IL, Similo S, et al. Obliterative bronchiolitis after lung and heart–lung transplantation: an analysis of risk factors and management. *J Thorac Cardiovasc Surg.* 1995;110:4–13.
12. Husain AN, Siddiqui MT, Holmes EW, et al. Analysis of risk factors for the development of bronchiolitis obliterans syndrome. *Am J Respir Crit Care Med.* 1999;159:829–33.
13. Jaramillo A, Smith MA, Phelan D, et al. Development of ELISA-detected anti-HLA antibodies precedes the development of bronchiolitis obliterans syndrome and correlates with progressive decline in pulmonary function after lung transplantation. *Transplantation.* 1999;67:1155–61.
14. Schulman LL, Weinberg AD, McGregor CC, et al. Influence of donor and recipient HLA locus mismatching on development of obliterative bronchiolitis after lung transplantation. *Am J Respir Crit Care Med.* 2001;163:437–42.

15. Estenne M, Hertz MI. Bronchiolitis obliterans after human lung transplantation. *Am J Respir Crit Care Med.* 2002;166:440–4.
16. Estenne M, Maurer JR, Boehler A, et al. Bronchiolitis obliterans syndrome 2001: an update of the diagnostic criteria. *J Heart Lung Transplant.* 2002;21:297–310.
17. Palmer SM, Davis RD, Hadjilladis D, et al. Development of an antibody specific to major histocompatibility antigens detectable by flow cytometry after lung transplant is associated with bronchiolitis obliterans syndrome. *Transplantation.* 2002;74:799–804.
18. Daud SA, Yusen RD, Meyers BF, et al. Impact of immediate primary graft dysfunction on bronchiolitis obliterans syndrome. *Am J Respir Crit Care Med.* 2007;175:507–13.
19. Knoop C, Estenne M. Chronic allograft dysfunction. *Clin Chest Med.* 2011;32:311–26.
20. Sims KD, Blumberg EA. Common infections in the lung transplant recipient. *Clin Chest Med.* 2011;32:327–41.
21. Van Delden C, Blumberg EA. Multidrug resistant gram-negative organisms in solid organ transplant recipients. *Am J Transplant.* 2009;9(suppl 4):S27–34.
22. Garzoni C. Multiply resistant gram-positive bacteria, methicillin-resistant, vancomycin-intermediate and vancomycin-resistant Staphylococcus aureus (MRSA, VISA, VRSA) in solid organ transplant recipients. *Am J Transplant.* 2009;9(suppl 4):S41–9.
23. Humar A, Snydman D. Cytomegalovirus in solid organ transplant recipients. *Am J Transplant.* 2009;9(suppl 4):S78–86.
24. Ettinger NA, Bailey TC, Trulock EP, et al. Cytomegalovirus infection and pneumonitis. Impact after isolated lung transplantation. Washington University Lung Transplant Group. *Am Rev Respir Dis.* 1993;147:1017–23.
25. Ison MG, Michaels MG. RNA respiratory viral infections in solid organ transplant recipients. *Am J Transplant.* 2009;9(suppl 4):S166–72.
26. Pappas PG, Silveira FP. Candida in solid organ transplant recipients. *Am J Transplant.* 2009; 9(suppl 4):S173–9.
27. Singh N, Husain S. Invasive Aspergillosis in solid organ transplant recipients. *Am J Transplant.* 2009; 9(suppl 4):S180–91.
28. Martin SI, Fishman JA. Pneumocystis pneumonia in solid organ transplant recipients. *Am J Transplant.* 2009;9(suppl 4):S227–33.
29. Straathof KC, Savoldo B, Heslop HE, et al. Immunotherapy for post-transplant lymphoproliferative disease. *Br J Haematol.* 2002;118:728–40.
30. Robbins HY, Arcasoy SM. Malignancies following lung transplantation. *Clin Chest Med.* 2011; 32:343–55.
31. Paranjothi S, Yusen RD, Kraus MD, et al. Lymphoproliferative disease after lung transplantation: comparison of presentation and outcome of early and late cases. *J Heart Lung Transplant.* 2001; 20:1054–63.
32. Yusen RD, Edwards LB, Kucheryavaya AY, et al. The registry of the International Society for Heart and Lung Transplantation: thirty-first adult lung and heart–lung transplant report—2014; focus theme: retransplantation. *J Heart Lung Transplant.* 2014;33:1009–24.

Index

Page numbers followed by f refer to figures; page numbers followed by t refer to tables.